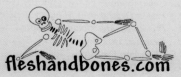

Commissioning Editor: Timothy Horne
Project Development Manager: Janice Urquhart
Project Manager: Nancy Arnott
Designer: Erik Bigland
Illustrator: Jon White, Evi Antoniou

Notes on
Medical
Microbiology

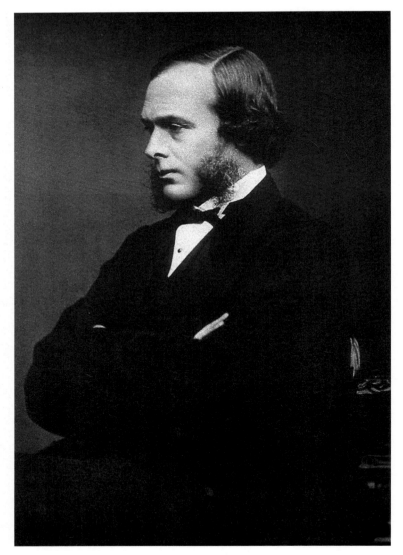

LORD LISTER
Professor of Surgery in Glasgow Royal Infirmary from 1861 to 1869, applied Pasteur's observations to show that wound sepsis could be prevented by using an antiseptic technique with carbolic acid.

Notes on Medical Microbiology

Morag C. Timbury
Formerly Director, Central Public Health Laboratory, Public Health Laboratory Service, Colindale, London, UK

A. Christine McCartney
Deputy Director, Central Public Health Laboratory, Public Health Laboratory Service, Colindale, London, UK

Bishan Thakker
Consultant Microbiologist and Honorary Clinical Senior Lecturer, Glasgow Royal Infirmary and the University of Glasgow, Glasgow, UK

Katherine N. Ward
Consultant and Honorary Senior Lecturer, Department of Virology, Royal Free and University College Medical School, University College London, London, UK

CHURCHILL
LIVINGSTONE

EDINBURGH LONDON NEW YORK PHILADELPHIA ST LOUIS SYDNEY TORONTO 2002

CHURCHILL LIVINGSTONE
An imprint of Elsevier Science Limited

First published 2002

This book uses material from Timbury M C 1998 *Notes on Medical Virology* 11th edn., Churchill Livingstone and Sleigh J D, Timbury M C 1998 *Notes on Medical Bacteriology* 5th edn., Churchill Livingstone

ISBN 0 443 07164 0

British Library Cataloguing in Publication Data
A catalogue record for this book is available from the British Library

Library of Congress Cataloging in Publication Data
A catalog record for this book is available from the Library of Congress

Note
Medical knowledge is constantly changing. As new information becomes available, changes in treatment, procedures, equipment and the use of drugs become necessary. The authors, contributors and the publishers have taken care to ensure that the information given in this text is accurate and up to date. However, readers are strongly advised to confirm that the information, especially with regard to drug usage, complies with the latest legislation and standards of practice.

ELSEVIER SCIENCE your source for books, journals and multimedia in the health sciences

www.elsevierhealth.com

The publisher's policy is to use paper manufactured from sustainable forests

Printed in China

Preface

This book aims to give a concise account of medical microbiology. It is based on the earlier "Notes" books on medical bacteriology and virology which have been combined, extensively revised and updated. Clinical aspects of microbiology are given prominence and the technical side has been reduced to the minimum required for understanding the basis of the work of a microbiology laboratory. Short accounts of mycology and parasitology are included. Three new authors have replaced Professor Sleigh who has now retired. We thank Professor Sleigh for his encouragement in the project.

We are grateful to colleagues who have helped us with invaluable advice and with revision of some chapters. These include Drs Peter Chiodini, Elizabeth Johnson, Henry Smith, Mr Peter Hoffman and Miss Pia Kirkpatrick. Thanks are due to Mr Jon White for his skilled art work for the diagrams and figures.

We thank Miss Jennifer Buchanan and Mrs Sheila Culkin for their help and expertise in the preparation of the typescript.

Morag C. Timbury
A. Christine McCartney
Bishan Thakker
Katherine N. Ward

London and Glasgow

Contents

1 Introduction to medical microbiology

Microbiology is the study of the organisms or microbes that cause infection.

There are four main types of infectious agent:

- *Bacteria:* unicellular, prokaryotic – i.e. the nucleus is not organized and the circular double-stranded DNA lies loose in the cytoplasm – with a rigid peptidoglycan cell wall; divide by binary fission;
- *Viruses:* smaller than bacteria, contain either DNA or RNA as the genome; metabolically inert but capable of replication by taking over the synthetic machinery of a susceptible cell;
- *Fungi:* eukaryotic, with a rigid cell wall; replicate sexually but also asexually; exist as unicellular, round yeast-like forms or filamentous branching forms bearing conidia or spore-like structures;
- *Parasites:* either unicellular, eukaryotic *Protozoa* or multicellular *helminths* (worms); replication often complex, especially with helminths, the lifecycle often involving intermediate animal hosts.

HISTORY

Since Biblical times it has been known that some diseases can spread from person to person, i.e. that they are infectious. However, it was centuries later before the causes were identified.

Some pioneers in microbiology:

Antony van Leeuwenhoek, a Dutch draper who built a microscope and in 1675 observed 'animalculi' in water, soil and human material.

Edward Jenner showed in 1796 that smallpox could be prevented by inoculation with the related disease cowpox, although he did not discover the nature of the infectious agents involved.

Louis Pasteur, the founder of modern microbiology; from 1867 to 1888 developed methods of culturing bacteria and propagated the virus of rabies in animals; he also established the principles of the preparation of vaccines against infectious diseases.

Robert Koch, a German general practitioner, discovered and cultured the bacteria that caused several diseases, including tuberculosis, during the latter part of the 19th century; he used solidifying agents such as agar – allegedly on the advice of Frau Hesse, the wife of a colleague – to prepare solid media on which bacteria could be grown in individual colonies and therefore in pure culture. He laid down the famous criteria for confirming an organism as the cause of a specific disease:

Koch's postulates

1. It must be found in all cases of the disease and its distribution must correspond to that of the lesions observed.
2. Able to be cultured outside the body for several generations.
3. Should reproduce the disease on inoculation into susceptible animals.
   Nowadays a fourth postulate would be added:
4. Antibody to the organism develops during the course of the infection.

Note: many infectious diseases of which the causal organism is clearly identified do not fulfil the third and fourth, nor even occasionally the second, postulates.

Joseph Lister, Professor of Surgery in Glasgow Royal Infirmary, applied Pasteur's observations to show in 1867 that wound sepsis could be prevented by using an antiseptic technique with carbolic acid.

Dmitri Ivanovski in 1892 discovered and studied tobacco mosaic virus in plants and differentiated it from bacteria by showing that it passed through filters that retained the larger bacteria.

John Enders showed in 1949 that poliovirus could be propagated in monkey kidney cell cultures, and thus enabled the study of modern virology – and the development of polio and other virus vaccines.

THE HOST-PARASITE RELATIONSHIP

The relationship between the host and the parasite (the infecting organism) determines the outcome of an infection. However, many organisms can coexist without ill-effects on the host – usually as part of the body's normal flora.

THE HOST

The host defends itself against infection in two main ways:

- **Non-specific**: not directed at a particular organism
- **Specific**: mediated by the host's immune system and directed at a particular organism or species. The specific response operates in two main ways:
  - *Humoral* – due to specific antibody production
  - *Cell-mediated* – due to T lymphocytes and the cytokines they produce.

The defence mechanisms against infection with bacteria differ in some of their effects from those that operate to protect the body from viruses.

NON-SPECIFIC DEFENCE MECHANISMS

- *Skin:* a tough and impermeable barrier unless breached by injury, disease, or the insertion of prosthetic or other devices.
- *Normal flora:* the presence of harmless bacteria in various body sites can make it difficult for exogenous pathogens to invade and establish themselves.
- *Flushing effect:* tears, the flow of urine and the upward flow of mucus by ciliated epithelium all act to remove invading organisms, both bacteria and viruses.
- *Gastrointestinal tract:* the low pH of stomach acid helps to inactivate acid-labile viruses and, less effectively, ingested bacteria.

- *Vaginal secretions:* in young women these have a low pH owing to lactobacilli in the normal flora, and so have a protective effect against bacterial infection.

Phagocytosis

An important defence mechanism whereby both bacteria and viruses are ingested by two types of scavenging cell:

- *Neutrophil polymorphonuclear leukocytes*
- *Macrophages,* the mononuclear cells of the reticuloendothelial system. There are two types of these scavenger cells:
  - *Free* macrophages in lung alveoli and the peritoneal cavity;
  - *Fixed* macrophages in lymph nodes, spleen, liver (Kupffer cells), connective tissue (histiocytes) and CNS (microglia).

Phagocytosis is enhanced by antibody (a specific immune mechanism) and complement: this effect is known as *opsonization*; macrophages 'activated' by cytokines released by T lymphocytes (also a specific immune mechanism) have increased phagocytic activity and are attracted by chemotaxis to the site of infection.

Complement: a complex of proteins produced in a cascade which becomes activated upon infection to enhance phagocytosis, lyse bacteria and increase vascular permeability.

SPECIFIC DEFENCE MECHANISMS – THE IMMUNE SYSTEM IN INFECTION

Humoral (antibody) response

Antibodies are immunoglobulins – proteins produced in the bloodstream by B (bone marrow-derived) lymphocytes which react with specific antigens on the surface of organisms:

- *B lymphocytes* have immunoglobulin on their surface which acts as a receptor for antigen on the invading organism; antibodies are somewhat less important in the defence against bacteria than of viruses: they neutralize the infectivity of the latter and produce specific and long-term immunity to viral infection. Encounter of B lymphocytes in spleen or bone marrow with antigen activates the lymphocytes and transforms them into antibody-secreting *plasma cells*. Antigen is presented by macrophages, dendritic cells and B cells and the involvement of T lymphocytes is required to initiate the immune response to many antigens.

- *Immunoglobulins* are Y-shaped: the stem is the *Fc* fragment which activates complement and binds to receptors on infected host cells; the two arms are the *Fab* fragments containing the antibody-combining sites.

Three immunoglobulins are mainly responsible for humoral immunity:

- *IgM*: the earliest antibody produced, appearing at a variable time after infection; persists for about 4–6 weeks; a pentamer of five immunoglobulin subunits;
- *IgG*: formed later than IgM but persists usually for years and conveys long-term immunity, especially to viruses;
- *IgA*: a dimeric molecule found in body secretions such as saliva, respiratory secretion, tears and gastrointestinal contents (as well as blood); the main antibody involved in immunity to respiratory and gut infections; 'secretory' IgA acquires a carbohydrate transport piece in extracellular fluids that is absent from serum IgA.

Note: Antibody is involved in *antibody-dependent cell-mediated cytotoxicity,* an important immune mechanism in viral infections.

Cell-mediated inmmune response

Mainly mediated by T, or thymus-derived, lymphocytes and includes the release of cytokines. Two main cell types are involved:

- **CD4 cells**: have the CD4 marker on their surface and act as *helper T cells*; require major histocompatibility complex (MHC) class II antigens to be present along with the target antigen for their activation; interact with B lymphocytes to induce antibody production;
- **CD8 cells**: have the CD8 marker on their surface and act as *cytotoxic T cells*; MHC Class I antigen-restricted; lyse target cells, such as virus-infected cells.

Lysis of infected cells is by two main mechanisms:

- *Non-antibody-dependent cytotoxicity* by cytotoxic T cells and natural killer cells.
- *Antibody-dependent cellular cytotoxicity* – infected cells are lysed by natural killer cells which have Fc receptors for IgG on their surface; these receptors bind to infected target cells coated with IgG produced by the infecting organism on the cell surface.

Cytokines

Small protein molecules which function as signals or mediators to activate, modulate and control the immune responses (and other activities) of various cells. There are numerous cytokines, for example interferon, which has important antiviral activity, interleukins and tumour necrosis factors (TNFs).

Among other functions, cytokines:

- *Inhibit* macrophage migration
- *Attract* lymphocytes, macrophages and polymorphonuclear leukocytes to the site of infection by chemotaxis
- *Increase* capillary permeability
- *Induce* mitogenic activity by stimulating the transformation of lymphocytes
- *Produce* IgE (the antibody responsible for allergic reactions) by mast cell activation.

PATHOGENIC MECHANISMS OF THE PARASITE

Infecting organisms vary in their *pathogenicity* or ability to produce disease. *Virulence* is a commonly used but ill-defined term which indicates the degree of pathogenicity.

BACTERIA

Bacteria have two basic pathogenic mechanisms:

- **Invasiveness**: the ability to spread within the body of the host, and this is principally due to the toxin production; other properties, such as the possession of a capsule, may enable the bacterium to evade defence mechanisms such as phagocytosis;
- **Toxin production**: bacteria produce two types, exotoxins and endotoxins, shown in Table 1.1.

Table 1.1   Bacterial toxins

	Exotoxins	Endotoxins
Composition	Protein	Lipopolysaccharide
Action	Specific	Non-specific
Effect of heat	Labile	Stable
Antigenicity	Strong	Weak
Produced by	Gram-positive; some Gram-negative bacteria	Gram-negative bacteria
Convertibility to toxoid*	Yes	No

* Toxoid is toxin treated, usually with formaldehyde, so that it loses toxicity but retains antigenicity.

VIRUSES

Viruses produce disease by:

- *Invasiveness*: viruses replicate within cells by taking over their metabolic activities and redirecting them to the synthesis of viral components, with subsequent assembly into new infectious virus particles; this usually (but not always) kills the cell, to produce lesions and disease within the tissue or organ to which the cell belongs. Sometimes virus-infected cells suffer damage from immune reactions.

FUNGI

- *Invasiveness*: fungi multiply in mucosal tissues and keratin, producing common superficial infections; fungi which have gained access to tissues cause subcutaneous infections; in the bloodstream they cause life-threatening systemic infections, especially in immunocompromised patients.
- *Toxin production*: ingestion of mouldy food in which fungal metabolites have been produced causes serious food poisoning.
- *Allergic reactions*: inhalation of fungal hyphae or spores causes hypersensitive reactions.

PARASITES

Parasites are much more complex than bacteria or viruses and cause infection by:

- *Ingestion*: consumption of food or water containing a life form of the parasite.

- *Transmission of infection via vectors*: injection into host by arthropod bite.

EPIDEMIOLOGY

Microbiology includes epidemiology or the study of the spread of infection, usually exogenously acquired, within a community or the population at large.

Epidemiology

Spread of an organism in a population depends on:

- *Reservoirs and sources*: these may be patients with active disease or symptomless carriers – important because usually unrecognized – but also animals or inanimate sources such as food, water, soil;
- *Routes of infection*: by inhalation, ingestion, inoculation, sexual or transplacental transmission;
- *Vectors*: many infections are spread by biting insects, a common route in tropical countries;
- *Herd immunity*: generally dependent on the level of protective antibody in the population; when this is low the organism can find many susceptible hosts to infect and multiply, and vice versa.

Measurements in epidemiology

Infectious disease is continuously monitored by epidemiologists and microbiologists; although infection cannot always be halted, preventive measures, promptly applied, may succeed in controlling an outbreak. Below are some of the measurements used in the surveillance of infectious disease:

- *Incubation period:* very variable, and in some diseases impossible to measure, but important to determine in order to identify sources of infection.
- *Incidence*: of infection or disease is the proportion of a population contracting that infection or disease during a specified period, usually a year; expressed as a ratio, e.g. per 1000, or per 100 000 in the population concerned.*

- *Prevalence*: refers to the proportion of a population infected (or sick or immune) at a specified point in time. Can be used only for states of relatively long duration, i.e. immunity, persisting infection or chronic disease.*
- *Attack rate*: the incidence of infection in a defined group, e.g. the inhabitants of an institution.
- *Secondary attack rate*: the number of cases appearing in contacts of the first or index case.
- *Mortality rate*: expressed as the ratio of:

$$= \frac{\text{No. of deaths from a disease in a given year}}{\text{Total population at mid year}}$$

- *Case fatality rate*: the proportion of patients with the disease who die from it.

*e.g. influenza – *incidence* of disease and *prevalence* of immunity.

Epidemics

These may be confined to one country or region but may also be seen worldwide, when they are known as pandemics: the AIDS epidemic is an example of the latter. Most are viral but some, such as cholera, and plague in former centuries, are bacterial.

Endemic infection is the constant presence of the infectious disease or its agent within a population.

Epidemics are recognized when the number of cases of infection rises above the expected level, or when a new infectious agent appears within the community concerned; the difference between *epidemics* and *outbreaks* – the latter implying a lower number of cases than in an epidemic – can be hard to determine.

BACTERIAL EPIDEMICS

Rarer than viral epidemics but still important. The most famous epidemic in history was the Black Death, i.e. bubonic plague, which spread from China through Europe in the 14th century, killing around one-third of the population. Nowadays cholera is in its seventh pandemic, which started in 1961; tuberculosis in association with HIV is at present epidemic in Africa. Dysentery, salmonella and campylobacter food-poisoning, and MRSA in hospitals are examples of bacterial diseases that remain out of control in many parts of the world, including developed western countries.

VIRUS EPIDEMICS

Many of these have been controlled or even eliminated by vaccination. HIV and its end-stage infection as AIDS is currently the most urgent problem facing the world today. Other epidemic virus diseases include influenza – which despite an available vaccine kills many thousands of patients in an epidemic year – and several of the vector or arthropod-borne infections, such as dengue and West Nile fever, which have both in the last few years spread beyond their traditional boundaries.

IMMUNIZATION

Without doubt, the advent of successful vaccines has had the most dramatic effect in all medicine on human health. Immunization has controlled diphtheria, tetanus, measles, mumps, rubella, yellow fever and, to a lesser extent, hepatitis B. Live attenuated virus vaccines are generally more effective than their bacterial equivalents, with the possible exception of the bacterial toxoids. Vaccination, together with appropriate control measures, succeeded in eliminating smallpox from the world altogether. Poliomyelitis is likely to follow soon.

Bacteria

2 Bacteria – structure, growth, nutrition and genetics

Bacteria form a heterogeneous group of unicellular organisms. Their cellular organization is *prokaryotic* (i.e. having a primitive nucleus) and differs from that of *eukaryotic* cells, in which the chromosomes are in a nucleus surrounded by a nuclear membrane, as in plants and animals.

Genome: the bacterial chromosome, or *genome*, is a single circular molecule of double-stranded DNA with no nuclear membrane. Bacteria may from time to time harbour *plasmids* (smaller circular DNA molecules), which can code for certain accessory functions.

STRUCTURE

Shape: Bacteria have a rigid wall which determines their shape. They may be:

- spherical – cocci
- cylindrical – bacilli or rods
- helical – spirochaetes.

Arrangement: depends on the plane of successive cell divisions. Examples of different arrangements are chains, e.g. streptococci; clusters, e.g. staphylococci; diplococci, e.g. pneumococci; angled pairs or palisades, e.g. corynebacteria.

Gram's stain divides bacteria into Gram-positive or Gram-negative, an important step in classification and identification. The Gram staining reaction reflects the structure of the cell wall.

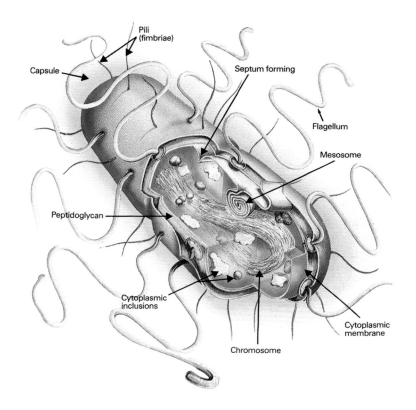

Fig. 2.1   Diagram of a bacterial cell.

A typical but composite bacterium is shown diagrammatically in Figure 2.1. Bacteria have a rigid cell wall which surrounds the *protoplast*, a cytoplasmic membrane enclosing internal components and structures, such as ribosomes and the bacterial chromosome.

External structures

Structures that protrude from the cell into the environment are present in many bacteria:

1. **Flagella**: long filaments; produce motility by rotation and are composed of subunits of the protein *flagellin*.
2. **Fimbriae or pili**: finer, shorter filaments extruding from the cytoplasmic membrane and also composed of protein (*pilin*).

Two types: *common fimbriae* responsible for attachment and adhesion, and *sex pili* associated with conjugation when genes are transferred from one bacterial cell to another.

3. **Capsules**: amorphous material which surrounds many bacterial species as their outermost layer; usually polysaccharide, occasionally protein. They often inhibit phagocytosis and so corrrelate with virulence in certain bacteria.

Cell wall

This confers rigidity upon bacteria and protects against osmotic damage. It is porous and permeable to substances of low molecular weight.

Chemically, the rigid part of the cell wall is *peptidoglycan*: this is a mucopeptide composed of strands of alternating *N*-acetyl-glucosamine and *N*-acetylmuramic acid residues. Structural rigidity is conferred by interstrand peptide cross-links between *N*-acetylmuramic acid molecules.

Structure: differs in Gram-positive and Gram-negative bacteria; this is illustrated diagrammatically in Figure 2.2.

Gram-negative cell wall: differs from that of Gram-positive bacteria by an *outer membrane* containing lipopolysaccharide (LPS), as well as specific proteins (outer membrane proteins) such as pore-forming proteins (porins) – through which hydrophilic molecules are transported – and proteins that are receptor sites for phages and bacteriocins. The lipid is embedded in the outer membrane, whereas the polysaccharide is anchored to the lipid and projects from the cell surface. The *periplasmic space* separates the peptidoglycan layer from the cytoplasmic membrane.

Gram-positive cell wall: the peptidoglycan layer of the cell wall of Gram-positive bacteria is much thicker than in Gram-negative bacteria. There is no periplasm and the peptidoglycan is closely associated with the cytoplasmic membrane.

Teichoic or *teichuronic acids* are part of the cell wall of Gram-positive bacteria and maintain the level of divalent cations outside the cytoplasmic membrane.

Antigens: the cell wall may contain antigens, such as the polysaccharide (Lancefield) and protein (Griffith) antigens of streptococci.

Cytoplasmic membrane: a trilaminar structure formed of proteins buried in a phospholipid bilayer which acts as a semiper-meable membrane through which there is uptake of nutrients by passive diffusion. It is also the site of numerous enzymes involved

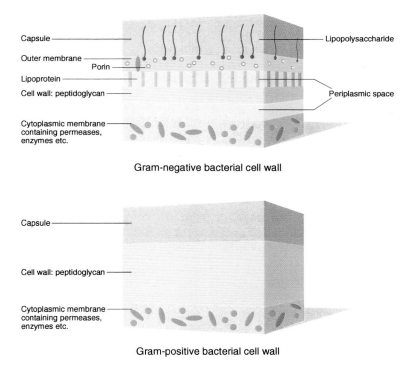

Fig. 2.2 Diagram showing the structure of Gram-negative and Gram-positive bacterial cell walls.

in the active transport of nutrients and in various other cell metabolic processes. Chemically, bacterial cytoplasmic membranes lack the sterols usually found in their eukaryotic cell equivalents.

Mesosomes: convoluted invaginations of the cytoplasmic membrane, often at sites of septum formation, and involved in DNA segregation during cell division. They are the site of respiratory enzyme activity, and may perform a function similar to that of mitochondria in eukaryotic cells.

Nuclear material: the single circular chromosome which is the bacterial genome or DNA undergoes semiconservative replication bidirectionally from a fixed point, the *origin*. Chromosomal DNA is condensed into about 50 supercoiled domains associated with an RNA core. DNA-binding proteins (histone-like) regulate supercoiling and influence expression.

Ribosomes: the sites of protein synthesis and distributed throughout the cytoplasm; composed of RNA and proteins and organized into two subunits: 30s and 50s.

Cytoplasmic inclusions: sources of stored energy, e.g. polymetaphosphate (volutin), poly-β-hydroxybutyrate (lipid), polysaccharide (starch or glycogen).

Spores: produced by the genera *Bacillus* and *Clostridium* to enable them to survive adverse environmental conditions. Spore production is triggered by a process analogous to differentiation in higher cells, and takes place within and at the expense of the vegetative cell. Dense and dehydrated, they contain a high concentration of calcium dipicolinate and are resistant to heat, desiccation and disinfectants. Often remaining associated with the cell wall of the bacillus from which they develop, and described as 'terminal', 'subterminal' etc. When growth conditions become favourable, they germinate to produce vegetative cells.

Taxonomy

Taxonomy consists of:

1. **Classification**: the division of organisms into ordered groups.
2. **Nomenclature**: the labelling of the groups and of individual members within groups.

Bacterial taxonomy is currently undergoing considerable change, organisms now being grouped to reflect the genetic information in their cells, determined by molecular analysis. Although species are generally now defined in terms of DNA–DNA relatedness, for identification purposes simple phenotypic characteristics are used, which often correlate with the genotype.

Phenotypic characteristics include:

• morphology
• staining
• cultural characteristics
• biochemical reactions
• antigenic structure

Antigenic differentiation:

• *Serotype*: a single bacterial strain or type, defined by antigenic structure
• *Serogroup*: a group of serologically related organisms

- *Serovar*: term sometimes used interchangeably with, or instead of, 'serotype', on the basis of individual preference.

NUTRITION AND GROWTH OF BACTERIA

Like all cells, bacteria require nutrients for the maintenance of their metabolism and for cell division. Fast-growing bacteria divide approximately every 30 minutes.

Chemically, bacteria consist of:

- protein
- polysaccharide
- lipid
- nucleic acid
- peptidoglycan.

Bacterial growth requires:

- materials for the synthesis of structural components and for cell metabolism
- energy.

NUTRITIONAL REQUIREMENTS

Some bacteria can synthesize all they require from the simplest elements. Others – including most pathogenic bacteria – are unable to do this: they need a ready-made supply of some of the organic compounds required for growth. Other necessary compounds can be synthesized from breakdown products of complex macromolecules (e.g. proteins, nucleic acids) which are taken into the cell and degraded by bacterial enzymes. These processes are illustrated diagrammatically in Figure 2.3.

Elements

Bacterial structural components and the macromolecules for cell metabolism are synthesized from the elements shown in Table 2.1, all of which are necessary for bacterial growth – whether available simply as elements or as part of complex molecules. The four most important are:

1. hydrogen
2. oxygen
3. carbon
4. nitrogen.

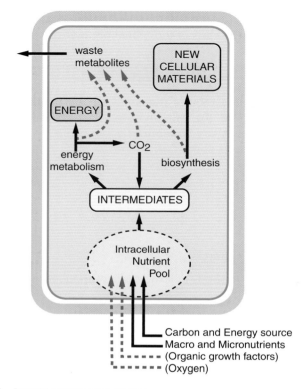

Fig. 2.3 Bacterial nutrition and metabolism.

Hydrogen and oxygen: obtained from water – essential for the growth and maintenance of any cell. Water must be available for there to be potential for bacterial growth.

Carbon and nitrogen: the principal elements for which an external source must be found. The main source of carbon is carbohydrate (usually sugars) degraded by either oxidation or fermentation (i.e. without oxygen). This provides energy in the form of adenosine triphosphate (ATP), the universal energy storage compound. The main source of nitrogen is ammonia, usually in the form of an ammonium salt: salts are either available in the environment or are produced by the bacterium as a result of the deamination of amino acids released from proteins.

Organic growth factors: are organic compounds that cannot be synthesized by many bacteria; an exogenous supply is therefore required, although often only in small amounts. Some examples are:

Table 2.1   Essential elements required for bacterial growth

Group	Element	Role
I Elements required for the synthesis of structural components	Carbon Hydrogen Oxygen Nitrogen Phosphorus Sulphur	Required for synthesis of carbohydrate, lipid, protein, nucleic acid
II Elements required for other cellular functions	Potassium	Major cation; activates various enzymes
	Calcium	Enzyme cofactor (e.g. proteinases): key role in spore formation
	Magnesium	Multienzyme cofactor: stabilizes ribosomes, membranes, nucleic acid; required for enzyme substrate binding
	Iron	Electron carrier in oxidation – reduction reactions; many other functions
III Trace elements	Copper Cobalt Manganese Molybdenum Zinc	Activators and stabilizers of a wide variety of enzymes

- **Amino acids**: required by many bacterial species which cannot synthesize them. Bacteria possess enzymes that degrade proteins to amino acids; these form an intracellular pool from which the appropriate amino acid is withdrawn to become incorporated into bacterial proteins.
- **Purines and pyrimidines**: the precursors of nucleic acids and coenzymes. In bacteria that require them they are converted into nucleosides and nucleotides before incorporation into DNA and RNA.
- **Vitamins**: many pathogenic bacteria lack the ability to synthesize vitamins, most of which are required for the formation of coenzymes.

Nutrient uptake: most nutrients are small molecules which diffuse freely across the bacterial cytoplasmic membrane to enter the cell. Some are at a higher concentration within the bacterial cell than in the external environment, so their uptake is an energy-dependent process.

- *Sugars* are nutrients of relatively large size, and therefore diffuse slowly into the bacterial cell.
- *Enzymes,* which facilitate the rapid uptake of larger nutrient molecules, are present in many bacteria. Usually associated with the cell membrane and energy dependent, they may be:
   inducible, i.e. produced only in the presence of the substrate, or
   constitutive, i.e. produced constantly and independently of the substrate.

ENVIRONMENTAL CONDITIONS GOVERNING GROWTH

Water: an absolute requirement for the growth of all bacteria: at least 80% of the bacterial cell consists of water.

Oxygen: bacteria differ in their need for molecular oxygen for growth or – in the case of anaerobic bacteria – in their need for its exclusion.

Carbon dioxide: required by all bacteria and usually available as a product of metabolism. Slow-growing or fastidious organisms may not generate enough carbon dioxide, so this must be supplied exogenously; this requirement may become increased by environmental change, as when bacteria are transferred from growth in vivo to culture in vitro.

Temperature: most medically important species are mesophiles, and grow best at temperatures around 37°C (i.e. body temperature).

Hydrogen ion concentration: not surprisingly, the optimal pH for bacteria that have evolved in association with humans is similar to physiological pH, i.e. 7.2–7.4.

BACTERIAL GROWTH AND DIVISION

Bacterial growth is the result of a balanced increase in the mass of cellular constituents and structures. The biosynthetic processes on which this increase depends are fuelled by energy, usually from ATP. *Cell division* is initiated when the increase in cellular constituents and structures reaches a critical mass. Bacteria divide by *binary fission.*

BACTERIAL GENETICS

Genetics is the study of inheritance and variation. Except in the case of RNA viruses, all inherited characteristics are encoded in DNA. *Bacteria* show exceptional ability to undergo genetic change.

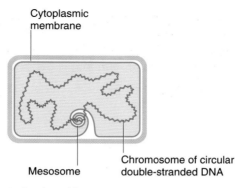

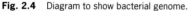

Fig. 2.4 Diagram to show bacterial genome.

Bacteria have two types of DNA that contain their genes:

- Chromosomal
- Extrachromosomal (e.g. plasmid).

The *bacterial chromosome* is

- circular, double-stranded DNA
- attached to the bacterial cell membrane (Fig. 2.4).

Genetic information is encoded in the sequence of purine and pyrimidine bases of the nucleotides that make up the DNA strand. Three bases comprise one *codon,* and each triplet codon codes for one amino acid or a regulatory sequence, e.g. 'start' and 'stop' codons. In this way, the sequence of bases in genes determines the amino acids which form the protein that is the gene product.

GENETIC VARIATION IN BACTERIA

This can be due to:

- mutation
- gene transfer.

MUTATION

Mutation: mutants are variants in which one or more bases in their DNA are changed: the change is heritable and irreversible (unless there is backmutation to the original sequence). The gene defect may result in alteration in:

• transcription
• amino acid sequence of the protein that is the gene product.

Mutation can involve any gene in the bacterial DNA: many are never detected, because the mutation does not affect a recognizable function (e.g. causing antibiotic resistance); others are lethal and therefore also undetected.

Molecular basis of mutation: involves change in the sequence of bases in DNA. Change of a single base alters the genetic code so that the triplet involved codes for a different amino acid, which then becomes substituted for the original amino acid in the protein gene product.

There are three types of mutation:

1. **Base substitution**: change of a single base to one of the three other bases, with consequent alteration in the triplet of the code. This may be *transition*, in which purine/pyrimidine orientation is preserved, e.g. GC changes to AT, or *transversion*, with altered purine/pyrimidine orientation, e.g. GC changes to CG.

2. **Deletion**: loss of a base affects the reading of subsequent triplets – *frame-shift* mutation (Fig. 2.5). Deletion sometimes involves several bases rather than a single base.

3. **Insertion** of an additional base (Fig. 2.5) or a mobile DNA *insertion sequence* (see section on transposons below) also alters the reading frame of the DNA.

DNA base sequence ↓	**–CAT–ACT–GAG–GTT–AGT–**
	| | | |
transcription/translation ↓	| | | |
	| | | |
amino acid sequence	–his– thr– glu– val– ↓
Deletion mutation delete **C** in **ACT**	**–CAT–ATG–AGG–TTA–** –his– met– arg– leu– ↓
Insertion mutation insert **G** in **CAT**	**–CAG–TAC–TGA–GGT–** –glut– tyr– cys– gly–

Fig. 2.5 Mutation. The effect of the deletion and insertion of a single base on the amino acid sequence of the gene product.

GENE TRANSFER

Gene transfer is largely responsible for the exceptional capacity for rapid genetic variability seen in bacteria. This may be mediated by plasmids, phages (bacterial viruses) or transposons.

PLASMIDS

Plasmids are extrachromosomal small DNA molecules consisting of circular, double-stranded DNA. Replication is autonomous, i.e. plasmids multiply independently of the host cell, but also divide with the cell so that they are inherited by daughter cells. *Multiple or single copies* of the same plasmid may be present in each bacterial cell, and different plasmids often coexist in the same cell. In some genera the majority of strains are plasmid free.

Transmissibility: some plasmids (but not all) can transfer to other bacteria of the same (or other) species. Transfer takes place normally by *conjugation*, and the ability to transfer is mediated by the *tra* or transfer promotion genes. Maintenance of the plasmid in the cell requires the expression of other plasmid genes.

Plasmid coding: plasmids code for many functions and phenotypic charcters. The most important in medical microbiology are *R-plasmids*, which contain genes that code for antibiotic resistance.

PHAGES

Phages are bacterial viruses that adsorb specifically to receptors on the bacterial surface. Some are vegetative and are carried without replication by the bacterial cell. Others infect the cell, replicate within it and lyse it when released. Phages may be species specific or strain specific – a property which enables them to be used for typing for epidemiological purposes.

TRANSPOSONS

Sometimes called 'jumping genes', transposons are DNA sequences that can transpose or relocate, carrying plasmid or other genes into the bacterial chromosome. Transposons belong to a family of transposable elements that includes *insertion sequences* and, like them, are flanked by terminal repeat DNA sequences – either inverted or direct (Fig. 2.6). These terminal repeat sequences enable transposons to translocate and insert into DNA. Transposons do not exist in the free state, but only in integrated form within plasmid or chromosome.

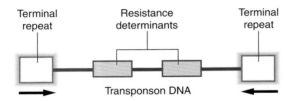

Fig. 2.6 Transposon. The structure of transposon DNA, with inverted terminal repeat regions.

There are four types of *gene transfer* which alter the DNA gene content of bacteria:

- Transformation
- Transduction
- Conjugation
- Transposition.

Transformation

The process by which fragments of exogenous bacterial DNA are taken up and 'absorbed' into recipient cells. Recombination with the bacterial chromosome takes place (Fig. 2.7) to *transform* the

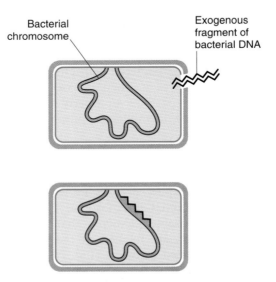

Fig. 2.7 Transformation. Gene transfer by the uptake and subsequent recombination of a fragment of exogenous bacterial DNA.

cell, which then expresses the new genes. Recombination depends on extensive DNA homology and on the function of a gene known as *recA*. The frequency of transformation in nature is low.

Transduction

Fragments of chromosomal DNA are transferred into a second bacterium by phage (bacterial virus). During phage replication a piece of bacterial DNA becomes accidentally enclosed within a phage particle in place of the normal phage DNA (Fig. 2.8). When this particle infects a second bacterial host cell, the DNA from the first bacterium is released and recombines into the chromosome of the second bacterium. Transduction is a relatively uncommon event in nature.

Plasmid DNA can also be transferred to the second bacterium by transduction. The donated plasmid can then function (and replicate) independently, i.e. without recombining with the chromosome of the bacterial cell. β-lactamase production in *Staphylococcus aureus* is plasmid mediated, and the responsible plasmids transfer between staphylococcal strains by transduction.

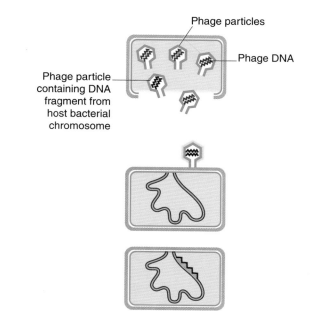

Fig. 2.8 Transduction. Gene transfer from one bacterium to another via phage.

Phage conversion: phage DNA (as distinct from plasmid DNA) becomes integrated into the bacterial chromosome and the phage genes cause changes in the phenotype of the host bacterium. Toxin production in *Corynebacterium diphtheriae* and the production of certain O antigens in salmonellae are examples of this. Integration of phage DNA into the bacterial genome acts as a switch, to cause the DNA expression of otherwise unexpressed bacterial genes. The continuing presence of the phage DNA is necessary for the maintenance of the altered phenotype.

Conjugation

This is the major way in which bacteria – particularly enterobacteria – acquire additional genes. In conjugation, plasmid DNA is transferred from donor to recipient bacterium by direct contact,

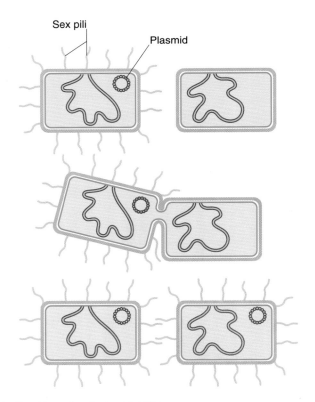

Fig. 2.9   Plasmid gene transfer by conjugation.

probably via a hollow-cored tube formed by a sex pilus (Fig. 2.9). The formation of the pilus is coded by plasmid *tra* genes.

Transposition

Transposons can move from plasmid to plasmid or from plasmid to chromosome (and vice versa). In this way, plasmid or other genes can be acquired by the chromosomal complement of genes. Unlike classic recombination in bacteria, transposition is independent of the *recA* gene. When transposons transfer to a new site it is usually a copy of the transposon that moves, the original transposon remaining in situ. For their insertion, transposons do not require extensive homology between the terminal repeat sequences of the transposon (which are responsible for integration) and the site of insertion in the recipient DNA, although certain sites are preferred. *Transposons code* for toxin production and for resistance to antibiotics, e.g. ampicillin, trimethoprim, as well as for other functions.

Transposition is therefore an additional mechanism that enables genetic flexibility among plasmids and bacterial chromosomes.

MEDICALLY IMPORTANT BACTERIA

3 Gram-positive bacteria

The medically important Gram-positive bacteria, classified on the basis of morphology and aerobic or anaerobic growth, are listed in Figure 3.1. This classification has been simplified and retains nomenclature still widely used in medical bacteriology.

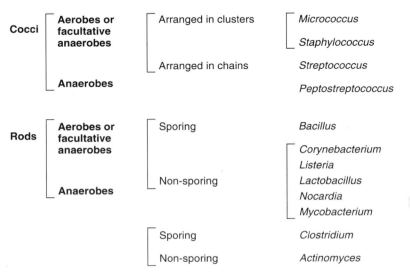

Fig. 3.1 Simplified classification of medically important Gram-positive bacteria.

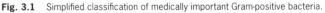

GRAM-POSITIVE COCCI

STAPHYLOCOCCUS

Gram-positive cocci arranged in grape-like clusters:

- *Staphylococci*: pathogenic or commensal parasites
- *Micrococci*: free-living saprophytes with little pathogenic potential
  – but are the occasional cause of opportunistic infections.

SPECIES

- *S. aureus* – the main pathogen – responsible for pyogenic
  infections; identified by a positive coagulase test.
- Other staphylococci are now rarely speciated – simply called
  coagulase-negative staphylococci (CNS): identified by a
  negative coagulase test. Commonest species *S. epidermidis*, a
  universal skin commensal: important pathogen of implanted
  metal and plastic devices and prostheses.
- Other important species *S. saprophyticus*, a cause of urinary
  tract infection in sexually active women.

  Habitat: the body surfaces and, by dissemination, air and dust.

- *S. aureus*: the nose – around 50–75% of healthy people carry it;
  less often, the skin (especially axilla and perineum), throat or gut.
- Coagulase-negative staphylococci: normally present in the
  resident skin flora. Also the gut or upper respiratory tract.

Laboratory characteristics

Morphology and staining: Gram-positive cocci, arranged in clusters
(Fig. 3.2).

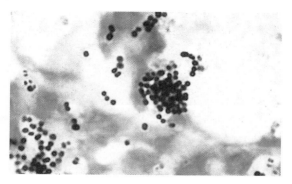

Fig. 3.2 Staphylococcal pus (approx. × 1000).

Culture: grow well on ordinary media aerobically and, although less well, anaerobically; optimal temperature 37°C.

Colonial appearance:

- *S. aureus*: typically golden, but pigmentation varies from orange to white.
- *Coagulase-negative staphylococci*: white colonies.

Selective media: staphylococci tolerate sodium chloride in concentrations of 5–10%. Salt-containing media are useful in isolating staphylococci from samples containing large numbers of other bacteria.

Identification of S. aureus: by the detection of *protein A* – commercial kits for detecting this surface protein have replaced traditional coagulase tests; confirm identity by test for DNA-ase (or coagulase – see Fig. 3.3).

Typing: strains of *S. aureus* can be distinguished by the pattern of their susceptibility to an internationally recognized set of over 20 bacteriophages (phages).

Toxins

S. aureus forms a large number of extracellular toxins and enzymes. Not all strains produce the whole range listed in Table 3.1; most of the products probably play a role in pathogenicity.

Coagulase-negative staphylococci: produce few toxins.

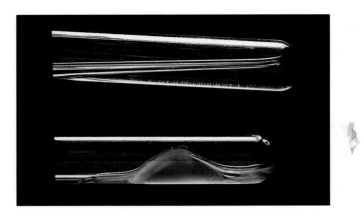

Fig. 3.3 Photograph of a positive tube coagulase test (bottom).

Table 3.1 Toxins and toxic components produced by *Staphylococcus aureus*

Toxin	Activity
Haemolysins α, β, γ and δ	Cytolytic; lyse erythrocytes of various animal species
Coagulase	Clots plasma
Fibrinolysin	Digests fibrin
Leukocidin	Kills leukocytes
Hyaluronidase	Breaks down hyaluronic acid
DNA-ase	Hydrolyses DNA
Lipase	Lipolytic (produces opacity in egg-yolk medium)
Protein A	Antiphagocytic
Epidermolytic toxins A and B	Epidermal splitting and exfoliation
Enterotoxin(s)	Causes vomiting and diarrhoea
Toxic shock syndrome toxin-1	Shock, rash, desquamation

Pathogenicity

S. aureus is an important pyogenic organism, causing:

- superficial infections: pustules, boils, carbuncles, abscesses, impetigo, sycosis barbae, conjunctivitis, wound infections (including postoperative sepsis)
- deep infections: septicaemia, endocarditis, pyaemia, osteomyelitis, pneumonia
- toxic food poisoning
- toxic shock syndrome
- skin exfoliation: toxic epidermal necrolysis (Ritter–Lyell's disease).

Antibiotic sensitivity

S. aureus readily appears in multiply resistant form, especially in hospitals.

Antibiotics active against *S. aureus* are:

- Penicillin (50% of domiciliary and 80% or more of hospital strains are now resistant)
- Flucloxacillin (stable to β-lactamase produced by penicillin-resistant strains)
- Macrolides (e.g. erythromycin)
- Fusidic acid
- Glycopeptides (e.g. vancomycin)
- Cephalosporins
- Lincomycins (e.g. clindamycin)
- Linezolid.

Antibiotic resistance

Penicillin resistance is due to the production of *β-lactamase*, which breaks down the β-lactam ring of penicillin. The β-lactamase is plasmid coded and transferred by transduction via bacteriophage.

MRSA (methicillin-resistant *Staphylococcus aureus*): strains of *S. aureus* resistant to methicillin (and related penicillins) have now spread to many hospitals in Britain and elsewhere. They are also often resistant to a variety of other antibiotics, e.g. fusidic acid, erythromycin, and sometimes also gentamicin. Although the infections caused by MRSA are not necessarily more severe than those due to other staphylococci, some strains (E-MRSA) possess the capacity to spread with ease and have caused hospital epidemics which have been difficult to control. Serious MRSA infections require treatment with glycopeptides or linezolid. The topical antibiotic mupirocin, as a nasal ointment, is frequently used to reduce nasal carriage of MRSA. Resistance to this agent is increasing.

Coagulase-negative staphylococci are often resistant to penicillin and many of the other antistaphylococcal antibiotics. Vancomycin and teicoplanin are particularly useful.

Micrococci have little pathogenic potential: occasional cause of opportunistic infections.

Anaerobic Gram-positive cocci

These are considered with the other anaerobic cocci (see Chapter 4).

Streptococcus, enterococcus and pneumococcus

CLASSIFICATION

This is complex, with many species described. An important basis for classification is the type of haemolysis produced around colonies growing on blood agar (Table 3.2).

The main classes are:

1. *Pyogenic streptococci*: this class includes the most pathogenic human species: the main pathogen is *Streptococcus pyogenes*. Pyogenic streptococci have polysaccharide Lancefield group antigens in their cell wall: *S. pyogenes* is in Lancefield group A; other common pyogenic streptococci belong to Lancefield groups B, C and G.

Table 3.2 Classification of streptococci, enterococci and pneumococci, based on haemolysis

Haemolysis	Appearance	Designation	Streptococcal class
Complete	Colourless, clear, sharply defined zone	β	Pyogenic streptococci
Partial	Greenish discoloration	α	'Viridans' streptococci
Partial	Greenish discoloration	α	Pneumococci
None	No change	γ or non-haemolytic	Enterococci

Note: Some strains produce variable haemolysis.

2. **Enterococci**: all enterococci have the same glycerol-teichoic acid group antigen of Lancefield group D. Their normal habitat is the gut.

3. **'Viridans' streptococci**: a heterogeneous group, sometimes called 'indifferent' or 'other' streptococci: some strains may possess one of a variety of Lancefield group antigens (A, C, E, F, G, H, K, M, O or Q) or none at all.

4. **Pneumococci**: important invasive pathogens. Bacteria are arranged in pairs or short chains and are surrounded by a capsule.

Laboratory characteristics

Morphology and staining: Gram-positive spherical or oval cocci, in pairs or chains (Fig. 3.4).

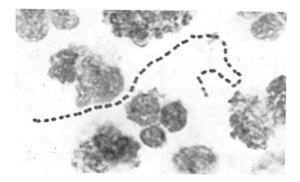

Fig. 3.4 Streptococcal pus (approx. $\times$ 1000).

Culture: grow well on blood agar; enrichment of media with blood, serum or glucose may be necessary. Incorporation of an aminoglycoside antibiotic inhibits other bacteria in a mixed culture, but permits growth of streptococci. Growth may be enhanced by 10% CO_2.

Haemolysis: see Table 3.2.

Biochemical reactions: streptococci can be characterized by their biochemical activities, and commercial systems, e.g. the API kit which comprises 32 tests, is useful in identification, particularly of species belonging to the 'viridans' group.

Serology: identifies *Lancefield groups*: 20 are recognized, designated A–H and K–V. The antigens that define the groups are either polysaccharide or teichoic acid. Serology performed by slide agglutination using commercially prepared kits.

The main medically important Lancefield groups, with the species usually responsible for human disease, are as follows:

Group A: *S. pyogenes*
Group B: *S. agalactiae*
Group C and group G: now classified as one species, *S. dysgalactiae* subsp. *equisimilis*
Group D: *Enterococci*.

PYOGENIC STREPTOCOCCI

STREPTOCOCCUS PYOGENES (LANCEFIELD GROUP A STREPTOCOCCI)

The most pathogenic member of the genus: produces a large number of powerful enzymes and toxins.

Habitat: present as a commensal in the nasopharynx of a variable proportion of healthy adults and, more commonly, children. The carriage rate in children is about 10%.

Laboratory characteristics

Culture: blood agar with small, typically matt or dry colonies surrounded by β-haemolysis. Strains that produce a hyaluronic acid capsule have mucoid colonies.

Capsule: some strains produce a hyaluronic acid capsule during the logarithmic phase of growth, and develop mucoid colonies on blood agar.

Toxins: the following extracellular products have been characterized:

1. *Streptokinase*: a protease that lyses fibrin.
2. *Hyaluronidase*: attacks hyaluronic acid – the cement of connective tissue – causing increased permeability. Antibodies to this enzyme are produced after infection.
3. *DNA-ases (deoxyribonucleases)*: four immunologically distinct types, A, B, C and D; B enzyme is the most common. Antibodies to DNA-ase – especially B enzyme – are demonstrable in most patients after recent infection with *S. pyogenes*.
4. *NADase (nicotinamide adenine dinucleotidase)*: kills leukocytes. Antibody formed after infection.
5. *Haemolysins*: two *streptolysins* (toxins which lyse erythrocytes) are produced.
6. *Erythrogenic toxin*: produced as a result of the presence of a lysogenic phage in the streptococci. Responsible for the characteristic erythematous rash in scarlet fever.
7. Other exotoxins and enzymes are produced and include *leukocidin, protease, amylase*.

Note: All these enzymes and toxins probably contribute to the invasiveness and pathogenicity of *S. pyogenes*.

Serotypes: *S. pyogenes* (Lancefield group A) can be subdivided into *Griffith* and *Lancefield* types, depending on three surface protein antigens:

- *M*: type-specific, i.e. there is a distinct M antigen for each strain. All group A streptococci carry M proteins. M antigens impede phagocytosis and antibody to them enhances phagocytosis. More than 100 distinct M serotypes have been identified. Immunity to infection with *S. pyogenes* is specific for each individual M type.
- *R*: the same R antigen can be found in different strains of group A streptococci.
- *T*: T antigens may be associated with different M types.

Pathogenicity

S. pyogenes causes:

- Tonsillitis and pharyngitis
- Peritonsillar abscess (quinsy)
- Scarlet fever
- Otitis media
- Mastoiditis and sinusitis
- Wound infections; may lead to cellulitis, lymphangitis, and necrotizing fasciitis.

- Impetigo
- Erysipelas (an acute lymphangitis of the skin)
- Puerperal sepsis.

Post-streptococcal complications: rheumatic fever, glomerulo-nephritis, septic arthritis or reactive arthritis in adults.

Antibiotic sensitivity

The drug of choice is penicillin. In patients hypersensitive to penicillin, use erythromycin or clindamycin. Resistance to erythromycin is currently ~ 10% and increasing globally.

LANCEFIELD GROUP B STREPTOCOCCI

Group B contains only one species, *S. agalactiae*, an important human (especially neonatal) pathogen. Three main types, with subdivisions, are recognized: human strains (mainly type I) are distinct from animal strains.

Habitat: commensal of female genital tract; usually secondary to anorectal carriage. Common in animals – especially cattle, in which it causes bovine mastitis.

Pathogenicity

An important pathogen in neonates, causing septicaemia, meningitis and also associated with septic abortion and puerperal or gynaecological sepsis.

Antibiotic sensitivity

Penicillin, erythromycin.

LANCEFIELD GROUP C STREPTOCOCCI

Can cause human disease: primarily veterinary pathogens.

S. dysgalactiae subsp. *equisimilis* is the most common species isolated from humans.

Toxins: elaborate a number of extracellular substances antigenically similar to those of *S. pyogenes*.

Note: Some strains of *S. milleri* (see under 'viridans' streptococci) may cross-react with group C streptococcal grouping reagents.

Pathogenicity

Low pathogenicity for humans. Occasionally cause tonsillitis (especially in closed institutional communities) and, rarely, endocarditis, septicaemia, meningitis or skin infections.

Antibiotic sensitivity

Penicillin.

LANCEFIELD GROUP G STREPTOCOCCI

A heterogeneous group: classified as *S. dysgalactiae* subsp. *equisimilis*. Share a number of characteristics with Lancefield groups A and C streptococci.

Habitat: human throat, gut and vagina.

Pathogenicity

As for group C streptococci. More common cause of human infection than group C.

ENTEROCOCCI (LANCEFIELD GROUP D STREPTOCOCCI)

Formerly classified as faecal streptococci, these organisms have now been placed in a separate genus, *Enterococcus*. The two medically important species are *E. faecalis* and *E. faecium*. Most infections are caused by *E. faecalis*.

Habitat: human and animal gut.

Laboratory characteristics

Morphology: oval cocci, usually in pairs; do not readily chain.

Culture: grow on ordinary and bile-containing media: heat-resistant and able to grow at 45°C; also able to grow in the presence of 6.5% sodium chloride.

Pathogenicity

Urinary and biliary tract infections, abdominal wound infection, endocarditis.

Antibiotic sensitivity

Enterococci are usually sensitive to ampicillin, moderately resistant to penicillin, and resistant to the cephalosporins. Vancomycin-resistant enterococci (VRE) are a problem in hospitals.

'VIRIDANS' OR 'OTHER' STREPTOCOCCI

Taxonomically complex group. Most human strains are commensals of the upper respiratory tract. Opportunistic pathogens in the immunocompromised.

Clinical laboratories do not usually differentiate species, but simply report *S. viridans*. Species identification within the 'viridans' group depends on the results of a range of biochemical tests. Species do not possess a characterizing Lancefield group antigen.

The principal species are listed in Table 3.3.

STREPTOCOCCUS PNEUMONIAE (PNEUMOCOCCUS)

The most common and the most important pathogen among the streptococci: also known as pneumococcus.

Habitat: normal commensal of the upper respiratory tract.

Table 3.3	'Viridans' or 'other' streptococci			
Species	**Haemolysis on blood agar**	**Lancefield group antigens**	**Habitat**	**Disease**
S. mitior	α (β or none)	none		Endocarditis
S. sanguis	α (β or none)	H or none	Human oropharynx	Endocarditis
S. mutans	None	none		Endocarditis; dental caries
S. salivarius	None	K or none		Rarely, endocarditis
S. milleri group	None (α or β)	A,C,F,G or none	Human oropharynx, gut, vagina	Abscesses (deep abdominal, liver, lung, brain)
S. bovis	α (or none)	D	Animal, sometimes human, gut	Endocarditis

Note: The *S. milleri* group (now called *S. anginosus* group) is recognized as an important cause of sepsis, and is sometimes classified with the pyogenic streptococci. ( ) = less common reactions.

Laboratory characteristics

Morphology: lanceolate diplococci (Fig. 6.3) arranged longitudinally in pairs, with the pointed ends outwards. Normally capsulated with carbohydrate antigenic capsule, which is correlated with virulence.

Culture: blood agar, sometimes broth enriched with serum or glucose.

Colonies: α-haemolytic, typically 'draughtsmen', i.e. with sunken centre owing to spontaneous autolysis of older organisms.

Differentiation from other α-haemolytic streptococci by:

- sensitivity to optochin
- solubility in bile: addition of bile to broth cultures lyses pneumococci
- fermentation of inulin.

Antigenic structure:

Capsule: contains the polysaccharide carbohydrate antigen; type-specific; 84 capsular types are recognized. Virulence correlates with the presence of a capsule, probably because this prevents or inhibits phagocytosis.

Identification: by a variety of serological tests directed against the antigen. The standard reference method is capsule swelling – the *quellung reaction* – observed microscopically when pneumococci are mixed with specific antisera.

C substance: a cell wall-associated antigen common to all pneumococci: consists of choline teichoic acid.

Transformation: the transfer of DNA – and some of the genetic markers for which it codes – from one bacterial strain to another was first demonstrated in pneumococci by Griffiths in 1928.

Pneumococcal types: not all types are equally common. The majority of human infections are associated with the lower-numbered serotypes.

Common infecting types are included in the polyvalent vaccine used in prophylactic immunization. Some of the infecting types are particularly invasive and liable to cause serious infections, such as pneumonia and septicaemia (types 1 and 3) and meningitis (types 7 and 12). Types 6 and 18 are important in children.

Pathogenicity

Pneumococci are important pathogens and cause a considerable amount of both morbidity and mortality today, despite their sensitivity to penicillin. They may cause:

- lobar pneumonia
- acute exacerbation of chronic bronchitis (often with *Haemophilus influenzae*)
- meningitis
- otitis media
- sinusitis
- conjunctivitis
- septicaemia (especially in splenectomized patients).

Antibiotic sensitivity

In the UK almost all strains remain sensitive to penicillin, but penicillin resistance is a significant problem in some European countries. Resistance to erythromycin, tetracycline and trimethoprim is more commonly encountered in the UK.

GRAM-POSITIVE BACILLI

BACILLUS

Members of the genus *Bacillus* are aerobic, sporing, Gram-positive, chaining bacilli. *Bacillus* species are ubiquitous soil saprophytes, but one, *B. anthracis*, is an important pathogen responsible for anthrax in animals and humans. Anthrax is now rare in developed countries.

BACILLUS ANTHRACIS

Habitat: infected animals, but spores are found in soil and pasture contaminated with vegetative cells from dead and dying animals.

Laboratory characteristics

Morphology: large, non-motile rectangular bacilli usually arranged in chains. Spores – oval and central – are not formed in tissue, but develop after the organism is shed or if it is grown on artificial media. The bacilli are capsulated in the animal body and on laboratory culture under certain conditions: the capsule consists of a polypeptide of D-glutamic acid.

Staining: Gram-positive; spores can be stained by modified Ziehl–Neelsen method.

McFadyean's reaction is used to demonstrate *B. anthracis* in the blood of animals, in a heat-fixed film stained with polychrome methylene blue.

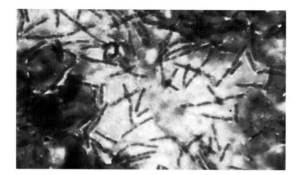

Fig. 3.5 *Bacillus anthracis*: McFadyean's reaction (approx. × 1000).

Observe: blue bacilli surrounded by purplish-pink amorphous material, due to disintegrated capsules and indicating a positive reaction: diagnostic of *B. anthracis* (Fig. 3.5).

Culture: aerobe and facultative anaerobe; grows readily on ordinary media over a wide temperature range. Characteristic colonial morphology the so-called 'medusa head' of 'curled hair lock' appearance.

Antigenic structure: the antigenic components described include a complex group of toxins and the capsular polypeptide.

Pathogenicity

The cause of anthrax. A wide range of animal hosts is susceptible. Infection is characteristically septicaemic, with splenic enlargement. Humans are infected from animals or animal products.

Viability: vegetative cells are readily destroyed by heat, but spores demonstrate a variable, often high, level of heat resistance – in the dry state, up to 150°C for 1 hour. Spores can remain viable for many years in contaminated soil.

Antibiotic sensitivity

B. anthracis is susceptible to many antibiotics: penicillin is the drug of choice.

OTHER BACILLUS SPECIES

Many species are recognized:

Habitat: saprophytes in soil, water, dust and air, and on vegetation.

The spores of certain bacilli, e.g. *B. stearothermophilus*, *B. megaterium*, are used as a test of the efficiency of sterilization by steam under pressure (i.e. in autoclaves), by ethylene oxide or by ionizing radiation.

B. cereus is a cause of food poisoning (e.g. when contaminating rice). A number of species may cause opportunistic infections.

Lactobacillus

Members of this genus are widely distributed as saprophytes in vegetable and animal material (e.g. milk, cheese); others are common human and animal commensals.

Classification is complex. Lactobacilli attack carbohydrates to form abundant acid, and are tolerant of an acid environment (pH 3.0–4.0). The best-recognized species is *L. acidophilus*.

LACTOBACILLUS ACIDOPHILUS

Habitat: present in the mouth, gastrointestinal tract and female genital tract – most vaginal lactobacilli (Döderlein's bacilli) seem to be *L. acidophilus*.

Laboratory characteristics

Morphology and staining: large, Gram-positive bacilli; non-branching, non-motile, non-sporing.

Culture: grows best, but slowly, under microaerophilic conditions in the presence of 5% CO_2 and at pH 6.0. Acid media, e.g. tomato juice agar (pH 5.0), support the growth of lactobacilli but inhibit many other bacteria.

Pathogenicity

Lactobacilli are associated with dental caries.

CORYNEBACTERIUM AND RELATED BACTERIA

CORYNEBACTERIUM

Gram-positive bacilli with a characteristic morphology; non-sporing; non-capsulate; non-motile.

Widely distributed in nature: several human and animal species are important pathogens.

CORYNEBACTERIUM DIPHTHERIAE

Habitat: the throat and nose of humans.

Laboratory characteristics

Morphology and staining: pleomorphic Gram-positive rods or clubs. Adjacent cells lie at different angles to each other, forming V, L and W shapes – a so-called *Chinese-character* arrangement; may also be parallel to one another, in *palisades*.

Culture: an aerobe and facultative anaerobe; optimum temperature 37°C. Does not grow well on ordinary agar. Selective media containing blood or serum are required.

• *Blood tellurite agar* (e.g. Hoyle's): after 48 h incubation corynebacteria produce characteristic grey-black colonies owing to their ability to reduce potassium tellurite to tellurium.

Colonial appearance: three colonial types are recognized: *gravis*, *intermedius* and *mitis*, so named from the type of clinical disease they were most likely to cause. Other corynebacteria also grow on tellurite media, to form colonies that can be confused with those of *C. diphtheriae*.

Identification: by biochemical tests and demonstration of toxin production. Other corynebacteria may mimic *C. diphtheriae* in films and on culture. Some isolates of *C. diphtheriae*, especially *mitis* strains, are not toxigenic and are therefore non-virulent.

Biochemical reactions: acid production from a range of carbohydrates and other biochemical tests is used to differentiate *C. diphtheriae* from other corynebacteria. *Gravis* (but not *intermedius* or *mitis*) strains ferment starch and glycogen.

Typing: serotyping, phage typing and bacteriocin typing have all been used to subdivide strains of *C. diphtheriae* for epidemiological studies.

Toxin: responsible for virulence; can be demonstrated by a gel precipitation test or a rapid immunochromatographic strip test.

Gel-precipitation (Elek) test: a filter-paper strip previously immersed in diphtheria antitoxin is incorporated into serum agar before it has set. The strain of *C. diphtheriae* under investigation is then streaked on to the agar at right-angles to the strip. Incubate at 37°C.

Observe: after 24 h and 48 h for lines of precipitation, indicating toxin–antitoxin interaction (Fig. 3.6).

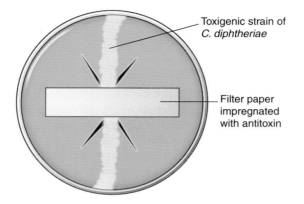

Fig. 3.6 Elek test for demonstration of toxin production by *Corynebacterium diphtheriae*. The toxin combines with antitoxin to produce antigen–antibody complexes which form visible lines of precipitation in the agar.

NB. Guinea pig inoculation is no longer used in the UK to detect toxin.

Diphtheria toxin: the exotoxin of *C. diphtheriae* is produced only by strains carrying a bacteriophage: its formation in vitro is stimulated in culture media with low iron content. The toxin interferes with protein synthesis in mammalian cells by splitting the molecule of NAD (nicotinamide adenine dinucleotide), an essential cofactor for the transferase involved in peptide bond formation by ribosomes. It acts locally on the mucous membranes of the respiratory tract to produce a grey, adherent pseudomembrane consisting of fibrin, bacteria, and epithelial and phagocytic cells. After absorption into the bloodstream it acts systemically on the cells of the myocardium, the nervous system (only motor nerves are affected) and the adrenal glands. The toxin can be rendered non-toxic but still antigenic by treatment with formaldehyde: the *toxoid* so formed is used in prophylactic immunization.

Pathogenicity

C. diphtheriae is the cause of diphtheria. Usually the mucous membranes of the upper respiratory tract are affected, but sometimes, especially in tropical countries, skin lesions are produced. The serious systemic manifestations follow absorption of the exotoxin.

Antibiotic sensitivity

C. diphtheriae is sensitive to penicillin, erythromycin and other antibiotics.

OTHER CORYNEBACTERIA

CORYNEBACTERIUM ULCERANS

May be responsible in humans for diphtheria-like throat lesions, but usually with little evidence of toxaemia.

Laboratory characteristics

Biochemical reactions distinguish it from *C. diphtheriae*.

Toxins: two are produced – one immunologically identical to the toxin of *C. diphtheriae*, the other identical to the toxin of *C. pseudotuberculosis*, an important animal pathogen.

HUMAN COMMENSALS

There are many so-called *diphtheroid bacilli*, e.g. *C. hofmannii* in the throat and *C. xerosis* in the conjunctiva.

Habitat: normally present in the skin (especially within sebaceous ducts) and mucous membranes.

Laboratory characteristics

Morphology and staining: less pleomorphic and more strongly Gram-positive than *C. diphtheriae*; metachromatic granules are few or absent. Tend to be arranged in palisades, with less pronounced Chinese lettering than *C. diphtheriae*.

Culture: grow well on ordinary agar.

Pathogenicity

Occasional opportunistic pathogens, causing, for example, endocarditis on prosthetic valves, infection in implanted artificial joints, peritonitis in patients receiving continuous ambulatory peritoneal dialysis (CAPD).

CORYNEBACTERIUM JEIKEIUM

A skin commensal diphtheroid with a particular ability to cause opportunistic infections. Notable because of its resistance to many antimicrobial agents: sensitive to glycopeptides and linezolid.

PROPIONIBACTERIUM

Gram-positive, non-sporing anaerobic bacilli, formerly classified as anaerobic corynebacteria. A differential feature from other similar bacteria is that they produce propionic acid as the major end-product from glucose fermentation: this can be detected by gas–liquid chromatography.

There are two main species *P. acnes* and *P. granulosum*.

Habitat: the human skin.

Pathogenicity

Association with the skin disease acne vulgaris.

ERYSIPELOTHRIX

ERYSIPELOTHRIX RHUSIOPATHIAE

A slender, Gram-positive non-motile bacillus of uncertain classification. Aerobe and facultative anaerobe.

Habitat: healthy pigs, but widely distributed in other animals and birds; found on the skin and scales of fish; causes swine erysipelas.

Pathogenicity

Responsible in humans for erysipeloid, a rare skin infection.

LISTERIA

Six species are recognized, but almost all human infections are due to *Listeria monocytogenes*.

LISTERIA MONOCYTOGENES

Morphologically similar to erysipelothrix and diphtheroids, but flagellated below 33°C. Non-motile at 37°C, but exhibits active tumbling motility at 25°C in young broth cultures.

Habitat: wild and domestic animals; ubiquitous in the environment, and found throughout the food chain.

Laboratory characteristics

Culture: aerobic and facultatively anaerobic; optimal temperature 37°C, but will survive and grow at 6°C.

Colonies on horse-blood agar are non-pigmented and surrounded by a narrow zone of complete (β)-haemolysis with an indistinct margin.

Typing: on the basis of O and H antigenic structure 13 serotypes are recognized, but almost all infections are caused by three of these serotypes, type 4b being the commonest.

Pathogenicity

Causes listeriosis in humans and animals.

Antibiotic sensitivity

Sensitive in vitro to a number of antibiotics. Ampicillin is usually used in treatment, often in combination with gentamicin.

CLOSTRIDIUM

Clostridia are anaerobic, sporing Gram-positive bacilli. Most species are soil saprophytes, but a few are pathogens. The most important, together with some of their principal properties, are listed in Table 3.4.

Table 3.4 Pathogenic properties of the main medically important species of clostridia

Species	Disease
C. perfringens	Gas gangrene, food poisoning
C. novyi	Gas gangrene
C. septicum	Gas gangrene, neutropenic enterocolitis
C. histolyticum	Secondary role in gas gangrene
C. sordellii	Secondary role in gas gangrene
C. difficile	Antibiotic-associated colitis
C. sporogenes	Doubtful pathogenicity in gas gangrene
*C. tetani**	Tetanus
C. botulinum	Botulism

* Forms round, terminal spores; the other species have oval, central, subterminal or terminal spores.

Habitat: human and animal intestine; soil; water; decaying animal and plant matter.

Laboratory characteristics

Morphology and staining: large Gram-positive rods, sometimes pleomorphic; filamentous forms are common.

Spores: all species form endospores, which may be 'bulging', i.e. wider than the bacterial body; sometimes useful in identification, e.g. *C. tetani*. Note that *C. perfringens* (the most common human pathogen) forms spores with difficulty.

Culture:

Blood agar anaerobically; in mixed culture the addition of an aminoglycoside makes an excellent selective medium for clostridia.

Biochemical activity:

Saccharolytic: many species ferment sugars; this produces reddening of the meat particles in Robertson's meat medium, with a rancid smell.

Proteolytic: production of enzymes that digest proteins is a common property of many clostridia: this causes blackening and digestion of the meat particles in Robertson's meat medium, with a foul smell.

Toxins: medically important clostridial species produce several toxins: the exotoxins of *C. tetani* and *C. botulinum* are among the most toxic substances known. Clostridial toxins are often lethal for laboratory animals.

Classification: the range of saccharolytic and proteolytic activity; tests for lecithinase and lipase activity; and detection of the fatty acid end-products of glucose metabolism (by gas chromatography) are used in classification.

Identification: often difficult; the characteristics and identification of four important pathogenic clostridia – *C. perfringens*, *C. tetani*, *C. botulinum* and *C. difficile* – are described below.

Antibiotic sensitivity

Sensitive to penicillin, metronidazole, clindamycin, tetracycline, erythromycin.

Resistant to aminoglycosides.

CLOSTRIDIUM PERFRINGENS (CLOSTRIDIUM WELCHII)

Laboratory characteristics

Morphology: a stubby bacillus in which spores are hardly ever seen.

Culture: most strains grow well on blood agar anaerobically, producing β-haemolytic colonies, but some strains are non-haemolytic.

Biochemical activity: mainly saccharolytic: in tube cultures of litmus milk a characteristic 'stormy clot' is formed owing to the production of acid and large amounts of gas.

Typing: *C. perfringens* can be divided into five types – A, B, C, D and E – on the basis of the 12 toxins formed; all five types produce α toxin. Type A is the human pathogen; the other types are important pathogens of domestic animals.

Toxins:

1. *Alpha (α) toxin*: an enzyme, phospholipase C, which causes cell lysis as a resulting of lecithinase action on the lecithin in mammalian cell membranes.

2. *Other toxins*: include collagenase, proteinase, hyaluronidase, deoxyribonuclease. Several have haemolytic activity: some are described as 'necrotizing' or 'lethal', from their effects on laboratory animals.

Identification: the *Nagler reaction* identifies *C. perfringens* by neutralization of α toxin with specific antitoxin (Fig. 3.7).

Pathogenicity

- *Gas gangrene*: wounds associated with the necrosis of muscle may become infected with *C. perfringens* and other clostridia,

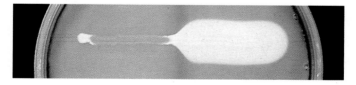

Fig. 3.7 Nagler reaction. The α toxin (a lecithinase) of *Clostridium perfringens* has produced opacity owing to degradation of lecithin in the medium on the right. This action has been neutralized by the antitoxin on the left of the plate.

causing a severe and life-threatening spreading infection of the muscles.
- *Food poisoning*: when ingested in large numbers some strains of *C. perfringens* produce an enterotoxin in the gut, causing diarrhoea and other symptoms of food poisoning.

CLOSTRIDIUM TETANI

Laboratory characteristics

Morphology: a longer, thinner bacillus than *C. perfringens*, with round terminal spores giving a characteristic 'drumstick' appearance (Fig. 3.8).

    Toxin: a protein, and exceedingly potent. There are two components:

- *Tetanospasmin*: neurotoxic – the true tetanus toxin
- *Tetanolysin*: haemolytic.

    Identification: by toxin neutralization tests.

Pathogenicity

The cause of tetanus – a classic toxin-mediated disease in which *C. tetani* in a wound elaborates the powerful neurotoxin, which spreads and acts on the central nervous system, causing severe muscle spasms.

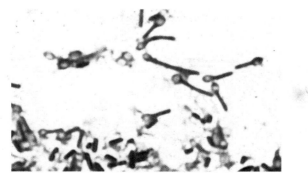

Fig. 3.8　*Clostridium tetani* (approx. × 1000).

CLOSTRIDIUM BOTULINUM

Laboratory characteristics

Toxin: protein, and even more potent than that of *C. tetani*, the toxin of *C. botulinum* is the most active known poison. It acts by preventing the release of acetylcholine at motor nerve endings in the parasympathetic system. Destroyed in 2 min at 60–90°C, depending on type. There are seven *toxin types* – A, B, C, D, E, F and G – with serologically distinct but pharmacologically similar toxins.

Human botulism is usually due to toxin types A, B and E.

Identification: by testing for the toxin in a culture, patient's serum or food sample. Mice, some of which are protected with antitoxin to A, B and E toxins, are injected with the suspect material: if toxin is present, mice inoculated with the appropriate antitoxin survive; the others become paralysed and die.

Pathogenicity

Produces a rare form of 'food poisoning' known as *botulism*, in which the symptoms are neurological rather than intestinal. It is caused by the ingestion of preformed toxin in food contaminated with the organism.

CLOSTRIDIUM DIFFICILE

Habitat: found in the faeces of 3–5% of healthy adults, and regularly present in the faeces of healthy infants. Found with its toxin in the faeces of patients suffering from antibiotic-associated colitis: in its severe form, this becomes pseudomembranous colitis.

Laboratory characteristics

Identification:
- *Isolation*: from faeces using selective media, e.g. cefoxitin–cycloserine–fructose agar; anaerobic incubation. Cultures produce a characteristic 'dung-like' aroma, and the irregular rough colonies fluoresce under ultraviolet light.
- *Demonstration of toxin* by inoculation of cell cultures (e.g. human embryo fibroblasts) with filtrate of broth culture of

C. difficile: cell cultures containing antitoxin are also inoculated. *Observe*: cytotoxicity, which is neutralized in the cultures containing *C. sordellii* antitoxin. All enteropathogenic isolates of *C. difficile* are toxigenic.

Note: This test can be carried out on faeces, to demonstrate directly the presence of toxin.

Typing: a molecular typing scheme, using a PCR (polymerase chain reaction) method, is available: of value in investigating hospital outbreaks.

ACTINOMYCES AND NOCARDIA

Actinomyces and nocardia are morphologically similar Gram-positive branching rods and filaments. Actinomyces are micro-aerophilic or anaerobic on primary isolation, although some species grow in air after a few subcultures. Nocardia are aerobic organisms.

ACTINOMYCES

Most actinomyces are soil organisms but some – and these are the potentially pathogenic species – are commensals of the mouth in humans and animals (Table 3.5).

Species are identified by colonial appearances, the ability to grow aerobically, and by biochemical tests.

ACTINOMYCES ISRAELII

Laboratory characteristics

Morphology and staining: Gram-positive bacteria which grow in filaments that readily break up into rods and may show branching.

Table 3.5 Some *actinomyces* species

Species	Host/habitat	Disease association
A. israelii	Oropharynx and gut of humans	Human actinomycosis
A. naeslundii A. viscosus A. odontolyticus	Oropharynx of humans	Dental plaque and caries; human actinomycosis
A. bovis	Oropharynx of cattle	Lumpy jaw in cattle

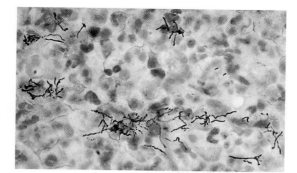

Fig. 3.9 Actinomycotic pus (approx. × 1000).

Non-motile, non-sporing, not acid-fast. In tissue, colonies develop to form diagnostic yellowish 'sulphur granules', which are visible to the naked eye and which are found in pus discharged through draining sinuses (Fig. 3.9).

Culture: small, white to cream adherent nodular colonies on blood or serum glucose agar incubated anaerobically at 37°C for 7 days or more; growth is enhanced by 5% CO_2.

Isolation of this exacting microorganism from clinical material is difficult, especially as the pus usually contains other, faster-growing bacteria. Presumptive diagnosis is made by the demonstration of typical Gram-positive branching filaments in a sulphur granule. Whenever possible, a washed, crushed sulphur granule should be cultured in preference to pus.

Pathogenicity

Actinomycosis is a mixed infection: *A. israelii* is the most important actinomycete involved. The infection is endogenous in origin, and results in a chronic granuloma with abscess formation: profuse pus discharges by draining through sinuses. Infection probably starts after local trauma, e.g. the extraction of carious teeth, appendicectomy. The typical sites of the disease are cervicofacial (65% of cases); abdominal (usually ileocaecal; 20% of cases); and, rarely, thoracic, affecting the lung.

Intrauterine contraceptive devices, especially those made of plastic, may be colonized with *A. israelii*. The significance of this is uncertain but, perhaps in association with other organisms, a low-grade intrauterine infection may result (Fig. 3.10).

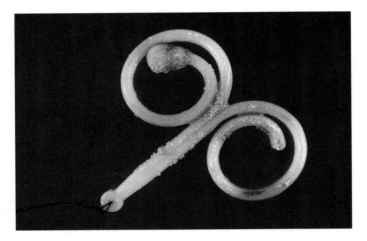

Fig. 3.10 Intrauterine contraceptive device heavily contaminated by *A. israelii* after a long period in situ.

Antibiotic sensitivity

Sensitive to penicillin, clindamycin, tetracycline, erythromycin.

NOCARDIA

Habitat: the majority of species are soil saprophytes; a few are pathogenic to humans.

Laboratory characteristics

Morphology and staining: similar to actinomyces, but some species are partially acid-fast.

Culture: wrinkled, rosette- or star-shaped colonies, initially white, then yellow and finally pink or red. Slow-growing aerobic organisms produced after 5–14 days' incubation on nutrient agar.

Pathogenicity

Generally cause chronic granulomatous suppurative infections.

NOCARDIA ASTEROIDES

Affects the lungs, sometimes with secondary spread to other organs, e.g. the brain. Pulmonary nocardiosis usually develops as an opportunistic infection in immunocompromised patients.

NOCARDIA MADURAE AND NOCARDIA BRASILIENSIS

Madura foot or *mycetoma* is a tropical form of nocardiosis which affects the skin, subcutaneous tissue and bones of the foot to produce a destructive infection with multiple discharging sinuses. The bacteria are implanted by contaminated thorns or splinters.

Antibiotic sensitivity

Sensitive to sulphonamides and to co-trimoxazole. Treatment may have to be continued for many months.

MYCOBACTERIUM

For simplicity, mycobacteria which stain poorly with Gram stain are included in this chapter.

Mycobacteria are referred to as *acid-fast* bacilli. Their cell wall has a high lipid content owing to the presence of mycolic acid: acid fastness is the result of the formation of complexes between the concentrated carbol fuchsin of the Ziehl–Neelsen stain and mycolic acid, one of the cell wall lipids. After decolonization with 20% sulphuric acid and alcohol the bacilli retain the bright red colour of the stain (see Fig. 14.2). Nowadays, tubercle bacilli are detected on slides using an auramine stain under fluorescent microscopy (Fig. 3.11)

The main medically important mycobacteria, together with some of their properties, are listed in Table 3.6.

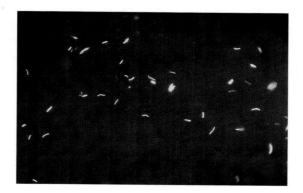

Fig. 3.11   Tubercle bacilli stained with auramine and viewed under ultraviolet light. Photograph courtesy of Dr Brian Watt.

Table 3.6   The main medically important species of *Mycobacteria*.

Species	Habitat and source	Disease	Cultural characteristics on Löwenstein–Jensen medium
M. tuberculosis	Infected humans	Tuberculosis	Rough, dry, yellow colonies: slow grower
M. bovis	Infected cattle	Tuberculosis	White, smooth colonies (inhibited by glycerol): slow grower
M. africanus	Infected humans	Tuberculosis	Colonies like those of M. bovis
M. leprae	Infected humans	Leprosy	No growth
Mycobacteria other than tuberculosis bacilli (MOTT)	Mainly soil, water; sometimes birds, animals	Pulmonary infection, cervical adenitis, skin ulcers	Colonies often pigmented: some grow slowly, others rapidly; may exhibit unusual temperature requirements

MYCOBACTERIUM TUBERCULOSIS

The cause of tuberculosis, a slowly progressive chronic infection, usually in the lungs, but many other organs and tissues can be infected. The incidence of tuberculosis is increasing worldwide, but especially in AIDS cases. Multiple drug resistance is now a significant problem.

Morphology: slender non-sporing bacilli.

Culture: do not grow on ordinary media. Grow well on Löwenstein–Jensen medium (contains egg, asparagine, glycerol and, to inhibit contaminants, malachite green). Growth takes a minimum of 2–3 weeks' incubation at 37°C. Figure 3.12 shows typical rough, tough and buff colonies on Löwenstein–Jensen medium. Cultures can be performed more rapidly using a radiometric BacTec.

MYCOBACTERIUM BOVIS

The main cause of tuberculosis in cattle: humans can become infected by ingestion of milk containing *M. bovis*. Can cause tuberculosis of the bones, joints and kidneys. Rare in UK now because of eradication of the disease in cattle.

Morphology: slender non-sporing bacilli.

Culture: grows poorly on Löwenstein–Jensen medium.

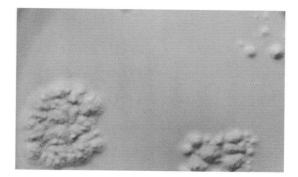

Fig. 3.12 *Mycobacterium tuberculosis:* culture showing 'rough, tough and buff' colonies.

Antibiotic sensitivity

Both *M. tuberculosis* and *M. bovis* are sensitive to a wide range of drugs (see Chapters 14 and 19). Because of the emergence of resistant variants therapy must always comprise a combination of drugs. Multiple-drug resistant (MDR) strains of *M. tuberculosis* are now a significant problem.

MYCOBACTERIUM LEPRAE

The cause of leprosy – still a scourge in many parts of the world today.

Culture: does not grown in vitro. Culture by inoculation into foot-pads of mice: slow-growing granulomas develop at the site of injection.

Antibiotic sensitivity

Sensitive to dapsone, rifampicin, clofazimine.

MOTT (MYCOBACTERIA OTHER THAN TUBERCULOSIS BACILLI)

A group of miscellaneous mycobacteria of low pathogenicity for humans. Sometimes are 'passengers' accompanying tuberculosis. However, they are a major problem in AIDS cases, especially *M. avium* complex. Often resistant to several of the standard anti-tuberculosis drugs.

Table 3.7 MOTT (mycobacteria other than tuberculosis bacilli)

Species	Disease

M. avium complex:
   M. avium
   M. intracellulare
   M. scrofulaceum
	Pulmonary; lymphadenopathy; disseminated infection in AIDS patients

M. fortuitum	Pulmonary
M. marinum	Granulomatous ulcers of skin
M. kansasii M. malmoense M. xenopi	Pulmonary

Table 3.7 lists the principal species, together with the diseases they can cause.

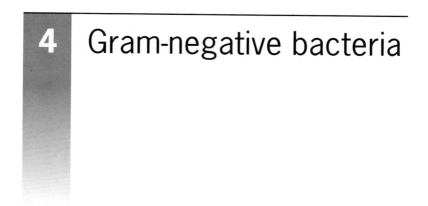

4 Gram-negative bacteria

The medically important Gram-negative bacterial genera classified on the basis of morphology and aerobic or anaerobic growth are listed in Figure 4.1. Note that this classification has been simplified and retains nomenclature still widely used in medical bacteriology.

GRAM-NEGATIVE COCCI

NEISSERIA

The neisseriae are Gram-negative diplococci: the two pathogenic species, *N. gonorrhoeae* (the gonococcus) and *N. meningitidis* (the meningococcus), have exacting growth requirements.

NEISSERIA GONORRHOEAE

Habitat: the human urogenital tract.

Laboratory characteristics

Morphology and staining: Gram-negative cocci, characteristically (when intracellular) in pairs (see Fig. 13.1).

Culture: requires an enriched medium (e.g. chocolate agar) and incubation in a moist aerobic atmosphere containing 5–10% CO_2 for 48 h. Selective media are necessary to inhibit other bacteria, e.g. Thayer–Martin medium.

Colonies: grey, glistening colonies after 24 h incubation, becoming larger, opaque and somewhat irregular at 48 h.

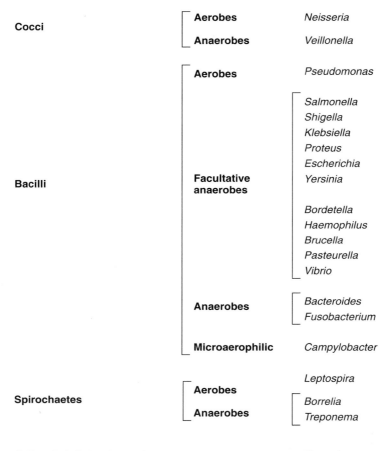

Fig. 4.1 Classification of Gram-negative bacteria.

Identification: Colonies are oxidase positive: rapidly turn dark purple on addition of the 'oxidase reagent' (Fig. 4.2). *Biochemical tests*: ferment glucose only. Serological tests, e.g. ELISA, coagglutination with monoclonal antibodies used as confirmatory tests.

Molecular methods: DNA amplification-based tests, e.g. ligase chain reaction (LCR) are rapid but expensive.

Typing: for epidemiology, by auxotyping (analysis of nutritional requirements), serotyping and molecular typing.

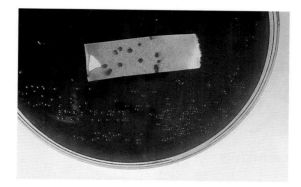

Fig. 4.2 Oxidase-positive colonies of *N. gonorrhoeae*.

Pathogenicity

The cause of the sexually transmitted disease gonorrhoea.

Viability: Dies rapidly outside the human host, but may remain viable in pus for some time.

Antibiotic sensitivity

Resistance increasing. Test strains against ampicillin, tetracycline, macrolides (e.g. azithromycin), spectinomycin, ceftriaxone and fluoroquinolones, e.g. ciprofloxacin.

NEISSERIA MENINGITIDIS

Habitat: the human nasopharynx: present in 10–25% of normal people.

Laboratory characteristics

Morphology and staining: as for *N. gonorrhoeae*. Films of the CSF in meningococcal meningitis have a similar appearance to that of genital tract exudate in gonorrhoea, but organisms are scantier.

Culture: requirements similar to those of *N. gonorrhoeae*, although somewhat less exacting. Selective media are not required for isolation, as organism is present in CSF or blood in pure culture.

Identification: by biochemical tests: ferments both maltose and glucose.

Antigenic structure: there are three main groups (A, B, C) and 10 subsidiary groups (X, Y, Z, D, E, W-135, H, I, K and L). Not all isolates are groupable. Groups B and C are the most common in the UK. Group B strains are poorly immunogenic.

Pathogenicity

Cause of meningococcal meningitis and/or septicaemia.

Viability: dies quickly at room temperature outside the human host.

Antibiotic sensitivity

Test strains against penicillin, ceftriaxone, chloramphenicol, ciprofloxacin and rifampicin.

COMMENSAL NEISSERIAE – *N. SICCA, N. LACTAMICA, N. CINEREA*

Habitat: regularly present in the mucous membranes of the mouth, nose and pharynx; less frequently in the genital tract. Rarely cause infections.

MORAXELLA

Gram-negative cocci or short bacilli arranged in pairs: strictly aerobic, non-motile, oxidase, catalase and DNase positive. *M. catarrhalis* is the main human pathogen. *M. lacunata* and *M. nonliquefaciens* are associated with ocular infections.

MORAXELLA CATARRHALIS

Formerly classified as *Neisseria catarrhalis* and (more recently) as *Branhamella catarrhalis*, this bacterium shares many characteristics with the commensal neisseriae and grows well on ordinary media.

Laboratory identification

By biochemical tests.

Pathogenicity

This nasopharyngeal organism is now recognized as a cause of otitis media and sinusitis in children, infective exacerbations of chronic obstructive pulmonary disease in adults, and pneumonia in the elderly.

Antibiotic sensitivity

The majority of clinically significant strains are β-lactamase producers and are resistant to ampicillin. Strains should be tested against co-amoxiclav, trimethoprim, cefuroxime, clarithromycin, tetracycline and ciprofloxacin.

ACINETOBACTER

Gram-negative coccobacilli (microscopic morphology may be confused with neisseria *but* oxidase negative). Precise classification of species not yet established. *A. calcoaceticus*, *A. lwoffi* and *A. baumannii* are the main 'species' associated with clinical infections.

Habitat: widely distributed in nature.

Laboratory characteristics

Isolation: grows well on routine media; aerobic.
Identification: by biochemical tests.

Pathogenicity

Generally an opportunistic pathogen seen in hospitalized patients, particularly those in intensive care units, e.g. ventilator-associated pneumonia, catheter-related septicaemia. Readily colonizes wards and specialist units, e.g. burns units, often requiring closure.

Antibiotic resistance

Usually resistant to many antibiotics, including those used to treat other forms of serious hospital sepsis.

KINGELLA

Gram-negative coccobacilli, often confused with neisseria.
Habitat: nasopharynx: present mainly in children.

Laboratory characteristics

Isolation: slow growing and fastidious.
Identification: oxidase positive, catalase negative, and by biochemical tests.

Pathogenicity

Most infections due to *K. kingae*. Causative agent of bone and joint infections in children and endocarditis in adults (HACEK organisms, see p. 205).

GRAM-NEGATIVE BACILLI

Gram-negative bacilli can be considered under six main groups:

- Pseudomonas and related bacteria
- Enterobacteria
- Campylobacter, Helicobacter, Vibrio and related bacteria
- 'Parvobacteria'
- Legionella
- Anaerobic.

PSEUDOMONAS, STENOTROPHOMONAS AND BURKHOLDERIA

These Gram-negative motile aerobic bacilli have very simple growth requirements and limited fermentation activity.

Several of the human pathogens formerly classified in the genus *Pseudomonas* have been reclassified (see Table 4.1).

PSEUDOMONAS AERUGINOSA

Habitat: human and animal gastrointestinal tract, water, soil and sewage. Moist environments are important reservoirs in hospitals; able to survive and multiply in some aqueous antiseptics, saline and 'sterile' water in hospitals.

Table 4.1 Reclassification of pathogenic aerobic Gram-negative bacilli

Genus	Species
Pseudomonas	P. aeruginosa
	P. fluorescens
	P. putida
Stenotrophomonas	S. maltophilia
Burkholderia	B. cepacia
	B. mallei
	B. pseudomallei

Laboratory characteristics

Morphology and staining: Gram-negative bacilli, motile; non-sporing; non-capsulate.

Culture: a strict aerobe; grows readily on routine media over a wide temperature range.

Colonies: often (but not always) large and irregular, with a fluorescent, greenish appearance owing to the production of *pyocyanin* (blue-green) and *fluorescein* (yellow) pigments, and with a characteristic 'fruity' odour. Strains isolated from the sputum of patients with cystic fibrosis often give rise to large mucoid colonies, owing to the formation of extracellular polysaccharide slime: such colonies may fail to produce pyocyanin.

Identification: colonial morphology and pigment production.

Biochemical tests: does not ferment, but oxidizes carbohydrates (e.g. API 2O NE tests).

Typing: several typing methods available: *serology*: based on O (somatic) and H (flagellar) antigens. RFLP (restriction fragment length polymorphism) of chromosomal DNA and DNA amplification typing are more sensitive techniques.

Pathogenicity

A major opportunistic pathogen causing hospital-acquired infections in debilitated patients, such as those with burns or malignancy, or as a result of therapeutic procedures:

- Complicated urinary tract infection; also common with indwelling catheters
- Wound infections, including pressure sores and varicose ulcers
- Septicaemia
- Lower respiratory tract infections:
  - in cystic fibrosis
  - in patients on ventilators
- Eye infections, secondary to trauma or surgery
- Chronic otitis media and otitis externa.

Antibiotic sensitivity

Resistant to many antibiotics; the main antipseudomonal drugs are:

- Aminoglycosides e.g. gentamicin
- Certain β-lactams: piperacillin, ticarcillin, ceftazidime, imipenem, aztreonam

- Fluoroquinolones: e.g. ciprofloxacin
- Polymyxin (colistin).

PSEUDOMONAS FLUORESCENS AND PSEUDOMONAS PUTIDA

These fluorescent pseudomonads are similar to *P. aeruginosa* but of lower pathogenicity. Their ability to grow at 4°C has occasionally caused the contamination of blood and other stored fluids.

STENOTROPHOMONAS MALTOPHILIA

Habitat and laboratory characteristics: as *P. aeruginosa*, but colonies are oxidase negative or weakly positive.

Pathogenicity

Important agents of opportunistic infections in immunocompromised patients: pneumonia, septicaemia, urinary tract infections. Administration of broad-spectrum antibiotics a predisposing factor.

Antibiotic sensitivity

Inherently resistant to carbapenems, e.g. imipenem, and often multiply antibiotic resistant. Also poor correlation between in vitro sensitivity and clinical outcome. Co-trimoxazole is the antibiotic of choice.

BURKHOLDERIA CEPACIA

Habitat and laboratory characteristics: as *S. maltophilia*.

Pathogenicity

Colonization and pneumonia in patients with cystic fibrosis.

Antibiotic sensitivity

Multiply resistant strains make antibiotic therapy difficult. In addition to antipseudomonal antibiotics, co-trimoxazole, chloramphenicol and minocycline may be effective.

BURKHOLDERIA PSEUDOMALLEI AND BURKHOLDERIA MALLEI

B. pseudomallei (Whitmore's bacillus) causes melioidosis, a disease of animals and humans endemic in southeast Asia. Most human cases are asymptomatic, but there may be pulmonary consolidation, skin lesions and fatal septicaemia. The organism is a saprophyte of certain soils and waters, often with a large animal reservoir locally.

B. mallei causes glanders in horses. Rarely, human infections are acquired from animals or from laboratory work with the organism.

ENTEROBACTERIA

Gram-negative bacilli which belong to the tribe *Enterobacteriaceae*. Often called *coliforms*, they are intestinal parasites of humans and animals: many are human pathogens. Table 4.2 lists the main medically important species.

Laboratory characteristics

Morphology and staining: Gram-negative bacilli. Non-motile, or motile by peritrichous flagella (Fig. 4.3). Non-sporing.

Culture: grow well on ordinary media, e.g. blood agar, CLED agar; aerobic and facultatively anaerobic; grow in a wide range of temperatures.

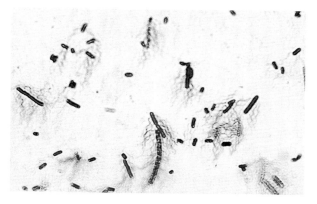

Fig. 4.3   Flagella. Peritrichous flagella demonstrated by a silver-impregnation staining method (× 2000).

Table 4.2 Medically important enterobacteria

Genus	Species	Principal diseases
Escherichia	E. coli	Urinary infection, gastroenteritis, septicaemia
Shigella	S. dysenteriae S. flexneri S. boydii S. sonnei	Dysentery
Salmonella	S. typhi S. paratyphi A, B, C	Enteric fever
	S. typhimurium Many other serotypes	Food poisoning
Klebsiella	K. pneumoniae K. oxytoca	
Morganella	M. morgani	
Proteus	P. mirabilis P. vulgaris	Urinary infections, other forms of sepsis
Providencia	P. stuartii P. rettgeri P. alcalifaciens	
Yersinia	Y. pestis Y. pseudotuberculosis Y. enterocolitica	Plague, septicaemia, enteritis, mesenteric adenitis
Enterobacter	E. cloacae E. aerogenes	
Serratia	S. marcescens	Wide range of nosocomial infections
Citrobacter	C. freundii	

Identification:

- *Lactose fermentation* on indicator media assists initial identification: e.g. CLED medium contains lactose and a pH indicator, so that lactose-fermenting colonies are yellow.
- *Biochemical tests* are used to identify species of enterobacteria, usually by means of test kits, e.g. API systems or automated machines.
- *Serological tests* for somatic and flagellar antigens are used mainly for the final identification of *Salmonella* and *Shigella* species. A diagram of the sites of the main antigens in enterobacteria is shown in Figure 4.4.

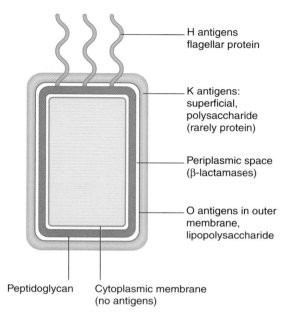

H antigens
flagellar protein

K antigens:
superficial,
polysaccharide
(rarely protein)

Periplasmic space
(β-lactamases)

O antigens in outer
membrane,
lipopolysaccharide

Peptidoglycan

Cytoplasmic membrane
(no antigens)

Fig. 4.4   Antigenic structure of Gram-negative bacteria.

Typing: strains within a species can also be identified by bacteriophage typing, RFLP typing of bacterial DNA, or DNA amplification methods.

Toxins:

Endotoxins: (O antigens) cell-wall lipopolysaccharides consisting of sugars and lipid A (see Chapter 2) are liberated when the bacterial cells lyse, and are responsible for many pathological effects of enterobacterial infection.

Exotoxins: are *proteins* liberated extracellularly from the intact bacterium by some species of enterobacteria.

Antibiotic sensitivity

Unpredictable, because enterobacteria readily acquire resistance-coding plasmids which can spread to other strains. Hospital strains are often multiply antibiotic resistant.

The *main antibiotics* used against enterobacteria are:

- Amoxycillin/co-amoxiclav
- Aminoglycosides
- Acylureidopenicillins, e.g. piperacillin
- Carbapenems
- Fluoroquinolones
- Cephalosporins
- Trimethoprim*
- Nitrofurantoin*
- Nalidixic acid.*

Note: drugs marked* are used only for urinary tract infections.

ESCHERICHIA COLI

Habitat: a normal inhabitant of the human and animal intestine.

Laboratory characteristics

Isolation: grows well as large lactose-fermenting colonies after overnight incubation.

Identification: biochemical tests.

Typing is rarely required, but phage typing is available for certain serogroups, e.g. 0157.

Pathogenicity

E. coli is a frequent cause of some common bacterial infections:

- Urinary tract infection
- Respiratory tract infections: aspiration, ventilator-associated pneumonia
- Surgical infections: peritonitis, wound, hepatobiliary tract (often polymicrobial, including anaerobes)
- Septicaemia
- Neonatal meningitis
- Enteric infections: a common cause of diarrhoea:
  - infantile gastroenteritis
  - tourist diarrhoea
  - haemorrhagic diarrhoea:
    - haemorrhagic colitis
    - haemolytic uraemic syndrome.

SHIGELLA

There are four species, most with several serotypes:

- *S. dysenteriae*
- *S. boydii*
- *S. flexneri*
- *S. sonnei* (one serotype).

Habitat: human intestine.

Laboratory characteristics

Isolation: grow well on routine media: do not ferment lactose; *S. sonnei* is an important exception, which ferments lactose slowly.

Enrichment culture of faeces in selenite F broth, with subsequent subculture on to MacConkey agar, improves isolation.

Identification:

- Non-motile
- *Biochemical tests*: produce acid, but not gas, from carbohydrates
- *Determination of O antigens*.

Pathogenicity

The cause of dysentery: *S. dysenteriae* type 1 causes the severe illness *shiga dysentery*. Dysentery due to other shigellae tends to be milder. *S. sonnei* is the cause of most dysentery in Britain.

SALMONELLA

Classification: all pathogenic isolates belong to a single species, *S. entericia*, which is subclassified into seven subspecies (based on DNA hybridization). *S. enterica* subspecies *enterica*, has over 2000 serotypes which are pathogenic for humans. *S. enterica* subspecies *arizonae* are also – but rare – human pathogens. For simplicity, serotypes can be abbreviated e.g. *S. enterica* subsp. *enterica* serotype Enteritidis to *S. Enteritidis*.

Habitat: the gut of domestic animals (especially cattle) and poultry. Foodstuffs from animals are therefore important sources of infection. *S.* Typhi and *S.* Paratyphi differ from the other serotypes in that humans and other primates are the only natural hosts.

Laboratory characteristics

Isolation: from faeces, on appropriate indicator and selective media: non-lactose fermentors.
  Identification:

- *Motile*: except *S.* Gallinarum-pullorum
- *Biochemical tests*: salmonellae generally produce acid and gas from carbohydrates, except for *S.* Typhi, which does not produce gas
- *Serology*: by identification of antigens (see Fig. 4.4):
  - O: somatic
  - H: flagellar
  - Vi: a surface antigen possessed by a few species, notably *S.* Typhi.

More than 2000 serotypes ('species') are recognized: sharing of O and H antigens is common and identification is complex, depending on detection of several antigens (Table 4.3). A single strain can possess two different sets of H antigens at different times (*phase variation*), and so both sets must be analysed for identification.
  Typing: bacteriophage typing of particular serotypes can be carried out to trace outbreaks, e.g. *S.* Typhi, *S.* Enteritidis, *S.* Typhimurium.

Pathogenicity

Enteric fever is due to *S.* Typhi or *S.* Paratyphi A, B, C. Most other salmonella serotypes cause gastroenteritis or food poisoning.

Table 4.3 Selected salmonellae showing antigenic profiles (Kauffman–White scheme)

Serotype ('species')	Group	O antigens	H antigens Phase 1	H antigens Phase 2
S. Paratyphi A	A	1.2.12.	a	–
S. Paratyphi B	B	1.4.5.12.	b	1.2
S. Agona	B	4.12.	f.g.s.	–
S. Typhimurium	B	1.4.5.12.	i	1.2
S. Paratyphi C*	C	6.7.	c	1.5
S. Typhi*	D	9.12.	d	–
S. Enteritidis	D	1.9.12.	g.m.	–

* Also possess Vi antigen.

Some types (e.g. *S.* Dublin, *S.* Virchow, *S.* Cholerae suis) have a particular tendency to cause septicaemia.

Rarely, salmonellae cause osteomyelitis, septic arthritis and other purulent lesions. Patients with HIV infection have a significantly increased risk.

KLEBSIELLA

Habitat: human and animal intestine. Some strains are saprophytes in soil, water and vegetation.

Laboratory characteristics

Isolation: grow well on ordinary media, producing lactose-fermenting colonies which are often large and mucoid because of prominent polysaccharide capsules.

Identification: non-motile and biochemical tests.

Typing: useful in hospital outbreaks: based on K antigenic analysis of the capsular polysaccharides. More than 80 serotypes recognized.

Pathogenicity

Most infections due to *K. pneumoniae*:

- Urinary tract infection
- Pneumonia: hospital and community acquired
- Septicaemia: secondary to urinary, respiratory and wound infections
- Meningitis (especially in neonates)
- Chronic upper respiratory tract infections (rare)
  - rhinoscleroma: due to *K. rhinoscleromatis*
  - atrophic rhinitis: due to *K. ozaenae*.

PROTEUS

There are two important species:

- *P. mirabilis*
- *P. vulgaris*.

Habitat: human and animal intestine.

Laboratory characteristics

Isolation: grow well on routine media, highly motile; produce a swarming type of growth on ordinary media.

Identification: swarming growth allows presumptive identification. Biochemical tests: produce a potent urease. *P. mirabilis* (indole negative); *P. vulgaris* (indole positive).

Pathogenicity

P. mirabilis is the most frequently isolated species, causing:

- Urinary tract infection: urinary urea is 'split' by the bacterial urease to produce ammonium salts: this results in alkaline urinary pH, which promotes renal stone formation.
- Often isolated from the mixed flora of wounds, burns, pressure sores, chronic discharging ears – generally a low-grade pathogen in such circumstances.
- Septicaemia: hospital-acquired (secondary to urinary, wound, respiratory infections). Mainly due to *P. vulgaris*.

YERSINIA

Habitat: yersinia are found in animals and sometimes – although rarely – cause disease in humans.

Laboratory characteristics

Isolation: on ordinary media. Colonies are often small and prolonged incubation of cultures is necessary.

Identification: small bacilli, which may show *bipolar* staining (i.e. darker at both ends of the bacillus). Biochemical tests permit formal identification, the reactions being more reproducible at 22–27°C than at 37°C.

Pathogenicity

- Plague: *Y. pestis* (formerly called *Pasteurella pestis*) causes bubonic and pneumonic plague ('the Black Death').

Y. pseudotuberculosis and *Y. enterocolitica* cause:

- Enteritis
- Mesenteric adenitis, sometimes associated with terminal ileitis – clinically, can closely mimic appendicitis

• A septicaemic illness similar to typhoid fever.

ENTEROBACTER; SERRATIA; PROVIDENCIA; MORGANELLA; CITROBACTER

These members of the enterobacteria can conveniently be considered together. The most frequently isolated species are *Enterobacter cloacae, E. aerogenes; Serratia marcescens; Providencia rettgeri, P. stuartii; Citrobacter freundii; Morganella morgani.*

Habitat: human and animal intestine, but some strains are saprophytes. Moist environments in hospitals are important reservoirs.

Laboratory characteristics

Isolation: grow well on routine media.

Identification: biochemical tests.

Pathogenicity

• Urinary tract infections (complicated)
• Wounds, skin lesions and respiratory infections in hospitalized patients
• Septicaemia.

Some species have been responsible for outbreaks of infection in intensive care areas, burns units and other special units.

VIBRIO, AEROMONAS, PLESIOMONAS, CAMPYLOBACTER AND HELICOBACTER

An important group of pathogenic Gram-negative bacilli which, like *Pseudomonas*, are oxidase positive.

VIBRIO

Widespread in nature, mainly in water: one species, *V. cholerae*, is the cause of cholera.

VIBRIO CHOLERAE

Habitat: water contaminated with faeces of patients or carriers.

Laboratory characteristics

Morphology and staining: Gram-negative slender bacilli, sometimes comma-shaped with a pointed end. Often arranged in pairs or short chains, giving a spiral appearance. Actively motile by one long polar flagellum; non-capsulate; non-sporing.

Culture: facultative anaerobe; grows readily on ordinary media as glistening colonies over a wide temperature range (optimum 37°C). Optimal growth is at pH 8.0–8.2.

Enrichment medium: alkaline peptone water (pH 8.6) promotes the rapid growth of *V. cholerae* from mixtures of other bacteria.

Selective medium: TCBS medium – thiosulphate citrate bile sucrose agar, pH 8.6.

Observe: for large yellow sucrose-fermenting colonies.

Identification: by biochemical tests and slide agglutination with specific antisera.

Antigenic structure

O antigens: 139 O serogroups are recognized. Epidemic cholera is caused by *V. cholerae* serogroup O1, which is divided into three serotypes, *Ogawa*, *Inaba* and *Hikojima*. However, antigenic structure (and therefore serotype) may change within the human gut.

Biotypes: two biotypes of *V. cholerae* O1, classic and El Tor, can be differentiated (biotyping is the distinguishing of different bacterial strains within a species by various biological and biochemical reactions). Any serotype can be of either classic or El Tor biotype.

Non-O1 vibrios, deficient in the O1 antigen, were classified as non-cholera vibrios – but a cholera epidemic in Bangladesh in 1992 was due to serogroup O139.

Toxins: endotoxins (cell-wall lipopolysaccharide) and exotoxins are recognized. The enterotoxin is an exotoxin which stimulates persistent and excessive secretion of isotonic fluid by the intestinal mucosa.

Pathogenicity

V. cholerae O1 (and O139) cause cholera in humans. Strains in serogroups O2–O138 – non-cholera vibrios – may be associated with milder diarrhoeal illness.

Viability: readily killed by heat and drying; dies in polluted waters but may survive in clean stagnant water (especially if alkaline) or sea water for 1–2 weeks.

Antibiotic sensitivity

Test against macrolides (e.g. erythromycin), ciprofloxacin, tetracycline and co-trimoxazole. Resistant strains of *V. cholerae* (including ciprofloxacin) have emerged in endemic areas.

VIBRIO PARAHAEMOLYTICUS

V. parahaemolyticus is a halophilic (i.e. salt-tolerant) marine vibrio isolated from shellfish, particularly in countries with warm coastal water, e.g. southeast Asia. It causes an acute gastroenteritis in which vibrios are excreted in large numbers in the stools. Faecal samples plated on TCBS agar yield large blue-green colonies typical of *V. parahaemolyticus*, which fails to ferment sucrose.

VIBRIO VULNIFICUS

V. vulnificus is a halofilic marine vibrio isolated from shellfish and crabs. It causes a severe necrotizing cellulitis and/or septicaemia, with a case fatality rate of 25%.

Antibiotic sensitivity

Treatment of choice is tetracycline. Ciprofloxacin and ceftriaxone are also effective.

V. alginolyticus, a halofilic vibrio, is associated with less severe cellulitis and ear infections in swimmers.

AEROMONAS AND PLESIOMONAS

Gram-negative bacilli; aerobes, facultative anaerobes; motile; oxidase positive.

Habitat: fresh and brackish water.

Aeromonas hydrophila and *Plesiomonas shigelloides* are the medically important species, but infections are rare and are usually in patients with some other serious disease; occasionally isolated from blood, CSF and wounds. Aeromonas wound infections are a recognized complication following the use of medicinal leeches in reconstructive plastic surgery. Both organisms are associated with diarrhoeal disease.

CAMPYLOBACTER

Strictly microaerophilic vibrios. Species that cause human or animal diarrhoeal illness are thermophilic, growing best at 43°C. The main human pathogenic species is *C. jejuni*. Other species occasionally found in human gastrointestinal disease include *C. coli* and *C. lari*.

Habitat: various animal species, including chickens, domestic animals and seagulls (*C. lari*).

Laboratory characteristics

Morphology and staining: small, Gram-negative, curved or spiral rods (Fig. 4.5). Highly motile, by a single flagellum at one or both poles.

Culture: microaerophilic; grow readily on simple media in an atmosphere of 7% O_2 and 10–15% CO_2, with the remainder nitrogen. Growth is optimal at 43°C after 24–48 h incubation. For isolation from faeces use selective medium containing antibiotics to which campylobacters are resistant.

Observe: effuse colonies that look like spreading fluid droplets.

Identification: by Gram-film appearance, motility, growth temperature requirements (25°C: no growth; 37°C: growth; 43°C: enhanced growth) and positive oxidase test.

Antibiotic sensitivity

Most strains are sensitive to macrolides (e.g. erythromycin), ciprofloxacin and chloramphenicol.

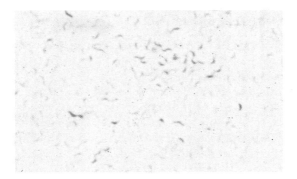

Fig. 4.5 Campylobacter (approx. × 1000).

HELICOBACTER

Helicobacter pylori is found closely associated with gastric mucosa and causes chronic active gastritis: it plays a role in gastric and duodenal ulceration, gastric cancer and gastric lymphoma.

Laboratory characteristics

Morphology and staining: small, Gram-negative spiral rods; motile by multiple polar flagella.

Culture: on blood or chocolate agar in a moist microaerophilic atmosphere. For isolation from clinical specimens use campylobacter-selective medium (see above). Small colonies grow after 3–7 days at 37°C.

Biochemical reactions: catalase positive; oxidase positive; strongly urease positive.

Typing: a variety of nucleic acid methods have been developed, but there is no agreed typing scheme.

Antibiotic sensitivity

Usually sensitive to amoxycillin, tetracycline, metronidazole, clarithromycin and bismuth salts. Strains resistant to metronidazole and clarithromycin have emerged.

PARVOBACTERIA

Parvobacteria (parvus = small) is a convenient but old-fashioned name for a number of quite different, small Gram-negative bacilli which generally require enriched media for isolation and culture. This heterogeneous group contains several important human pathogens which cause a wide variety of diseases. They are unrelated and classified in separate genera; consequently, the term 'parvobacteria' lacks taxonomic respectability.

The following genera are considered here as parvobacteria:

- *Haemophilus*
- *Brucella*
- *Bordetella*
- *Pasteurella*
- *Francisella*
- *Actinobacillus*
- *Cardiobacterium*
- *Eikenella*

• *Gardnerella*
• *Streptobacillus.*

HAEMOPHILUS

Habitat: mainly the respiratory tract: often part of the normal flora, but may also cause respiratory disease, usually as a secondary invader. Some species are associated with other mucosal surfaces, e.g. conjunctiva, genital tract.

Laboratory characteristics

Morphology and staining: small, Gram-negative coccobacilli (see Fig. 6.3); non-sporing, non-motile.

Culture: optimum growth at 37°C and in an atmosphere with added CO_2. Enriched media are necessary because *Haemophilus* species need one or both of two growth factors:

• Heat-stable X factor – haemin or some other iron-containing porphyrin
• Heat-labile V factor – di- or triphosphopyridine nucleotide.

Requirement for growth factors can help to differentiate between species (Table 4.4).

Pathogenicity

The diseases caused by *Haemophilus* species are listed in Table 4.5.

HAEMOPHILUS INFLUENZAE

The main pathogenic species.

Habitat: the upper respiratory tract; most strains found in the normal flora are non-capsulated.

Table 4.4 Growth factors for *Haemophilus* species

Factor required	Species
X and V	H. influenzae, H. aegyptius, H. haemolyticus
X	H. ducreyi
V	H. parainfluenzae, H. parahaemolyticus

Table 4.5 Pathogenicity of *Haemophilus* species

Species	Disease
H. influenzae	Exacerbations of chronic bronchitis, pneumonia Sinusitis, otitis media, meningitis Epiglottitis
H. aegyptius	Conjunctivitis
H. ducreyi	Chancroid
H. parainfluenzae *H. haemolyticus* *H. parahaemolyticus*	Commensals of the upper respiratory tract; rarely cause disease

Laboratory characteristics

Morphology: small, Gram-negative coccobacillus; a minority of strains are capsulated.

Culture: on chocolate or blood agar: a streak of *Staphylococcus aureus* across the plate produces V factor and enlarges the size of adjacent colonies of *H. influenzae* – satellitism (Fig. 4.6).

Colonial morphology: small, translucent, non-haemolytic colonies: capsulated strains form larger iridescent colonies.

Selective medium: chocolate bacitracin agar facilitates the isolation of *H. influenzae* from sputum specimens by inhibiting the growth of other bacteria found in the upper respiratory tract.

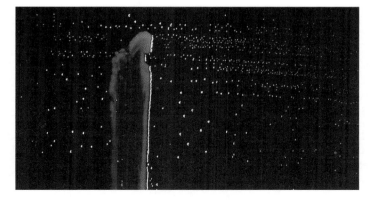

Fig. 4.6 Satellitism. A blood agar plate showing enhancement of growth of colonies of *Haemophilus influenzae* next to the streak of *Staphylococcus aureus* which supplies V factor.

Identification: by testing:

- on nutrient agar for growth requirements, using discs impregnated with X and V factors
- biochemical tests, e.g. API systems.

Serotypes of capsulated strains: six are recognized, on the basis of capsular polysaccharide antigens – Pittman types a, b, c, d, e, f. Type b is the main pathogen.

Pathogenicity

Non-capsulated strains are mainly responsible for exacerbations of chronic bronchitis and bronchiectasis.

Capsulated strains (predominantly type b) can cause various invasive infections, mainly in children from 2 months to 3 years old:

- Meningitis
- Acute epiglottitis
- Osteomyelitis
- Arthritis
- Cellulitis (orbital)

these infections are often accompanied by septicaemia

Vaccine

A vaccine (Hib) which protects against invasive *H. influenzae* type b infections was introduced into the UK schedule for childhood immunization in 1992 (see Chapter 39).

Antibiotic sensitivity

Test against the following antibiotics:

- Ampicillin
- Co-amoxiclav
- Clarithromycin
- Trimethoprim
- Ciprofloxacin
- Second- and third-generation cephalosporins.

Antibiotic resistance: resistance to ampicillin (due to β-lactamase production) and co-amoxiclav is now present in 20–30% of UK strains.

HAEMOPHILUS INFLUENZAE BIOGROUP AEGYPTIUS

Formerly called the Koch–Weeks bacillus.

Pathogenicity

Acute conjunctivitis and Brazilian purpuric fever.

HAEMOPHILUS DUCREYI

The cause of the sexually transmitted disease *chancroid*, or soft sore.

Laboratory characteristics

Morphology: slender, Gram-negative ovoid bacilli; slightly larger than *H. influenzae*; bacteria en masse from clinical specimens have the configuration of 'shoals of fish'.

Culture: on special enriched medium: incubate at 33°C for 3–5 days, with added moisture and CO_2. *Growth factors*: only X factor is required.

Molecular methods: DNA amplification by polymerase chain reaction may be useful.

Antibiotic sensitivity

Erythromycin, azithromycin, ceftriaxone and ciprofloxacin.

BRUCELLA

Predominantly infect domestic animals, from which infection may be transmitted to humans (Table 4.6).

There are three main species, *B. melitensis*, *B. abortus* and *B. suis*, each with a number of biotypes.

Habitat: chronically infected domestic animals.

Laboratory characteristics

Morphology and staining: short, slender, pleomorphic Gram-negative bacilli; non-motile, non-sporing, non-capsulate.

Table 4.6 Animal hosts and geographical distribution of *Brucella* species

Strain	Usual animal host	Geographical distribution
B. melitensis	Goats, sheep	Mediterranean countries
B. abortus	Cattle	Worldwide
B. suis	Pigs	Denmark and USA

Culture: in enriched medium, small transparent colonies develop after several days' incubation at 37°C in aerobic conditions. CO_2 is required for the growth of *B. abortus*.

Identification of the different species is done by a variety of biochemical and serological tests, and the ability of certain dyes to inhibit growth.

Antigenic structure: the three species share two antigens, A and M, but these are present in different proportions. Typical *melitensis* strains contain an excess of M antigen, whereas typical *abortus* and *suis* strains contain an excess of A antigen. Monospecific antisera can be prepared, and these are of use in identification.

Pathogenicity

The cause of 'undulant fever' or brucellosis.

Antibiotic sensitivity

Doxycycline in combination with streptomycin or rifampicin.

BORDETELLA

The important member of the genus is *B. pertussis*, the cause of whooping cough. *B. parapertussis* causes a milder form of whooping cough, which is uncommon in Britain. *B. bronchiseptica* is an animal pathogen.

BORDETELLA PERTUSSIS

Habitat: the human respiratory tract, usually associated with acute disease.

Laboratory characteristics

Morphology and staining: short, sometimes oval, Gram-negative bacilli; freshly isolated strains may be capsulated.

Culture: special enriched medium is required for primary isolation: the most widely used medium is charcoal blood agar.

Colonial morphology: colonies like 'split pearls' or 'mercury drops' appear after 3 or more days of incubation in a moist aerobic atmosphere at 35°C.

Identification is confirmed serologically by slide agglutination with a polyvalent antiserum reacting with all three main antigens.

Antigenic structure: surface antigens (agglutinogens) designated 1–6 are recognized: all freshly isolated strains possess agglutinogen 1.

Serotypes: there are three main serotypes, based on the presence of surface antigens: type 1,2; type 1,3; type 1,2,3.

Pathogenicity

The cause of whooping cough.

Antibiotic sensitivity

Erythromycin.

PASTEURELLA

PASTEURELLA MULTOCIDA

The main pathogenic member of the genus.

Habitat: respiratory tract of many animals, notably dogs.

Laboratory characteristics

Morphology: small, sometimes capsulated, ovoid Gram-negative bacilli, often showing bipolar staining.

Culture: on nutrient agar or blood agar, aerobically at 37°C. Does not grow on MacConkey agar – a differentiating feature from enterobacteria. Colonies are oxidase positive.

Pathogenicity

An important animal pathogen. In humans it may cause septic wounds after dog or cat bites.

Antibiotic sensitivity

Penicillin, tetracyclines, ciprofloxacin, second- and third-generation cephalosporins.

FRANCISELLA

FRANCISELLA TULARENSIS

The cause of tularaemia.
  Habitat: rodents and other small mammals.

Laboratory characteristics

Morphology: pleomorphic, capsulated, small Gram-negative coccobacilli, often showing bipolar staining.
  Culture: on blood agar enriched with cystine and glucose.

Pathogenicity

Tularaemia, a plague-like disease of rodents, is contracted by contact with animal hosts or their products. It is widespread in the USA and is occasionally seen in parts of Europe, but not yet in the UK.

Antibiotic sensitivity

Streptomycin or gentamicin are the drugs of choice. Tetracyclines are also generally effective.

ACTINOBACILLUS

Facultatively anaerobic, non-branching Gram-negative coccobacilli that can grow on nutrient agar. The type species *Actinobacillus lignieresi* is responsible for actinobacillosis in cattle and sheep, a disease that resembles actinomycosis in humans. *A. actinomycetemcomitans*, present in the normal oral flora of humans, is found along with *Actinomyces* species in 30% of human cases of actinomycosis. It also causes periodontal disease and infective endocarditis (HACEK organism; see Chapter 12).

CARDIOBACTERIUM

Cardiobacterium hominis: a capnophilic, small pleomorphic Gram-negative bacillus, present in the normal oral flora of humans. It grows slowly on blood or chocolate agar. It can cause infective endocarditis (HACEK organisms).

EIKENELLA

Eikenella corrodens: a slow-growing facultative anaerobic, Gram-negative bacillus present in the normal oral flora. Grows slowly on blood agar, forming pinpoint 'pitting' or 'corroding' colonies. Causes human bite infections and infective endocarditis (HACEK organisms).

GARDNERELLA

Gardnerella vaginalis: small, Gram-variable bacilli, non-motile, non-sporing. Facultative anaerobes requiring enriched media, producing small β-haemolytic colonies.

Biochemical tests: starch hydrolysis, demonstrated by a zone of clearing on dextrose–starch agar. Cause bacterial vaginosis in association with anaerobes, but asymptomatic vaginal carriage is present in about 60% of women. Sensitive to metronidazole.

STREPTOBACILLUS

Streptobacillus moniliformis: slender, filamentous, Gram-variable bacterium with slub-shaped ('moniliform') terminal swellings. Normal inhabitant of the nasopharynx of rats. Requires enriched media for growth. Causes one form of rat-bite fever in humans.

LEGIONELLA

Legionella is a genus of which the base composition of the DNA is distinct from that of other bacteria.

There are over 40 recognized species of legionellae, but *L. pneumophila* is by far the most important human pathogen.

LEGIONELLA PNEUMOPHILA

The most common infecting strain is serogroup 1.

Habitat: an environmental organism found in soil and water (including domestic water supplies and air-conditioning units).

Laboratory characteristics

Morphology and staining: slender rods. Gram-negative, but legionellae sometimes do not stain well.

Culture: requires media with iron and cysteine for isolation. *Incubate* for 21 days at 35–37°C in 5% CO_2; colonies usually appear in 3–5 days.

Identification: by direct immunofluorescence.

Diagnosis is most often serological; however, better culture media are now increasing the rate of isolation from clinical material.

Pathogenicity

L. pneumophila serogroup 1 is the major cause of Legionnaires' disease – a severe form of pneumonia – and of the less serious respiratory disease Pontiac fever. Other species also cause pneumonia, most often in immunocompromised patients.

Antibiotic sensitivity

Sensitive to macrolides, e.g. erythromycin; fluoroquinolones, e.g. ciprofloxacin and rifampicin.

ANAEROBIC GRAM-NEGATIVE BACILLI

The classification of these organisms is complex and there have been many revisions. Until recently, the genus *Bacteroides* included organisms now placed in the genera *Prevotella* and *Porphyromonas*. For the sake of simplicity, and to conform with current terminology in clinical practice, the term 'bacteroides' is used elsewhere in this book as an all-embracing term for non-sporing Gram-negative anaerobic bacilli.

Habitat:

• *Colon*: Gram-negative anaerobic bacilli are present in enormous numbers in the faeces (10^{10}/g or more). The majority belong to the genus *Bacteroides*, mostly *B. vulgatus*, *B. distasonis* and *B. fragilis*.

• *Female genital tract*: Gram-negative anaerobic bacilli are common in the cervix and vaginal fornices: prevotella, mostly *P. melaninogenica*, predominate; porphyromonas is also common.

• *Mouth*: always found in large numbers in the normal mouth. Most are prevotella, the commonest species being *P. oralis*; fusobacteria and leptotrichia are also present.

Laboratory characteristics

Morphology and staining: small, ovoid or short Gram-negative, non-motile, non-sporing bacilli. Fusobacteria and leptotrichia tend to be long and spindle-shaped, but pleomorphism is common.

Culture: strict anaerobes: require enriched media. Fluid media, e.g. Robertson's cooked meat broth, and selective media aid isolation of anaerobes.

Incubate: anaerobically with 10% CO_2 (which enhances growth) for a minimum of 48 h.

Identification: most anaerobes can be identified to generic level by the examination of a Gram-stained smear, colonial morphology, growth inhibition by bile salts, antibiotic resistance, and gas chromatographic analysis of the fatty acid end-products of glucose metabolism. Species differentiation is time-consuming and costly, requiring biochemical tests, and is rarely attempted by routine diagnostic laboratories.

Pathogenicity

The most common isolate from clinical specimens is *B. fragilis*, and thus this species seems to have a special pathogenic potential.

Gram-negative anaerobic bacilli are important in abdominal and gynaecological (including puerperal) sepsis: they are usually found along with other organisms, notably coliforms. It appears that these combinations of anaerobic and aerobic bacteria potentiate the ability of each other to cause infection – *pathogenic synergy*.

Gram-negative anaerobic bacilli are also responsible for dental, periodontal and oropharyngeal disease.

Vincent's infection (see Fig. 6.2) is caused by *Borrelia vincenti* in association with a variety of Gram-negative anaerobic bacilli, including one or more of *Prevotella intermedia*, *Fusobacterium nucleatum* and *Leptotrichia buccalis*.

Antibiotic sensitivity

Like other anaerobes, these organisms are sensitive to metronidazole. Many are also sensitive to clindamycin, chloramphenicol and cefoxitin.

Bacteroides are penicillin resistant owing to β-lactamase production, but many strains of the other genera are penicillin sensitive. There is uniform resistance to the aminoglycosides.

VEILLONELLA

Gram-negative anaerobic cocci: metronidazole sensitive but resistant to vancomycin. Have many similarities to *Peptostreptococci* (anaerobic Gram-positive cocci, vancomycin sensitive).

Habitat: commensals in the skin, oropharynx, colon and female genital tract.

Pathogenicity

Local sepsis, in mixed infections with anaerobic Gram-negative bacilli and aerobes.

SPIROCHAETES

Spirochaetes are a group of helical organisms that share many properties with Gram-negative bacteria.

Habitat: most are free-living and non-pathogenic, but a few are causes of important human disease.

Laboratory characteristics

Morphology and staining: unique helical structure, with a central protoplasmic cylinder bounded by a cytoplasmic membrane and cell wall of similar structure to that of Gram-negative bacteria (Fig. 4.7). Between a thin peptidoglycan layer and the outer membrane run the *axial filaments*, now regarded as internal flagella. These are fixed at the extremities of the organism and meet to

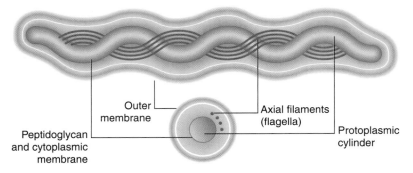

Fig. 4.7   The structure of a spirochaete.

overlap in the middle of the cell. They constrict and distort the bacterial cell body to give rise to the typical helical structure.

The larger spirochaetes (e.g. *Borrelia* species) are Gram-negative. Others stain poorly or not at all by the usual methods. Spirochaetes are too slender and weakly refractile to be seen with the ordinary light microscope, but can be rendered visible by dark-ground microscopy (Fig. 4.8), by staining with heavy metals (e.g. silver), or by immunofluorescence.

GENERA

Three genera contain human pathogenic species:

1. Treponema
2. Borrelia
3. Leptospira.

TREPONEMA

The main treponemes are:

- *T. pallidum*
- *T. pertenue*
- *T. carateum*.

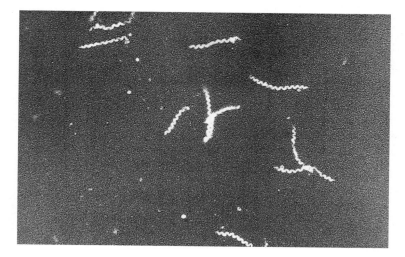

Fig. 4.8 Dark-ground photomicrograph of *Treponema pallidum*. (Reproduced with permission from Abbott Laboratories *Slide Atlas of Infectious Diseases*, 1982, Gower Medical Publishing, London. Photograph courtesy of Dr R. D. Caterall.)

Morphologically indistinguishable from, and antigenically similar to, each other; cannot be cultivated in vitro, but can be propagated by inoculation of rabbit testes.

Other treponemes are found as commensals in the mouth, genital secretions and intestine.

TREPONEMA PALLIDUM

Habitat: the lesions of primary and secondary syphilis.

Laboratory characteristics

Morphology: long, slender filamentous helices.

Identification: in material from primary and secondary clinical lesions, by dark-ground or phase-contrast microscopy.

Serology: diagnose by detection of antibody (see Chapter 13).

Pathogenicity

Cause of the sexually transmitted disease syphilis.

Viability: a strict parasite that dies rapidly outside the body; it is very sensitive to drying and to heat.

Antibiotic sensitivity

Penicillin.

TREPONEMA PALLIDUM, SUBSPECIES PERTENUE

The cause of yaws, a chronic relapsing non-venereal treponematosis widespread in the tropics: characterized by ulcerative and granulomatous lesions in skin, mucous membranes and bone.

TREPONEMA CARATEUM

The cause of pinta, a non-venereal treponematosis with lesions confined to the skin. It affects dark-skinned people in Central and South America, causing hyperkeratosis and depigmentation of skin.

OTHER TREPONEMES

A number of species are found as commensals in the mouth, genital secretions and intestine. Some grow in vitro anaerobically.

BORRELIA

BORRELIA VINCENTI

Habitat: the oropharynx, as a commensal and potential pathogen.

Laboratory characteristics

Morphology and staining: large spirochaetes with three to eight irregular open coils; Gram-negative.

Culture: can be grown, with difficulty, in serum-enriched media; a strict anaerobe.

Identification: in exudates from clinical lesions by morphology, in Gram-stained film (see Fig. 6.2).

Pathogenicity

In association with anaerobic fusiform bacilli (e.g. *Leptotrichia buccalis*), responsible for gingivostomatitis and Vincent's angina.

Antibiotic sensitivity

Penicillin.

BORRELIA BURGDORFERI

Habitat: ticks, small mammals, deer.
Spread: by ticks of the genus *Ixodes*.

Laboratory characteristics

Morphology: flexible helical spirochaete; Gram-negative.
Culture: microaerophilic, grows at 34°C in special medium.
Diagnosis: serological and DNA amplification by PCR.

Pathogenicity

The cause of Lyme disease.

Antibiotic sensitivity

Amoxycillin, doxycycline, ceftriaxone, macrolides, e.g. azithromycin.

BORRELIA RECURRENTIS

The cause of louse-borne relapsing fever.

BORRELIA DUTTONI AND OTHER SPECIES

The causes of tick-borne relapsing fever. Both diseases are encountered in parts of Asia, Africa and South America.

Relapsing fever is characterized by febrile episodes alternating with afebrile periods, and lasts for several weeks. Each relapse is the result of a change in the antigenic structure of the organism: antibodies already formed are ineffective against the new variants.

Antibiotic sensitivity

Tetracyclines, erythromycin, penicillin, chloramphenicol.

LEPTOSPIRA

The classification is complex and there has been a major revision. Modern molecular-based classification contains at least seven pathogenic species. To conform with present clinical practice the traditional serovar classification is retained.

Leptospira are traditionally classified into two species: *Leptospira interrogans*, which is divided into over 200 serovars (organized into 23 serogroups), and non-pathogenic *Leptospira biflexa*, containing 60 serovars (28 serogroups). *L. interrogans* contains several important human pathogenic serovars and their respective reservoirs: *L. interrogans* serovar *icterohaemorrhagiae* (rats), *hardjo* (cattle), *canicola* (dogs and cats) and *pomona* (pigs).

Habitat: Leptospires are found in moist environments. *L. biflexa* is a saprophyte present in pools, ditches and streams. *L. interrogans* is harboured in the kidneys of some rodents and domestic animals.

Laboratory characteristics

Morphology: spiral organisms with very numerous closely set coils and hooked ends.

Culture: obligate aerobes; grow in enriched fluid or semisolid media; optimum temperature is around 30°C.

Diagnosis: serological and DNA amplification methods using PCR.

Pathogenicity

L. interrogans is the cause of the zoonotic disease leptospirosis.

Viability: pathogenic strains may survive for days outside the animal body in moist surroundings, as long as they are not acid.

Antibiotic sensitivity

Penicillin, tetracyclines.

MYCOPLASMA

Mycoplasmas are bacteria that lack cell walls. They are bounded by the cytoplasmic membrane and resemble L forms of bacteria but, unlike them, are independent naturally occurring microorganisms.

Table 4.7 lists some of the better-known mycoplasmas and their habitats. T-strain mycoplasmas form minute colonies ('T' = tiny), and are now classified in the genus *Ureaplasma*. Some

Table 4.7 Mycoplasmas and related organisms

Genus, species	Habitat
M. pneumoniae	Human respiratory tract
M. orale *M. salivarium*	Human mouth
M. hominis *M. genitalium*	Human genital, and possibly respiratory, tracts
Ureaplasma urealyticum	Human genitourinary tract
Acholeplasma laidlawii	Soil, water

mycoplasmas with less exacting growth requirements have been assigned to a separate genus, *Acholeplasma*.

Laboratory characteristics

Morphology and staining: pleomorphic; several different forms exist, varying from small spherical shapes to longer branching filaments. Gram-negative, but stain poorly with Gram's stain.

Culture: on semisolid enriched medium; (incubate aerobically for 7–12 days with CO_2).

Observe: typical 'fried-egg' colonies, embedded in the surface of the medium.

Identification of isolates: by inhibition of growth round discs impregnated with specific antisera, or by immunofluorescence on colonies transferred to glass slides.

Pathogenicity

Mycoplasma pneumoniae: the main pathogenic member of the group; it is a major respiratory pathogen responsible for one form of atypical pneumonia, and also causes febrile bronchitis and milder upper respiratory infections.

Ureaplasma urealyticum (T-strain mycoplasma): implicated in, although not the major cause of, non-specific urethritis, vaginitis and cervicitis. Rarely, can cause respiratory disease in preterm infants owing to transfer of infection from the mother.

Mycoplasma hominis: has been implicated in some cases of gynaecological or postpartum sepsis. An unusual cause of atypical pneumonia.

Antibiotic sensitivity

Sensitive to tetracycline – the drug of choice for treatment – and also to erythromycin. Mycoplasmas are resistant to antibiotics that interfere with bacterial cell wall synthesis, e.g. penicillin.

5 Laboratory diagnosis of bacterial disease

The main techniques used in bacteriology laoratories are:

- microscopy
- culture
- bacterial identification
- antibiotic sensitivity tests
- serology
- molecular methods.

MICROSCOPY

Light microscopy: smears of clinical samples (e.g. sputum, pus) or from bacterial cultures are stained and examined for the types of bacteria present. Light microscopy of stained films with the oil-immersion objective gives a magnification of about × 1000.

Wet (unstained) microscopy: routinely used for examination of fluids, e.g. urine and CSF; useful for cell counts.

Fluorescence microscopy: bacteria stained with auramine or other fluorescent dyes become visible as bright objects against a dark ground under ultraviolet light.

Stains

Gram's stain: the most widely used stain; it classifies bacteria into two categories, Gram positive and Gram negative, and also shows their shape and size. Gram-positive bacteria retain the purple colour of crystal violet with iodine after decolorization with acetone or alcohol; Gram-negative bacteria decolorize and show up pink with carbol fuchsin counterstain.

Ziehl-Neelsen: for tubercle bacilli; these are acid and alcohol fast and resist decolorization with acid (and alcohol) after staining with heated carbol fuchsin; auramine–phenol, which renders the bacilli fluorescent, is now often used to detect tubercle bacilli.

Other stains: many other special stains are used in bacteriology, such as Albert's or Neisser's stains to demonstrate volutin granules in diphtheria bacilli, and other stains to show capsules, spores, spirochaetes or flagella.

Immunofluorescence

This uses antibody labelled with a fluorescent dye (e.g. fluorescein isothiocyanate, lissamine rhodamine) to detect specific antigens and so identify bacteria.

CULTURE

Bacteria grow well in vitro on artificial media but differ in their growth requirements so that many different kinds of media must be used. Most pathogenic bacteria grow on blood agar, the mainstay of diagnostic bacteriology.

Media

Culture media contain:

• water
• sodium chloride and other electrolytes
• peptone (a protein digest)
• meat or yeast extract
• blood (usually defibrinated horse blood).

Solid media: solidified to the consistency of a jelly with agar, a setting agent that allows sterilization when liquid at 90°C but does not set until 40°, so that heat-sensitive components such as blood can be added. Dispensed in plastic Petri plates.

Plating: specimens (or cultures of bacteria) are stroked out on the medium with a wire loop so as to ensure a reducing concentration of the inoculum (Fig. 5.1). This ensures that, after incubation, separated colonies develop each derived from a single bacterium. Bacteria so isolated can often be identified by their colonial morphology.

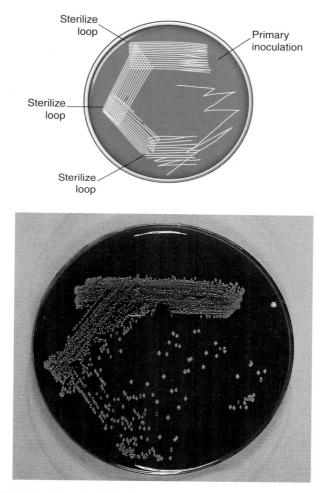

Fig. 5.1 Plating. The method of inoculating a plate of solid medium with bacteria to achieve separated colonies, and a blood agar plate inoculated in this way after overnight incubation.

Selective media: are solid media that contain ingredients to inhibit unwanted contaminants (e.g. from the normal flora) but which allow certain pathogens to grow.

Liquid media: in tubes or screw-capped bottles. Growth is recognized by turbidity; simple media consist of peptone water or nutrient broth. *Robertson's meat medium* (nutrient broth with minced meat) supports the growth of both aerobic and anaerobic bacteria.

Enrichment media: fluids which encourage the preferential growth of a particular bacterium and contain inhibitors for contaminants.

Blood cultures: two bottles, each with a perforated cap, are inoculated by injection of blood, collected aseptically using a syringe, through the cap. One bottle contains a broth for the growth of aerobes, the other a medium designed for anaerobes.

Transport medium: to preserve delicate pathogens during transit to the laboratory, e.g. *Stuart's transport medium*, a semisolid non-nutrient agar with thioglycollic acid (as reducing agent), electrolytes, and sometimes pieces of charcoal.

Incubation

Atmosphere: most human pathogens grow in air, sometimes supplemented with 10% carbon dioxide for the isolation of some species.

Anaerobic bacteria require incubation without oxygen: use a sealed jar from which the air is removed and in which hydrogen and carbon dioxide are liberated using a commercial gas-generating system; the remaining oxygen combines with the hydrogen in the presence of a catalyst to form water. Most laboratories now use a cabinet capable of handling a large number of plates in which anaerobic conditions are maintained.

Temperature: the optimal temperature for most pathogens is body heat, 37°C.

BACTERIAL IDENTIFICATION

Bacteria isolated by culture are identified by:

1. *Colonial and microscopic morphology*
2. *The conditions required for growth*
3. *Biochemical tests*: these test the ability of the bacterium to metabolize particular substrates. Often performed on a number of substrates, presented in a commercially prepared kit, and can be automated.
4. *Recognition of enzymes*: although enzyme production is the basis of most of the reactions included in the biochemical tests, some bacteria can be identified primarily by the production of a characteristic enzyme. For example, coagulase is characteristic of *Staphylococcus aureus* and lecithinase of *Clostridium perfringens*.

5. *Antigenic structure*: serology depends mainly on the recognition of antigens in flagella, cell wall or capsule, or liberated from the bacteria as toxins. Particularly useful for the large numbers of biochemically similar enterobacteria (e.g. salmonella).

6. *Typing of bacterial strains*: by testing for different characteristics to identify individual strains or types within a bacterial species and so aid the tracing of epidemic spread of an organism. Often more than one method employed:

- *Biotyping* and *auxotyping*: based on biochemical tests and the organism's ability to utilize chemicals
- *Serotyping*: differences in antigenic structure
- *Bacteriophage typing*: differences in the susceptibility of the bacterium to a series of bacterial viruses (bacteriophages)
- *Molecular typing*: rapidly replacing traditional methods. A variety of methods analysing either *proteins* or, more commonly, *nucleic acids*: genomic or plasmid DNA or ribosomal RNA, many based on amplification methods, e.g. polymerase chain reaction (PCR).

ANTIBIOTIC SENSITIVITY TESTS

Sensitivity tests

One of the most important functions of a diagnostic bacteriology laboratory, and a large part of the day-to-day workload.

Disc diffusion: the most widely used method. Paper discs impregnated with antibiotic solutions (at a concentration related to blood or urine levels attained by the drug) are placed on the surface of a plate inoculated with either the specimen or the bacterial culture under test. After incubation the plate is examined for zones of inhibition round the discs. The following methods are available:

- *Stokes' method*: the outside of the plate can be inoculated with a standard organism (e.g. the Oxford strain of *Staphylococcus aureus*). The zones round the discs can then be compared to those produced against the test organism in the middle of the plate (Fig. 5.2). Difficult to standardize.
- *British Society for Antimicrobial Chemotherapy (BSAC) method*: a standardized method based on correlation of zones of inhibition to minimum inhibitory concentration (MIC) – see below. Can be automated. Used mainly in the UK.

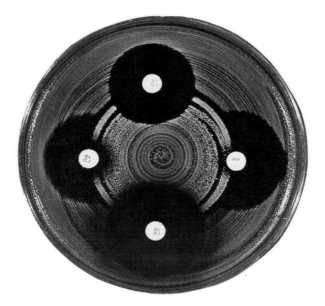

Fig. 5.2 Antibiotic sensitivity test – Stokes' method. The fully sensitive standard organism is on the outside. Reduced zones around two of the discs indicate resistance in the test organism.

- *Kirby–Bauer method*: a standardized method used widely throughout the world. Approved by the National Committee for Clinical Laboratory Standards (NCCLS) and WHO: interpretation based on relating zone diameter to the MIC by regression line analysis.

Tube dilution: laborious; only done in special circumstances.

Method: a series of tubes with doubling dilutions of the antibiotic in broth are inoculated with the bacterium under test. After incubation, the tube with the lowest concentration in which there is no growth represents the MIC or *minimum* (bacteriostatic) *inhibitory concentration.*

MBC or *minimum bactericidal concentration* is estimated by subculture from the tubes of an MIC test on to solid media; growth on subculture indicates the presence of surviving bacteria and that the concentration has not been bactericidal. MBC is the lowest concentration of antibiotic in which the bacteria have been killed.

E test® *(AB Biodisk)*: a simple, robust method for the determination of MIC: an antimicrobial gradient strip is placed on the inoculated plate and incubated. The MIC is read at the point where the inhibition ellipse intersects the scale (Fig. 5.3).

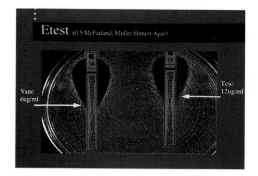

Fig. 5.3 E-test: showing increased MIC to glycopeptides in a strain of *S. aureus*. (Photograph courtesy of Professor C. G. Gemmell.)

Estimation of the level of antimicrobial agents in blood

Necessary to ensure that blood levels are at effective therapeutic levels but below those associated with toxicity.

Method: serum samples are taken before and after a dose of drug to estimate 'trough' and 'peak' levels, respectively, and tested by either:

- *Immunological assays*: fast, accurate and now widely used; run on computerized assay equipment with commercially prepared kits. Available for relatively few antibiotics – principally aminoglycosides and vancomycin, but these are the drugs most frequently in need of assay.
  or
- *Bioassay*: zones of inhibition produced by serum in wells in an agar plate inoculated with a suitable bacterial culture are compared to zones produced by standard concentrations of the drug to calculate the level in the serum.

SEROLOGY

Detection of antibody to an infecting bacterium is a classic method of diagnosing infection: still essential for some diseases.

Titre is the term for the highest dilution of serum at which antibody activity is demonstrable, usually expressed as the reciprocal of the serum dilution, e.g. 64 if antibody was detected at a final serum dilution of 1 in 64.

1. *Agglutination*: antibody is detected when it causes visible aggregation of suspensions of bacteria. *Indirect (Coombs')*

agglutination: some antibodies are incomplete and combine with bacteria but do not cause agglutination: later addition of rabbit antihuman globulin causes the antibody-coated bacteria to agglutinate.

2. *Precipitation*: antibody to antigen in soluble form is detected by the formation of a visible line of precipitate when they diffuse towards each other in an agar gel.

3. *Complement fixation*: reaction of antigen with antibody 'fixes' or uses up complement; absence of complement (i.e. a positive reaction) is detected by an indicator system (sheep erythrocytes coated with rabbit antibody) which is unable to haemolyse when added later.

4. *Immunofluorescence*: smears containing the organism (antigen) are treated with the patient's serum, followed by antihuman globulin labelled with a fluorescent dye. The labelled antihuman globulin attaches to antibody that has reacted with the organism and, after washing, the organisms fluoresce.

5. *Enzyme-linked immunosorbent assay (ELISA)*: similar in principle to immunofluorescence, but the antihuman globulin is tagged with an enzyme: reaction is detected by a colour change produced by the enzyme on addition of a suitable substrate.

MOLECULAR METHODS

These are being introduced into diagnostic bacteriology but more slowly than in virology. Basically, molecular methods are used to amplify and detect nucleic acid sequences and so to trace the organism responsible. The techniques used are exquisitely sensitive and, provided care is taken to avoid contamination, also extremely specific; they are described in more detail in Chapter 21.

Hybridization: detects specific nucleotide sequences either directly in situ in a clinical sample or in an extract of it using a radioisotope-labelled probe of DNA or RNA complementary to sequences in the bacterium sought.

Polymerase chain reaction (PCR): using a thermostable DNA polymerase, target DNA in a patient's sample is amplified yielding 10^5–10^6 copies.

Other amplification methods: are now being used, such as the ligase chain reaction (LCR), an alternative to PCR, and branched DNA assay which measures the amount of target DNA in the sample. New methods are under development and being introduced by several commercial companies which market increasingly reliable kits for this work.

SPECIMENS

Efficient diagnosis in the bacteriology laboratory depends on:

• *careful collection*: of appropriate specimens, accurately labelled, and containing adequate information for the staff to process the specimen correctly
• *rapid transport* to the laboratory.

Specimen collection

Urine: a midstream specimen, with precautions to avoid contamination.

Faeces: collect in a plastic container; if not available, take a rectal swab.

Sputum: a morning specimen in a wide-mouthed container; if tuberculosis is suspected, collect specimens on three consecutive mornings.

Serous fluids (e.g. pleural, synovial, ascitic fluids): collect in a sterile container.

Cerebrospinal fluid: collect by lumbar puncture into a sterile container.

Blood culture: blood, aseptically collected, is injected into each of two capped bottles (see above).

Clotted blood (for serological tests, antibiotic assays): 5–10 mL in a clean, dry container.

Swabs: widely used and extremely useful: usually a shaft (of wood, plastic or metal) with a cottonwool tip rubbed over the infected site or inserted into the lesion and replaced in a stoppered tube for transport to the laboratory. Essential for sampling some areas, e.g. throat, cervix. Where available, it is always better to collect *pus* into a sterile container.

Labelling: every specimen **must** be labelled with the patient's identification data and accompanied by a *request form* stating the nature of the specimen, clinical history, antibiotic therapy, date and time of collection.

Infectious hazard: specimens that could present a hazard to laboratory staff (such as blood samples positive for hepatitis B or HIV, sputum from a known case of open pulmonary tuberculosis) must be labelled '*Dangerous specimen*'. But all specimens should be handled as potentially hazardous.

Gloves: should always be worn when taking any specimen from a patient.

Transport: most specimens need to be sent to the laboratory without delay: some bacteria die off quickly outside the body; others can overgrow and give a false impression of their original numbers. If delay is unavoidable, store in a refrigerator, except blood cultures and CSF, which should be incubated at 37°C.

Stuart's transport medium: when looking for exceptionally delicate organisms such as gonococci, place swabs in this medium to preserve any present.

LABORATORY INVESTIGATION

Laboratory confirmation of the diagnosis of infection is therefore achieved by:

- *Culture*: isolation of the infecting organism – by far the best and most widely used method of diagnosis. Crucially, it allows the antibiotic sensitivity to be determined.
- *Direct demonstration*: presumptive diagnosis of some infections can be made morphologically by finding the causal organism in a stained smear: with immunofluorescence, detecting the causal organism not only confirms its presence in the material under examination but also identifies it serologically.
- *Serology*: demonstration of antibody to the causal organism: in general, less satisfactory for the diagnosis of bacterial infections than isolation. However, of great value in a few infections (e.g. syphilis, Legionnaires' disease, leptospirosis) in which the organism responsible is difficult to culture.

BACTERIAL
DISEASES

6 Bacterial infections of the respiratory tract

A very important cause of sickness, reckoned – together with virus infections – to account for a half of general practitioner (GP) consultations and a quarter of all absences from work due to illness.

Route of infection – inhalation. More frequent in winter time: close contact in school, at work and socially allows ready transfer of the causal agents – 'coughs and sneezes spread diseases'. *Direct spread* can also take place: hand-to-hand transfer of infected respiratory secretions. In family outbreaks infection is often introduced by the most susceptible member, usually a preschool or school-age child.

The same clinical syndrome may be produced by a variety of agents, and the same aetiological agent may produce a variety of clinical syndromes.

Respiratory infections can be classified into four groups:

1. Infections of throat and pharynx
2. Infections of middle ear and sinuses
3. Infections of trachea and bronchi
4. Infections of the lungs.

INFECTIONS OF THROAT AND PHARYNX

Sore throat is the commonest symptom, accompanied by a variable degree of constitutional upset. Typical throat appearances for the different aetiological agents are described below, but it is often impossible to decide on the cause of a sore throat by clinical examination alone. Over two-thirds of these infections are caused by viruses, often with a sore throat as part of the common-cold syndrome; the remainder are bacterial in origin, almost all due to *Streptococcus pyogenes*.

STREPTOCOCCAL SORE THROAT

Clinical features

Mild redness of the tonsils and pharynx may be the only sign, but the classic picture is of infection and oedema involving the fauces and soft palate with exudate – *acute follicular tonsillitis*. Infection is most common in 5–8-year-olds.

In severe cases the tonsillitis may be complicated by a peritonsillar abscess (*quinsy*) and extension of the infection to involve the sinuses and middle ear, producing *sinusitis* and *otitis media*. Systemic illness with fever is the rule, and the cervical lymph nodes may be enlarged.

Scarlet fever is a streptococcal infection – usually involving a sore throat – accompanied by an erythematous rash when the infecting strain of *S. pyogenes* produces erythrogenic toxin in a susceptible (i.e. non-immune) patient, usually a child.

Incubation period: 1–3 days.

Source: infection is acquired from either cases or carriers. After an acute attack, transient carriage for a few weeks is common. Throat carriers outnumber nasal carriers but the latter, who often have an associated sinusitis, are much more effective disseminators.

Treatment

Penicillin is the drug of choice. Therapy should be for 10 days, to prevent complications and further spread of the organism to contacts. Patients hypersensitive to penicillin are given erythromycin, although resistance is common. Recurrent infections should be treated with clindamycin or co-amoxiclav.

Late complications of streptococcal infections

Streptococcal infections, usually those causing sore throat, are sometimes followed by disease which appears to be immunologically induced. The disease is of two main kinds:

• Rheumatic fever
• Acute glomerulonephritis.

RHEUMATIC FEVER

Clinical features

Acute onset of fever, pain and swelling of the joints – and pancarditis on average 2–3 weeks, but up to 5 weeks after streptococcal sore throat. The most serious manifestation is involvement of the *heart*: patients commonly have myocarditis and sometimes, in addition, pericarditis and endocarditis. The disease has been said to 'lick the joints but bite the heart'.

Now relatively uncommon in the UK, it remains a major problem in developing countries and there has been a resurgence in the USA.

Prognosis: rheumatic fever usually clears up spontaneously, although it has a marked tendency to recur after subsequent episodes of pharyngitis in those predisposed to the disease. It may follow infection with almost any serotype (Griffith type) of *S. pyogenes*, although certain M types, e.g. 5, 18 and 24, are particularly associated with institutional outbreaks of the disease.

After the acute phase of rheumatic fever, patients later (often much later) develop, as the result of endocardial involvement, chronic valvular disease of the heart – usually stenosis, or incompetence of the mitral or aortic valves.

Pathogenesis: rheumatic fever appears to be the result of antibodies, produced against protein and polysaccharide cell-wall antigens of *S. pyogenes*, cross-reacting with connective tissue in the heart and elsewhere.

Diagnosis: can normally be made clinically (Jones criteria), but it is useful to check for the continuing presence of *S. pyogenes*:

- Throat swab
  - culture
  - rapid streptococcal antigen test
- Serology.

Specimen: serum: paired samples, a few weeks apart should be sent.

Examine: for antibody to streptolysin O (ASO), a haemolysin produced by *S. pyogenes*. An ASO titre of ≥200 units is regarded as significant; evidence of recent infection requires the demonstration of rising or falling titres. Tests are available to detect antibody to other streptococcal products, e.g. hyaluronidase, DNA-ase B – they may be positive when the ASO titre is not raised.

Use of antibiotics

Required to eradicate *S. pyogenes* from the throat. Thereafter, prophylaxis on a long-term basis is mandatory to prevent reinfection, with its risk of precipitating a recurrence. Penicillin is the drug of choice, and administration should be continued until adult life, when the natural incidence of infection falls.

ACUTE GLOMERULONEPHRITIS

Also an immunological complication which may follow streptococcal sore throat or, less often, skin infection, e.g. impetigo. It is particularly liable to follow infection with certain nephritogenic serotypes of *S. pyogenes*, e.g. in throat infections, type 12 and, in skin infections, type 49.

Clinical features

Acute glomerulonephritis presents 1–3 weeks after a streptococcal throat infection, with *haematuria, albuminuria* and *oedema*. The oedema affects the face on waking, causing a characteristic puffy appearance; as the day wears on, this disappears and oedema of the feet and ankles develops. Oliguria is common, and there may be hypertension.

Prognosis: good, especially in childhood – morbidity and mortality increase with age. Although the disease usually clears up spontaneously, it may cause permanent kidney damage and eventually progress to renal failure. Second attacks are uncommon.

Pathogenesis: the disease is the result of an immunological process, but the exact pathogenesis is unclear. Immune complexes (antibodies with streptococcal antigens) are deposited on to the glomerular basement membrane. The complexes activate complement with the release of toxic substances, which provoke an inflammatory reaction.

Diagnosis: usually made on clinical grounds, but attempts should be made to confirm past or present streptococcal infection, as described above for rheumatic fever. If impetigo or pyoderma present a swab or pus for the lesion should be cultured.

Complement estimations: the level of C3 in serum is reduced: this has been interpreted as evidence of immune complex formation.

Use of antibiotics

Eradicate *S. pyogenes* if the organism is still present at the site of infection; penicillin is the drug of choice. As recurrent episodes are rare, long-term prophylaxis is not recommended.

DIPHTHERIA

Cause: *Corynebacterium diphtheriae.*

A *severe disease* in which the primary site of infection is the throat; if untreated, there is a high case fatality rate.

Clinical features

Incubation period: 2–5 days.

Local symptoms: sore throat, due to inflamed fauces, with grey-white membrane due to serocellular exudate caused by locally produced toxin. Formerly, death was often due to suffocation caused by obstruction of the airways by membrane. Diphtheria sometimes affects the nose and other body sites, classically the skin, where signs of systemic disease may also be apparent. Milder forms of the disease are usually observed in vaccinated individuals.

Distant symptoms: due to circulating exotoxin; are of two types:

- *Cardiotoxic*: exotoxin affects the heart to cause heart failure, a common cause of death in diphtheria.
- *Neurotoxic*: exotoxin acts on nerves to cause cranial and peripheral nerve paralysis.

Pathogenesis

Classically, a disease with toxic effects at sites distant from the focus of primary infection. But note, severe effects are also due to exotoxin produced locally, with the formation of a suffocating membrane in the throat. *Gravis* and *mitis* strains of *C. diphtheriae* (see Chapter 3) can both cause severe disease.

Diagnosis:

Isolation: throat swab.

Culture: on tellurite media.

Observe: typical grey-black colonies of bacteria with distinct microscopic morphology, with Albert's (granules) or Gram stain.

Note: In view of the resurgence of the disease in Europe and other regions globally, most UK laboratories screen throat swabs for *C. diphtheriae*.

Demonstrate toxin production

Production of toxin can be demonstrated by Elek plate in vitro (toxin–antitoxin lines of precipitation in agar gel – see Chapter 3).

Treatment

Antitoxin: inject on suspicion of the diagnosis of diphtheria.
  Antibiotics: penicillin or erythromycin.
  Tracheotomy: may be necessary to relieve laryngeal obstruction.

Epidemiology

About 300 non-toxigenic and one to three toxin-producing strains are isolated annually in the UK. Diphtheria is uncommon in well-vaccinated developed countries, although occasional sporadic cases and small outbreaks are seen, usually due to infection imported from abroad. In 1991–2000 the former Soviet Union experienced a large epidemic of infection involving thousands of cases, apparently due to inadequate immunization programmes and increased population movement and other social factors. Large epidemics have also recently been described in southeast Asia and the eastern Mediterranean regions.

Source of infection is respiratory secretions from the throat – and also the nose – of cases and asymptomatic carriers. Spread is facilitated by close contact. Most at risk are those in poor health and those living in bad housing conditions, and also individuals with low levels of immunity.

Non-toxigenic C. diphtheriae are being increasingly isolated from throat cultures among UK patients with severe and recurrent episodes of pharyngitis. The predominant biotype is var. *gravis*; isolates of the biovar. *mitis* are commonly isolated from cases of cutanous infection. The apparent increase of non-toxigenic bio-types is of concern in view of the association with serious invasive diseases such as endocarditis, septic arthritis and bacteraemia. The overall global incidence of infections caused by these organisms is unknown.

C. ulcerans is a rare cause of mild pharyngitis. The organism has the ability to produce diphtheria toxin and can rarely cause diphtheria. It is usually associated with the consumption of unpasteurized dairy products.

CANDIDIASIS

Oral thrush caused by the yeast *Candida albicans* presents as white patches superimposed on red, raw mucous membrane, which may involve the throat as well as the more common site of the mouth (Fig. 6.1). It is particularly common in babies.

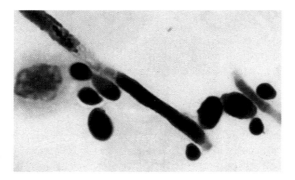

Fig. 6.1 *Candida albicans* in pus (approx. × 1000).

Source: endogenous. In adults candidiasis may be precipitated by antibiotic treatment, but the patient is often debilitated by disease, e.g. malignancy, diabetes.

Treatment

Locally applied nystatin, amphotericin B or miconazole. Oral fluconazole is used in immunocompromised patients.

VINCENT'S ANGINA

An *ulcerative tonsillitis* which causes much tissue necrosis: often an extension of similar disease of the gums and mouth (gingivostomatitis).

Source: endogenous. The causal organisms are a spirochaete, *Borrelia vincenti*, and a variety of Gram-negative anaerobic bacilli, found in small numbers in the normal mouth (Fig. 6.2).

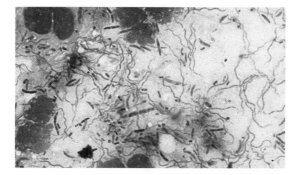

Fig. 6.2 Vincent's angina: film (approx. × 1000).

Overgrowth, to produce disease, is precipitated by dental caries or poor oral hygiene, nutritional deficiency, leukopenia (e.g. in leukaemia) and viral infections (e.g. herpes simplex, infectious mononucleosis).

Treatment

Penicillin and/or metronidazole.

DIAGNOSIS OF THROAT AND PHARYNGEAL INFECTIONS

Diagnosis depends on *isolation* and *demonstration* of the causal bacterium or antigen.

Specimen: a well-taken throat swab. Illumination of the throat and depression of the tongue are essential. The swab should be gently rubbed over the affected area, so that it collects a sample of any exudate present.

Gram-stained film: a mixed bacterial flora is always present, and the only findings of value are recognition of Vincent's organisms (Fig. 6.2) and yeasts (Fig. 6.1).

Note: This is the only method of diagnosing Vincent's infection – the causal organisms cannot be isolated by routine culture methods.

Culture: the swab is inoculated on to a variety of media selected to isolate *S. pyogenes, C. albicans* and *C. diphtheriae.*

Antigen detection tests: for rapid diagnosis of streptococcal pharyngitis.

INFECTIONS OF MIDDLE EAR AND SINUSES

Acute infection of the middle ear or sinuses is often due to secondary bacterial invasion following a viral infection of the respiratory tract: this may be a common cold or measles, of which otitis media is a frequent complication.

ACUTE INFECTIONS OF THE MIDDLE EAR AND SINUSES

Clinical features

Otitis media

An upper respiratory infection involving the middle ear by extension of infection up the eustachian tube. Predominantly a disease of infants and children: the main symptom is earache.

On examination the eardrum is red and the infection may progress to cause bulging, with eventual rupture of the tympanic membrane and discharge of pus from the ear. Recurrent attacks are common.

Sinusitis

Mild discomfort over the frontal or maxillary sinuses due to congestion is a frequent symptom in common colds. Severe pain and tenderness with purulent nasal discharge, however, indicate bacterial infection.

Causal bacteria

H. influenzae (non-capsulated strains), *S. pyogenes*, *S. pneumoniae*, *M. catarrhalis*.

Source

Endogenous spread of organisms from the normal flora of the nasopharynx.

Diagnosis

In the majority of cases of sinusitis and otitis media, specimens from the site of infection cannot be obtained. If the eardrum ruptures, or if myringotomy (incision of the tympanic membrane to release pus in the middle ear) is performed, collect a swab of exudate; if drainage or lavage of the sinuses is carried out, material should be collected and cultured in the same way as a sample of pus, on a range of suitable media.

Treatment

Amoxycillin or co-amoxiclav; alternatively, erythromycin. For penicillin-resistant *S. pneumoniae* use ceftriaxone.

CHRONIC INFECTIONS OF THE MIDDLE EAR AND SINUSES

Clinical features

Chronic suppurative otitis media

Two types: with and without cholesteatoma – an ingrowth of skin-containing sac into the middle ear. Both characterized by suppuration in the middle ear. Symptoms are of intermittent discharge (otorrhoea) and painless hearing loss. This is usually a long-standing disease, which can recur at intervals throughout childhood and into adult life.

Chronic sinusitis

Painful sinuses with headache are prominent symptoms; often associated with nasal obstruction and mucoid or purulent nasal discharge.

Cause: the same organisms as those implicated in acute infections. *Staphylococcus aureus*, 'coliform bacilli', pseudomonads, proteus and 'bacteroides' are also common in chronic ear discharges. Detection of anaerobes requires the careful laboratory examination of a well-taken specimen. The clinical significance of some of these organisms is uncertain.

Diagnosis: *culture*: of swabs of pus from the ear; lavage specimens from the sinuses – such saline washings are always contaminated by nasal flora. Examine as specimens of pus.

Treatment

Antibiotics often give disappointing results. If prescribed, therapy should be guided by the antibiotic sensitivities of isolated organisms, but treatment may have to be on a 'best-guess' basis. Topical antimicrobials (e.g. neomycin or framycetin, polymyxin, bacitracin) are often given in chronic otitis media because systemic drugs fail to penetrate to the site of infection, but there is conflicting evidence about their efficacy. Cholesteatoma requires surgery.

INFECTIONS OF TRACHEA AND BRONCHI

Laryngitis, tracheitis and bronchitis are usually associated with or follow a viral infection of the upper respiratory tract.

LARYNGITIS

Clinical features

Hoarseness and loss of voice: in more severe form, *croup* (or acute laryngotracheobronchitis) with croaking cough and stridor. In children, most often associated with parainfluenza virus infection; occasionally due to a rare but important bacterial infection, acute epiglottitis.

ACUTE EPIGLOTTITIS

Clinical features

Severe croup syndrome in children (usually under 5 years of age), which may rapidly progress to respiratory obstruction and death. The epiglottis is inflamed and oedematous.

Cause: capsulated strains of *H. influenzae* (almost always of type b).

Diagnosis: *H. influenzae* may be isolated from the epiglottis and from blood culture.

Treatment

Parenteral amoxycillin or ceftriaxone: tracheostomy may be necessary.

Vaccine: the recent introduction of Hib vaccination in infancy has dramatically reduced the incidence of this disease (see Chapter 39).

BRONCHITIS

Clinical features

A feeling of tightness in the chest ('tubes'); cough, initially dry and painful, later productive with expectoration of yellow-green sputum, most marked in early morning specimens; variable degree of fever and of constitutional upset. Abnormal chest signs, e.g. rhonchi, are found on auscultation.

Acute bronchitis

Acute bronchitis in a patient with a healthy respiratory tract is often a trivial complication of a viral upper tract infection: the initial viral attack damages respiratory mucous membrane, with paralysis of ciliary movement. Although viral acute bronchitis is usually mild and self-limiting, secondary bacterial infection often supervenes in more severe attacks, especially in patients with chronic cardiopulmonary disease. Other bacterial agents include

Bordetella pertussis (whooping cough, see below), *Chlamydophilia pneumoniae* and *Mycoplasma pneumoniae*. Infections with *M. pneumoniae* are mainly seen in young adults: the source is exogenous and spread is by the respiratory route. Cases are usually sporadic, but there may be family outbreaks and, occasionally, institutional epidemics. The frequency of infection in the community varies from year to year.

Treatment

In previously healthy subjects symptoms normally subside in 2–5 days and antibiotic therapy is not required. Appropriate antibiotic treatment should be used for specific pathogens.

Chronic bronchitis and acute infective exacerbations

Chronic bronchitis is defined as productive cough on most days for at least 3 months for 2 consecutive years. Incidence and prevalence are increasing, and it is fourth leading cause of death in the UK.

Chronic bronchitis is not itself due to infection – aetiological factors include low socioeconomic class, urban dwelling (atmospheric pollution) and tobacco consumption, especially cigarettes ('smoker's cough'). Exacerbations, however, are associated with bacterial infection. They commonly follow viral respiratory infections or a fall in atmospheric temperature with an increase in humidity (together causing foggy weather): all these factors are often present concurrently in winter. During exacerbations both the volume and the purulence of sputum increase.

Pathology

Pathological changes in chronic bronchitis are: (i) increase in the number of mucus-containing cells in the bronchi, with consequent hypersecretion of mucus; (ii) inflammation, fibrosis, collapse, dilatation and cyst formation in the bronchioles and alveoli. After exacerbations some changes may resolve but others do not, resulting in progressive irreversible damage.

Causal pathogens and source

1. *H. influenzae* (usually non-capsulated strains). The closely related organism *H. parainfluenzae* is sometimes isolated, but is of uncertain pathogenicity.

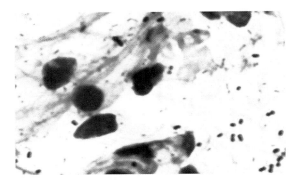

Fig. 6.3   Film of sputum with pneumococci and *H. influenzae* (approx. × 1000).

2. *S. pneumoniae* (pneumococcus).

3. *M. catarrhalis.*

All three organisms are present in the normal upper respiratory tract flora. The secondary bacterial invaders in bronchitis are therefore endogenous. Normal subjects have a sterile bronchial tree, but in chronic bronchitis the bronchi become colonized, especially with *H. influenzae*, even when the disease is quiescent. During exacerbations the concentration of *H. influenzae* in respiratory secretions increases, along with sputum purulence. Specific antibodies to *H. influenzae*, absent in non-smoking healthy adults, are present in the serum of two-thirds of chronic bronchitis cases. *H. influenzae* is now regarded as the prime pathogen in exacerbations of chronic bronchitis and is often found in the sputum, along with pneumococci (Fig. 6.3).

4. *M. pneumoniae* and viruses, e.g. influenza, parainfluenza, account for up to one-third of acute exacerbations.

5. 'Coliform' bacilli, *Pseudomonas aeruginosa* and *S. aureus* (including MRSA): found in patients with more severe disease.

Treatment

Antibiotic therapy may shorten the duration and reduce the severity of exacerbations but, unfortunately, does not prevent deterioration of respiratory function.

Drugs used must ideally be active against the three main pathogens:

- *H. influenzae*: strains resistant to amoxycillin are now common, and a significant number are also resistant to co-amoxiclav. Fully sensitive to quinolones.

- *Pneumococci*: resistance to penicillin is still rare in Britain (<5%), but many strains are now resistant to tetracycline and erythromycin.
- *M. catarrhalis*: most strains produce a β-lactamase and are therefore amoxycillin resistant.

Short-term (7–10 days) courses of treatment include:

1. *Amoxycillin*: bactericidal in action. Co-amoxiclav is indicated when the infecting strain is shown to be a β-lactamase producer.
2. *Tetracyclines*: bacteriostatic action; uncertain sputum penetration. An advantage is their activity against *M. pneumoniae*.
3. *Cephalosporins*: second- or third-generation agents, active against all three main pathogens. No activity against *M. pneumoniae*.
4. *Macrolides*: active against most pneumococci. Erythromycin has poor activity against *H. influenzae* compared to newer agents, e.g. clarithromycin. *M. pneumoniae* is also sensitive.
5. *Quinolones*: *ciprofloxacin* and other quinolones are effective in bronchitis, perhaps surprisingly, because although they are very active against *H. influenzae* and *M. catarrhalis*, pneumococci are not fully sensitive. Newer quinolones, e.g. moxifloxacin, are highly active against all respiratory pathogens, including pneumococci, and preliminary use is promising.

The ultimate choice of an appropriate antibiotic will depend on many factors, including cost.

Laboratory examination of sputum is essential if the patient fails to respond to an apparently adequate course of treatment.

Vaccines – *bacterial*: polyvalent pneumococcal polysaccharide vaccines are now available. They may be of value in preventing pneumococcal pneumonia in this 'at risk' group.

Diagnosis: see below in 'Diagnosis of bacterial chest infections'.

CYSTIC FIBROSIS

This inherited defect leads to the production of abnormally viscid mucus, which blocks tubular structures in many different organs. The most disabling obstructive changes affect the lungs, and chronic respiratory infection is a major problem. Thanks to improved management, more infants and children with this disease, transmitted as an autosomal recessive trait, survive to adult life than did formerly.

Causal bacteria

1. *S. aureus* (including MRSA) and *H. influenzae* initially, tending to be replaced by:

2. *P. aeruginosa*: the strains involved produce an extracellular alginate polysaccharide, which adheres to bronchial mucus, increasing respiratory obstruction. Isolates from sputum form mucoid colonies on culture.

3. *Burkholderia cepacia*: now recognized as an important cause of rapid clinical deterioration; can be acquired readily by direct or indirect person-to-person contact.

4. Enterobacteriaceae and *Stenotrophomonas maltophilia* can also colonize the lungs.

5. Fungi, e.g. *Aspergillus* spp. and *Mycobacteria*, can also cause infections in severe disease.

Treatment

Determined by bacteriological findings. Ciprofloxacin, although not recommended for children, is a useful antipseudomonal drug. Long-term administration may be required.

PERTUSSIS (WHOOPING COUGH)

Clinical features

An acute tracheobronchitis of childhood.

Onset is insidious – initially a catarrhal stage with common-cold symptoms, which lasts about 2 weeks, followed by a stage of paroxysmal coughing (2 weeks); residual cough persisting for a month or more is a common sequel; a marked lymphocytosis is common.

Paroxysmal cough is a diagnostic feature: it consists of repeated violent exhalations with a distressing, severe inspiratory whoop; the vehemence of the spasms can cause subconjunctival haemorrhage (Fig. 6.4). There is expulsion of tenacious, clear bronchial mucus, and vomiting is common.

Fatality is low, but morbidity may be high: there is a significant risk of developing subsequent chronic chest disease, e.g. bronchiectasis. Most acute deaths are in infants during the first year of life, especially in the first 6 months.

Cause: Bordetella pertussis (types 1,3; 1,2,3; and 1,2). During the 1970s and early 1980s type 1,3 was responsible for most

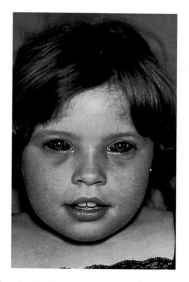

Fig. 6.4 Pertussis: subconjunctival haemorrhages caused by spasms of severe coughing. (Photograph courtesy of Dr A. K. R. Chaudhuri.)

infections, then for a few years type 1,2 predominated, before type 1,3 – now responsible for about two-thirds of cases – became common again, along with type 2,3. This is explained by the sharp decline in vaccine uptake in earlier years, followed by greatly increased acceptance: vaccine immunity protects best against strains containing agglutinogen 2.

B. parapertussis causes mild whooping cough and is relatively rare in Britain.

A similar syndrome may be caused by adenoviruses and by *M. pneumoniae*.

Epidemiology

Following the decline in the acceptance of immunization in the mid-1970s, there were three epidemics of whooping cough in the UK between 1977 and 1987. The 1989–1991 and 1994 outbreaks were much smaller, owing to the improvement in vaccine uptake, which is now about 90%.

Incubation period: 1–3 weeks: often about 10 days.

Source: patients – most infective during catarrhal stage, becoming non-infective at end of paroxysmal stage.

Spread: airborne, via droplets.

Diagnosis

Isolation, from infected clinical cases: this is not easy and diagnosis is usually based on symptoms. Organisms are much less numerous after the catarrhal stage (i.e. when typical symptoms develop) and in immunized patients.

Specimen:

- Pernasal swab: passed gently along the floor of the nose to sample nasopharyngeal secretions.
- Cough plate: held in front of mouth during a paroxysm of coughing; superseded by pernasal swabbing.

Inoculate: appropriate selective media.

Serology: ELISA for IgM; PCR is a rapid method of confirmation.

Treatment

Antibiotics are only of value within the first 10 days of infection, i.e. during the catarrhal stage, when the diagnosis may not be suspected. If secondary pneumonia develops it should be treated appropriately, guided by the antibiotic sensitivity of the causal organism.

Administration of erythromycin to the patient reduces the duration of infectivity, and this drug is a successful chemoprophylactic when given to close contacts (e.g. siblings).

Vaccine: see Chapter 39.

INFECTIONS OF THE LUNGS

PNEUMONIA

The most severe and life-threatening of respiratory infections, in which there is exudate in the alveolar spaces. Although antibiotic therapy has transformed the prognosis for many patients, pneumonia remains a significant cause of death – in infancy, in the elderly and in immunocompromised patients.

Clinical features

Onset: sometimes abrupt, but sometimes insidious when due to the extension of a pre-existing respiratory infection.

Symptoms: fever, rigors, malaise; respiratory symptoms include shortness of breath, rapid shallow breathing, cyanosis, cough, sometimes pleural pain; sputum may be tenacious and rusty initially, later becoming purulent. There is usually polymorphonuclear leukocytosis.

Clinical investigation

Investigate for signs of consolidation of lungs, i.e. dullness on percussion, reduced air entry, moist rales; assess respiratory function; *radiology* to indicate the site and extent of the consolidation.

Classification

Pneumonia may be classified as follows:

1. *Lobar (or segmental) pneumonia*: in which the consolidation is limited at least initially to one lobe or segment of the lung: the main type of pneumonia seen in previously healthy people.
2. *Bronchopneumonia*: usually bilateral; the consolidation is scattered throughout the lung fields, although it is mainly concentrated at the bases. The most common form of pneumonia, seen principally in the elderly and in patients with debilitating or chronic respiratory disease, such as chronic bronchitis, bronchiectasis.
3. *Primary atypical pneumonia*: patchy consolidation of the lungs, in which the walls of the bronchioles are thickened by an interstitial mononuclear cell infiltrate and the lumina contain exudate.
4. *Legionnaires' disease*: a severe pneumonia first recognized in 1976 among members attending an American Legion convention.

Causal agents

Table 6.1 lists the main organisms associated with the different types of pneumonia.

S. pneumoniae (pneumococcus)

The main cause of pneumonia.
   Source: human respiratory tract.

Table 6.1 Causes of pneumonia

Pneumonia	Main causal organisms
Lobar pneumonia	*Streptococcus pneumoniae*
Bronchopneumonia	*Streptococcus pneumoniae*
	Haemophilus influenzae
	Rarely: *Staphylococcus aureus*, coliforms
Primary atypical pneumonia*	*Mycoplasma pneumoniae*
	Coxiella burneti
	Chlamydophila psittaci
	Chlamydophila pneumoniae
Legionnaires' disease*	*Legionella pneumophila*

*These are multisystem diseases which affect other organs as well as the lungs.

Spread:

- Exogenous: droplet transmission of virulent strains (incubation period 1–3 days).
- Endogenous, owing to downward spread of pneumococci from the flora of the nasopharynx.

Treatment: recommended drugs: penicillin, macrolides, e.g. erythromycin. For penicillin/erythromycin-resistant strains: ceftriaxone, vancomycin or linezolid.

H. influenzae

Often underestimated as a cause of pneumonia: in infants, usually due to capsulated strains; in adults it is often (but not always) a complication of chronic respiratory disease. *Note*: in pneumonia following exacerbations of chronic bronchitis, the pneumococcus is the commonest bacterial cause.

Treatment: recommended drugs: amoxycillin, co-amoxiclav, ceftriaxone, ciprofloxacin.

S. aureus

A relatively uncommon cause of bronchopneumonia: probably most often seen in hospital patients; sometimes complicates influenza. The cause of severe secondary bacterial pneumonia, an increasing problem in intravenous drug users and in ventilator-associated pneumonia.

Treatment: recommended drug: cloxacillin, often combined with rifampicin or fusidic acid. Very few infecting strains are penicillin sensitive. Vancomycin or linezolid for MRSA strains.

Coliforms

Coliforms, e.g. *Escherichia coli*, *Proteus*, *Klebsiella* and *Pseudomonas* species are recognized causes of bronchopneumonia. Their isolation from sputum often indicates merely colonization of the respiratory tract, e.g. after a course of antibiotic, and must be interpreted cautiously. As a cause of pneumonia they are most often encountered in hospital patients, especially the immunocompromised or those on support ventilation under intensive care.

Friedländer's bacillus: a klebsiella of uncertain taxonomy; has been described as a cause of a rare pneumonia with much tissue destruction.

Treatment: recommended drugs: ceftriaxone, ciprofloxacin, piperacillin–tazobactam, often combined with an aminoglycoside.

Mycoplasma pneumoniae

Formerly known as Eaton agent: responsible for most cases of primary atypical pneumonia. Overall, second only to the pneumococcus as the commonest recognized cause of pneumonia. School-aged children and young adults are the groups most frequently affected.

Clinical features

Incubation period: 1–3 weeks.

Fever, dry hacking cough, often with severe headache, weakness and tiredness. X-ray changes of diffuse, patchy infiltrates are often out of proportion to the relatively mild degree of illness and the few clinical signs. Also causes febrile bronchitis and tracheitis, with upper respiratory symptoms such as pharyngitis, coryza and otitis media with bullous myringitis of the tympanic membrane.

Non-respiratory disease: *M. pneumoniae* pneumonia may be followed or accompanied by:

• *Erythema multiforme* (which may also be caused by herpes simplex virus): a skin rash of erythematous haloes surrounding pale, oedematous lesions; this may progress to Stevens–Johnson syndrome, with bullous involvement of the oral, conjunctival and genital mucosa.

- *Haemolytic anaemia*: possibly due to the development of haemagglutinins for human group O erythrocytes (active at 4°C).

Spread: respiratory (droplet) spread to involve individuals, families, and sometimes institutions (e.g. schools, military camps). The prevalence peaks every 4 years.

Treatment: Recommended drug: tetracycline. Other effective drugs: erythromycin, ciprofloxacin.

Coxiella burneti

The cause of the acute febrile disease Q fever (see Chapter 18): up to half of the patients have pneumonia – usually a patchy consolidation. The disease is a zoonosis, acquired from domestic animals – usually cattle and sheep – by the inhalation of infected dust, straw etc.

Treatment: recommended drug: tetracycline. Other effective drug: erythromycin.

Chlamydophila psittaci

Causes ornithosis and psittacosis in birds (see Chapter 17): may infect humans via inhalation of dried bird droppings. Produces an acute influenza-like illness, with patchy pneumonia.

Treatment: recommended drug: tetracycline. Other effective drug: erythromycin.

Chlamydophila pneumoniae (see also Chapter 17)

Spreads from person to person: no known animal association. Usually causes mild respiratory infections, but can be responsible for pneumonia. Antibodies are detectable in childhood and are found increasingly with age, indicating that infection is common.

Treatment: as for *Chlamydophila psittaci* infection.

Legionella pneumophila and related species

The result of infection varies from asymptomatic seroconversion to non-specific febrile illness (*Pontiac fever*) to pneumonia. The pneumonia, *Legionnaires' disease*, is now being increasingly recognized in middle-aged smokers, who are often in poor general health.

Clinical features

Symptoms: initially influenza-like, with abrupt onset. The illness may progress to a severe pneumonia, with purulent, sometimes bloodstained, sputum and sometimes with respiratory failure. Other prominent features are mental confusion, acute renal failure and gastrointestinal symptoms.

Source: environment: usually associated with water, in which the organism can survive for long periods.

Spread: by contaminated aerosols, e.g. via air-conditioning systems, water from storage tanks through showers and taps, etc. Person-to-person droplet spread has not been recorded.

Epidemiology: the majority of cases are sporadic, with the route of infection unconfirmed. Outbreaks are usually associated with large buildings (e.g. hotels, hospitals), and the origin can often be traced to a source within their complex water systems.

Treatment: recommended drug: erythromycin. Other effective drugs: rifampicin, ciprofloxacin, usually given in combination.

Virus causes of pneumonia

See Chapter 22.

TREATMENT OF PNEUMONIA

This is governed by the clinician's experience, in/outpatient therapy, national and local guidelines, and knowledge of what the infecting agent and its antibiotic sensitivity are likely to be. As a rule, treatment has to be started before laboratory results are available, and even after investigation the cause of pneumonia in some patients is never identified.

For community-acquired pneumonia the choices are:

- An aminopenicillin, e.g. amoxycillin or co-amoxiclav, with the addition of a macrolide, e.g. clarithromycin for 'atypical' organisms.
- A cephalosporin, e.g. ceftriaxone (with clarithromycin) for severe cases, and for penicillin-allergic patients.
- A new-generation quinolone, e.g. moxifloxacin.

Flucloxacillin should be considered if staphylococcal pneumonia is suspected. Treatment should be changed if laboratory investigation indicates a more appropriate antibiotic.

In hospital-acquired pneumonia consider the possibility that the causal organism is a coliform (give an extended-spectrum β-lactam or quinolone with the addition of an aminoglycoside). If aspiration pneumonia is suspected (see below), the causal organism may be an anaerobe (add metronidazole).

TUBERCULOSIS

Although tuberculosis is not considered in this chapter (see Chapter 14), in any long-standing chest infection the possibility of tuberculosis must *always* be considered.

ASPIRATION PNEUMONIA AND LUNG ABSCESS

Aspiration pneumonia follows the inhalation of vomit, or sometimes a foreign body, by an unconscious patient.

The causal organisms are commensals of the upper respiratory tract – principally *S. pneumoniae*, but 'coliform bacilli' and anaerobic organisms are also involved.

Lung abscess is nowadays rare. It is usually due to obstruction of a bronchus or bronchiole, e.g. by an inhaled foreign body, or to suppuration developing within an area of pneumonic consolidation. The infecting organisms are similar to those listed above, namely *S. pneumoniae* and anaerobic bacteria of the upper respiratory flora.

Diagnosis: the isolation of anaerobic organisms requires the examination of aspirated specimens. They are seldom isolated from sputum.

Treatment: recommended drugs: co-amoxiclav or ceftriaxone and metronidazole.

EMPYEMA

Literally, pus in the pleural space and nowadays a rare complication of pneumonia, or sometimes tuberculous. It is usually due to *S. pneumoniae* or *S. aureus*, with upper respiratory anaerobes sometimes being implicated.

Laboratory diagnosis requires aspiration.

Treatment involves drainage and removal of the infected fluid, and appropriate antibiotic therapy.

DIAGNOSIS OF BACTERIAL CHEST INFECTIONS

Diagnosis involves:

1. *Isolation of causal pathogen* from sputum or, less commonly, from the aspirate of a pleural effusion, lung abscess or area of pneumonic lung. Aspiration samples may be collected by the transtracheal route, via a fine catheter introduced through the cricothyroid membrane. Best to take specimens during bronchoscopy and bronchoalveolar lavage (BAL). In BAL, saline is injected through a bronchoscope and aspirated to sample an affected area of lung, so producing an excellent specimen to make an accurate diagnosis in difficult cases of pneumonia – especially in immunosuppressed patients. *Blood cultures* should also be taken, as the infecting bacterium is present in the blood of up to one-third of patients with pneumonia.
2. *Detection of bacterial antigen* in sputum or urine.
3. *Serology*: demonstration of specific antibody in patient's serum is only useful in cases of atypical pneumonia (see below).
4. *Molecular methods*: detection by amplification of bacterial DNA by PCR.

1. Isolation of pathogen from sputum

Specimen: early morning sputum: likely to be the most purulent.

   Collection: try to minimize salivary contamination – but the presence of some oropharyngeal flora is inevitable.

   Transport: send to laboratory without delay: in transit, delicate organisms (e.g. *H. influenzae*) die; robust bacteria (e.g. coliforms) multiply and overgrow.

Laboratory examination

Macroscopic: note naked-eye appearance.
   Microscopic:

1. *Gram film*: observe amount of pus, squamous epithelial cells (indicating buccal contamination) and nature of the bacterial flora: the presence of a predominant organism may allow an immediate provisional diagnosis. Figure 6.3 shows a typical Gram film of sputum from a patient infected with both pneumococci and *H. influenzae*.

2. *Ziehl–Neelsen or auramine film*: examine for acid- and alcohol-fast bacilli. If present, a presumptive diagnosis of tuberculosis can be made.

Culture

Bacteria are not distributed evenly throughout sputum: select a purulent portion. Alternatively, homogenize the specimen by treating with a liquefying agent: such treatment allows semiquantitative culture and makes evaluation of the results easier.

Inoculate: appropriate selective and non-selective media for isolation of respiratory pathogens.

Assessment of culture results: may be difficult because of contamination from the oropharyngeal flora. Viridans streptococci, neisseriae, coagulase-negative staphylococci, commensal corynebacteria etc. are normally regarded as upper respiratory tract commensals. Small numbers of haemophilus and pneumococci in a mixed growth may be part of the normal flora; larger numbers, especially if other bacteria are scanty, are regarded as pathogens.

The oropharynx of patients who have received antibiotics often becomes colonized with coliform organisms and yeasts, and under such circumstances undue significance should not be placed on their isolation.

Culture for Mycobacterium tuberculosis: should be carried out if indicated clinically. See Chapter 14.

2. Detection of bacterial antigen in sputum or urine

Pneumococcal capsular antigens can be detected by a variety of methods. A positive result may be obtained when culture of the same specimen failed to isolate *S. pneumoniae*, usually because the patient had received antibiotics before the sputum was collected.

In some patients with Legionnaires' disease a rapid diagnosis can be made by the demonstration of *L. pneumophila* in respiratory secretions using direct immunofluorescence. Legionella antigen may be detected in urine by an ELISA test.

Direct immunofluorescence has also been used as a method of detecting *C. pneumoniae* in sputum.

3. Serological tests

Atypical pneumonias (see Table 6.1) and Legionnaires' disease are difficult to diagnose by isolation of the causal organism. All suspected cases should be investigated serologically by detection of antibody in patient's serum. Often diagnosed by stationary high titres, although it is better to demonstrate a fourfold or greater rising titre in paired 'acute' and 'convalescent' specimens, collected a few weeks apart. The tests used are complement fixation, immunofluorescence and ELISA.

Molecular methods

Detection of bacterial DNA by amplification with PCR can provide a rapid diagnosis of slow-growing organisms, e.g. *Mycobacterium* spp., or organisms that are difficult to culture, e.g. legionella.

7 Bacterial gastrointestinal disease

This chapter describes bacterial infections acquired via the gastrointestinal tract and includes the main bacterial causes of diarrhoeal disease together with infective gastritis and the severe foodborne intoxication botulism. Diarrhoea remains a major cause of morbidity and infant death in developing countries, largely because of inadequate sewage disposal and contaminated water. Most (but not all) cases of diarrhoea are due to infection – bacteria, viruses and protozoa cause diarrhoea, but this chapter deals mainly with bacteria. Viral gastroenteritis is considered in Chapter 23.

Host: the young are most susceptible to diarrhoeal disease, and poor general health and nutrition also predispose to it.

Bacteria: factors such as the size of the infecting dose; enterotoxin and cytotoxin production; ability to adhere to gastrointestinal epithelium; and ability to invade the gut wall affect the ability of organisms to infect the gut and cause diarrhoea.

Epidemiology: prevention largely depends on sanitation (i.e. adequate disposal of sewage), clean food and a safe water supply. Personal hygiene (i.e. washing hands after defecation) is a remarkably effective means of preventing faecal–oral spread. The storage of food at room temperature *must* be avoided, as it permits rapid bacterial multiplication and, with some bacteria, the formation of toxins. Note that although refrigeration prevents bacterial multiplication, the bacteria are *preserved*, not killed, at 4°C.

INVESTIGATION OF DIARRHOEA

Key features to note in patient's history include:

- Clinical symptoms, duration etc.
- Recent foreign travel
- Food history, including symptoms in other consumers of suspect food
- Probable incubation period.

Specimens for laboratory examination

- Faeces (rectal swab if none available)
- The suspected food: strenuous efforts should be made to obtain samples; this is often difficult, as it has usually all been eaten or discarded
- Vomit
- Blood culture: in severe cases, especially the very young and the elderly.

Other investigations especially important in an outbreak include:

- Food-handling practices in the kitchen concerned
- Faecal samples from kitchen staff.

The main enteropathogenic bacteria, with some characteristics of the epidemiology of the diseases they cause, are listed in Table 7.1.

Table 7.1   Causal organisms and some features of the epidemiology of diarrhoeal diseases

Organism	Usual source	Common route, source of infection
Campylobacter species	Animal gut	Poultry, meat, milk
Salmonella species	Animal gut	Poultry and eggs, meat, milk
Shigella species	Human gut	Faecal–oral or food, fomites
Escherichia coli	Human gut Animal gut (VTEC)	Faecal–oral or food, water, fomites
Staphylococcus aureus	Septic lesions on food handlers	Cooked meats, dairy products
Clostridium perfringens	Animal gut	Stews, meat pies
Bacillus species	Environment (soil)	Rice
Clostridium difficile	Human gut	Overgrowth of strains already in colon, also faecal–oral fomites
Yersinia enterocolitica	Uncertain	Faecal–oral or food, personal contact
Vibrio cholerae	Human gut	Water, food

COMMON BACTERIAL CAUSES OF DIARRHOEAL DISEASE IN BRITAIN

- Campylobacter
- Salmonella
- *Escherichia coli*
- Shigella
- *Staphylococcus aureus*
- *Clostridium perfringens.*

The changing trends of the three commonest organisms is illustrated in Figure 7.1. The diseases all of these organisms cause are described below.

An important cause of diarrhoea in hospital patients is *Clostridium difficile*, and this is considered later in this chapter, along with the less common causes of diarrhoea. Cholera, once epidemic in Britain and still a major problem in the Third World, is described at the end of the chapter.

CAMPYLOBACTER

This organism is now the commonest cause of diarrhoea in Britain (see Fig. 7.1). It requires a high temperature for growth and its frequency and importance were only appreciated when special methods of culture and temperature of incubation were introduced.

Campylobacters are small vibrio-like organisms. The main cause of human infections are *C. jejuni* and *C. coli*.

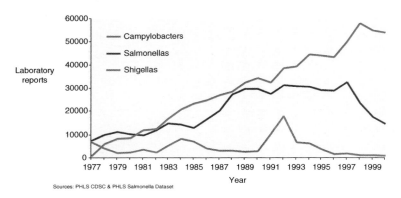

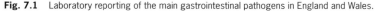

Fig. 7.1 Laboratory reporting of the main gastrointestinal pathogens in England and Wales.

Clinical features

There are two kinds of clinical presentation but, as in most intestinal infections, symptoms vary from mild (or even none) to a severe illness with prostration:

- With flu-like prodromal symptoms: fever, headache, backache, limb aches, nausea and abdominal pain; after 24 h, sometimes longer, diarrhoea develops.
- Without prodromal symptoms: acute onset of abdominal pain and diarrhoea.

Incubation period: 3–10 days.

Symptoms: diarrhoea: often severe, with blood and mucus in stools. Up to 20 stools a day may be passed, and there may be faecal incontinence. Abdominal pain is a prominent feature. Septicaemia, with fevers, rigor and malaise, is sometimes seen in severe cases, confirming the invasiveness of the causal organism.

Duration: often several days, and relapses are common.

Pathogenesis: typically an enterocolitis: infection involves the ileum but is not restricted to the small intestine, and there is often colitis also. Histology of gut biopsies suggests that campylobacters are invasive and penetrate beyond the mucosa.

Diagnosis: culture faeces on selective medium (containing antibiotics to which campylobacters are resistant) at 43°C. Observe for typical colonies.

Identification: by morphology: curved, slender Gram-negative bacilli, with characteristic darting motility, positive oxidase reaction and other features.

Treatment: usually self-limiting. Erythromycin reduces the duration of excretion and can relieve symptoms, but should be reserved for severe cases. An alternative drug is ciprofloxacin, but resistance to this drug is increasing, particularly with infections acquired abroad.

Epidemiology

Source of infection: farm animals – especially poultry – are probably the major source of human infection; milk and water have been incriminated in outbreaks; dogs and cats have also been reported as sources of campylobacters.

Route of infection: eating contaminated food, but note that campylobacters do *not* multiply in food at room temperature. Although uncommon, faecal–oral spread can occur, especially between children.

Sporadic infections seem to be the rule in the UK, but infections are so common that it may be that outbreaks are missed. Further developments in molecular typing methods, together with more epidemiological follow-up, may help identify outbreaks.

Control: food, clean water and personal hygiene. Control of infection in animals is not practicable, at present not least because the organisms are carried symptomlessly and do not harm the animals (usually poultry) concerned.

SALMONELLA

Formerly the commonest cause of diarrhoea in Britain – and still with a high incidence (see Fig. 7.1). Diarrhoea due to salmonella is traditionally called food poisoning, although this term is somewhat misleading.

The incidence of salmonella infections increased dramatically in the UK during the late 1980s: this was partly due to the emergence of *S.* Enteritidis phage type 4, and its appearance as the commonest cause of 'incidents' in poultry flocks.

There are more than 2000 serotypes of salmonella, but only about 14 are important or common causes of infection. In recent years the commonest serotype has been *S.* Enteritidis. Other common salmonellae are *S.* Typhimurium and *S.* Virchow. *S.* Typhi and *S.* Paratyphi A, B and C classically cause enteric fever, a septicaemic febrile illness in which diarrhoea is a late symptom (see Chapter 8). *S.* Paratyphi is intermediate in its pathogenicity, and can cause either mild enteric fever or a primarily diarrhoeal illness.

Habitat: for the common non-typhoidal salmonellae, domestic animals, especially poultry.

Clinical features

Asymptomatic infections and cases with only mild gastrointestinal disturbance are not uncommon.

Incubation period is short: around 12–36 h.

Main symptoms are acute onset of abdominal pain and diarrhoea, sometimes with fever and vomiting. Dehydration may require correction, especially in babies.

Septicaemia sometimes develops in severe cases, and is more common with certain serotypes (e.g. *S.* Dublin, *S.* Virchow).

Pathogenesis: site of infection is the small or large intestine. Many strains produce enterotoxins similar to those of toxigenic strains of *E. coli*. **NB**: The salmonella enterotoxins are still poorly defined. Other salmonellae invade the mucosa of the small intestine – like shigellae.

Diagnosis: *culture* faeces on MacConkey (indicator) medium and also on selective and enrichment media. Observe for pale, non-lactose-fermenting colonies on MacConkey medium, or typical morphology on other media. Identify initially by biochemical tests; then by serology.

Treatment: rarely necessary: rehydration may be required in babies: oral isotonic fluid replacement can be life-saving in infants with diarrhoea.

Antibiotics are contraindicated except in septicaemia cases: they do not affect symptoms and may prolong convalescent carriage of the organism; they also contribute to the emergence of antibiotic-resistant strains. In recent years the predominant *S.* Typhimurium strain, definitive phage type 104, has become multiply resistant.

Epidemiology: food derived from domestic animals and poultry is the main *source* – usually meat contaminated from viscera at slaughter. There have been numerous outbreaks owing to the contamination of eggs, especially if consumed raw or lightly cooked in sauces, desserts etc. Infection is transmitted from infected hens via the oviduct to the egg. Poultry- and egg-associated infection caused record numbers of food poisoning cases in the UK in the late 1980s. Occasional outbreaks due to contaminated milk, and sometimes therefore to cheese, have also been reported.

Food, especially meat and offal, is often contaminated in the raw state. If it is then inadequately cooked and stored for some time at a warm room temperature, surviving salmonellae can multiply. Alternatively – and perhaps more commonly – salmonellae from raw meat can contaminate other cooked foods by common use of kitchen tools and work-surfaces, with subsequent multiplication during storage.

Outbreaks of salmonella food poisoning are common: they often involve communal catering, e.g. weddings, large dinners etc., but may also be a problem in hospitals, especially in mental or geriatric units. Recently there has been an increase in infections carried by rarer salmonella serotypes, acquired from reptiles as a result of their increased popularity as pets.

Control: control of infection in domestic animals, especially intensively reared poultry flocks, with vaccines especially against

S. Enteriditis, has dramatically reduced human infections since 1997 (see Fig. 7.1).

Other control measures include:

- Good farming and abattoir practice; control of animal feedstuffs; restricted prescribing of antibiotics – especially to calves, because indiscriminate use results in selection of multiply resistant bacteria, which can then spread to human populations.
- Cooking to a temperature (i.e. boiling point) at which vegetative bacteria are killed.
- Rigorous hygiene in the kitchen, e.g. separation of cooked and raw foods, prompt and effective refrigeration of cooked food, thorough thawing of frozen poultry and meat before cooking.
- Good personal hygiene among food handlers.
- Exclusion of known human excretors from food handling.

ESCHERICHIA COLI

Although *E. coli* is part of the normal commensal gut flora, certain strains can be a cause of diarrhoea. Several mechanisms of enteric pathogenicity have been discovered in these strains.

E. coli diarrhoea

Mainly seen as three types of disease:

1. *Haemorrhagic colitis and haemolytic uraemic syndrome*: the most serious infections, now being recognized with increasing frequency in the UK.
2. *Infantile gastroenteritis*: largely confined to babies under 2 years of age.
3. *Travellers' diarrhoea*: mostly in adults recently arrived in a foreign country.

HAEMORRHAGIC SYNDROMES

Two important and sometimes life-threatening syndromes associated with bleeding tendency are due to strains of *E. coli* which produce toxins that have a cytopathic effect on Vero (monkey kidney) cells. There are two Vero cytotoxins, VT1 and VT2, which are antigenically distinct from each other. Vero cytotoxin-producing *E. coli* strains are known as **VTEC**. By far the most important VTEC in the UK is serogroup O157: Over 80 phage types of this serogroup can be distinguished.

Haemorrhagic colitis: a syndrome seen in children and adults, both in outbreaks and as sporadic infections. Deaths have been reported, especially in outbreaks among the elderly in residential homes.

Haemolytic uraemic syndrome (HUS): seen mainly in children aged 1–4 years, both as outbreaks and as sporadic cases. Children have a diarrhoeal prodrome, followed by uraemia, thrombocytopenia and haemolytic anaemia.

The syndrome is associated with various serogroups, notably O157, but others, belonging to non-O157 serogroups such as O26 and O111, are occasionally involved.

HUS due to VTEC O157 is one of the commonest reasons for renal dialysis in children, and has a significant (although low) case fatality rate.

Diagnosis: *culture* faeces on cefixime tellurite sorbitol MacConkey agar (CTSMAC). Observe for colourless colonies, as the vast majority of *E. coli* produce pink colonies. Identify by serology and biochemical tests.

Epidemiology: Cattle are often carriers of VTEC O157, and one of the main sources of infection is *beef*.

Several large outbreaks have been traced to hamburgers, inadequately cooked at barbecues, and milk. In addition to contaminated foods and water, VTEC O157 infection can be transmitted by direct or indirect contact with animals or their faeces, and also by person-to-person spread, as the infectious dose is very low. There have been several large outbreaks, some associated with deaths in the elderly in the UK in recent years. Figure 7.2 illustrates the rising in numbers of VTEC O157 in the UK and shows the different picture in Scotland, where there is a much higher incidence.

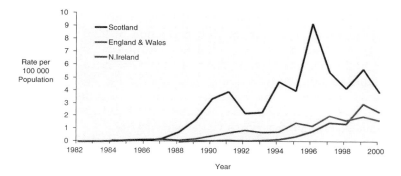

Fig. 7.2 Laboratory reporting of VTEC O157 infection in the UK.

ENTEROINVASIVE *E. COLI* (EIEC)

EIEC cause a disease like shigella dysentery in all age groups, and share the same invasive pathogenic mechanisms as shigellae. They are atypical in the laboratory in that they do not ferment lactose. They belong to several well defined serogroups, e.g. O124, O164.

INFANTILE GASTROENTERITIS DUE TO ENTEROPATHOGENIC *E. COLI*

Cause: generally enteropathogenic (EPEC) strains, e.g. serogroups O55, O111 (and also sometimes by enterotoxigenic (ETEC) strains, e.g. serogroups O6, O78). **NB**: O6 and O78 are associated with travellers' diarrhoea (see below).

Note: Rota and other viruses are also important causes of infantile gastroenteritis (see Chapter 23).

Clinical features

Acute diarrhoea, after an incubation period which varies from 1 to 3 days: the diarrhoea may lead to dehydration (Fig. 7.3) and acid–base imbalance. *Hypernatraemia* is a particular problem because of the disproportionate loss of water relative to sodium from the extracellular spaces.

Pathogenesis: most EPEC strains do not produce toxins and are non-invasive, but produce an attaching and effacing lesion in the small intestine.

Diagnosis: *culture* faeces on MacConkey medium. Observe for pink (lactose-fermenting) colonies, and pick several for further tests. Identify by biochemical tests and serology.

Treatment: rehydration, with correction of fluid loss and of electrolyte and acid–base imbalance. Antibiotic therapy is of doubtful value, although it may be useful in severe cases.

Epidemiology: Infection is sporadic in the community in Britain: previously the main problem in this country was outbreaks in institutions and nurseries. EPEC infections have declined very significantly since the early 1970s.

Overseas in countries with poor sanitation and housing, the disease is a major cause of infant mortality. Flies probably play a part in transmitting the infection. *Transmission*: faecal–oral, perhaps sometimes via food or contaminated milk.

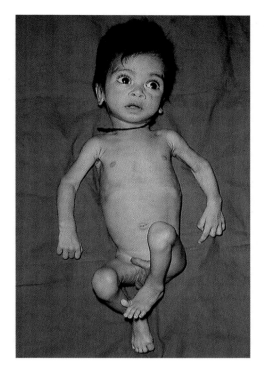

Fig. 7.3 Child with gastroenteritis. (Reproduced with permission from Abbott Laboratories *Slide Atlas of Infectious Diseases*, 1982, Gower Medical Publishing, London. Photograph courtesy of Professor H. Lambert.)

Control: scrupulous hygiene in nurseries and neonatal units is necessary. Outbreaks are controlled by: *prompt isolation* of cases and contacts; *screening* of staff to detect carriers of the epidemic strain; *closure* of the unit to new admissions. *Overseas*: control is only possible when clean water, sanitation and adequate housing can be provided.

TRAVELLERS' DIARRHOEA (TURISTA)

Also known as 'Delhi belly', 'Montezuma's revenge', 'Tokyo two-step' etc.

Causal organism: generally the enterotoxigenic strains of *E. coli* (ETEC). There are more than 100 O serogroups: important examples are O6, O78. Most cases are not investigated bacteriologically.

Clinical features

Diarrhoea, abdominal pain and vomiting: usually self-limiting and of a few days' duration; occasionally protracted.

Route of infection: via contaminated food and drinks; polluted water is the usual source of infection.

Pathogenesis: ETEC produce *heat-labile toxin (LT)* or *heat-stable toxin (ST)*, or both. They also possess *colonization factors*, which facilitate attachment of the organism to the epithelium of the small intestine.

Diagnosis: Laboratory facilities are often not available at tourist resorts: information about the cause of this major problem to the tourist industries of many countries has come from a few research studies.

Control: Public health measures, e.g. clean water supply; caution in diet by travellers.

SHIGELLA

Shigellae cause bacillary dysentery, 'the commonest of the unpreventable diseases'. A worldwide problem and an important cause of death and morbidity in young children, especially in developing countries.

The four species of *Shigella* are:

- *S. dysenteriae*
- *S. flexneri*
- *S. boydii*
- *S. sonnei* (one serotype: the main cause of dysentery in Britain).

All the species except *S. sonnei* contain several distinguishable serotypes.

Clinical features

Diarrhoea with blood, mucus and often pus in the stools, which varies from a severe life-threatening disease to a mild or symptomless infection.

Incubation period: 1–9 days.

Shiga dysentery

Due to *S. dysenteriae 1*: a severe, even life-threatening disease found only in tropical countries, with fever, abdominal pain and diarrhoea. The disease sometimes becomes septicaemic, indicating that, unlike other shigellae, *S. dysenteriae* has invasive properties. *S. dysenteriae* produces a powerful *neurological exotoxin*, but this probably does not play a role in Shiga dysentery. An enterotoxin and a cytotoxin are also produced: their role is uncertain, but they may be partly responsible for invasiveness. Shiga toxin, produced by *S. dysenteriae 1*, is very closely related to *E. coli* Vero cytotoxin 1 (VT1).

Dysentery due to other shigellae

This is generally a milder disease, which varies from asymptomatic excretion to a prostrating attack of diarrhoea with abdominal pain and (usually minimal) fever. The stools may contain blood, mucus and pus, but blood is unusual in cases of Sonné dysentery.

Sonné dysentery due to *S. sonnei* is worldwide. The disease is commonest in young children, and outbreaks in nursery schools are not uncommon. The disease is usually mild but in a few cases dehydration ensues, requiring emergency treatment. Epidemics of Sonné dysentery are also frequent in mental hospitals, and the infection may be difficult to eradicate.

S. flexneri was formerly quite common in Britain – still common overseas, mainly in tropical countries.

S. boydii is rare in Britain but is common in the Middle and Far East.

Diagnosis: *isolation*: *culture* faeces and rectal swabs on MacConkey medium and selective media. Observe for pale (non-lactose-fermenting) colonies, but note: *S. sonnei* is a late lactose fermenter and may produce pale pinkish colonies. Identify by biochemical tests, then serology.

Treatment: antibiotics are rarely necessary for Sonné dysentery: the more severe disease should be treated systemically, depending on the sensitivity of the organism isolated (multiply antibiotic-resistant strains are common). Antibiotics tend to prolong the excretion of shigellae. Ciprofloxacin is the antimicrobial of choice for treatment.

Epidemiology: *reservoir of infection* is the human gut: symptomless infections are common, with excretion of the organism in the faeces. After an acute attack some patients excrete shigellae for a considerable time (i.e. for weeks, sometimes months). Patients with acute dysentery are the most dangerous sources of infection, doubtless owing to the large numbers of shigellae excreted during the acute phase of the disease.

Route of infection is faecal–oral, either directly or via contaminated equipment, towels and lavatory seats (in nursery schools). The infectious dose is very low. Shigellae can remain viable for long periods of time in cool, moist environments.

Spread: 'food, flies, fomites' are the classic means of spread of dysentery; contaminated water can also be a source of infection.

Dysentery waxes and wanes in incidence over long periods of time: after two decades of high incidence which started in 1950, the disease waned in Britain in the late 1970s and early 1980s. This periodicity appears to be unrelated to improved sanitation or other public health measures. 1992 saw a dramatic rise in cases of Sonné dysentery in the UK, but with a return to lower levels in succeeding years.

Control: good sanitation with safe water; adequate sewage disposal. A high standard of personal hygiene is important, especially in children.

STAPHYLOCOCCUS AUREUS

A classic cause of toxic food poisoning, which is due to the ingestion of food contaminated with the enterotoxin of *S. aureus*. The disease is very rapid in onset because it is due to preformed toxin in food. About 40% of *S. aureus* strains produce several heat-stable enterotoxins – A, B, C, D, E. There are three types of enterotoxin C. Enterotoxin-producing strains mostly belong to phage group III.

Clinical features

Acute onset of nausea and vomiting within a few hours of eating the contaminated food, sometimes followed by diarrhoea. Self-limiting and rarely severe; dehydration is occasionally a problem in the uncommon severe case.

Pathogenesis: preformed toxin is ingested in contaminated food and has a local action on the gut mucosa. The toxin resists temperatures that kill *S. aureus*, so food may contain toxin but no viable staphylococci.

Diagnosis: *culture* the suspect food, vomit or faeces for *S. aureus* on ordinary media or a selective medium. Identify by commercial slide test; later, by phage typing to correlate identity of strains from food and patients.

Demonstration of enterotoxin: examine culture filtrate from a strain of *S. aureus* isolated from food or vomit by latex agglutination test.

Treatment: disease is short and self-limiting, so treatment is unnecessary.

Epidemiology: *source of infection*: usually a staphylococcal lesion on the skin, especially of the fingers of a food handler.

Route of infection: ingestion – enterotoxin-producing strains of *S. aureus* multiply in the food and liberate toxin which is relatively heat-stable and, unless the food is thoroughly heated afterwards, retains activity.

Food: cooked food is usually involved, although contamination most often takes place after initial cooking. Cold cooked meat is often implicated. Unless food is correctly stored at 4°C, staphylococci can multiply in the warm conditions of the kitchen, with consequent toxin production. Other foods which have been involved include milk and milk products, e.g. creams and custards.

Control: exclusion of food handlers with septic lesions; prompt refrigeration of food after preparation.

CLOSTRIDIUM PERFRINGENS

Diarrhoea or food poisoning due to *C. perfringens* is fairly common and is caused by the contamination of food by spore-bearing (and therefore heat-resistant) anaerobic organisms.

Classically, non-haemolytic strains of *C. perfringens* which have particularly heat-resistant spores are involved, but β-haemolytic strains with relatively heat-labile spores are also implicated.

Clinical features

Acute onset between 8 and 24 h after eating contaminated food. The predominant symptoms are diarrhoea and abdominal pain: vomiting is rare. The illness is self-limiting.

Pathogenesis: *heat-resistant spores* of *C. perfringens* survive 100°C for 30 min. During cooling after cooking, the spores germinate into vegetative bacilli. These multiply rapidly if food is stored at room temperature (the temperature range for growth of *C. perfringens* is 15–50°C) and if there are anaerobic conditions (e.g. within some deep meat pies).

Following ingestion of food contaminated with vegetative *C. perfringens*, sporulation takes place in the small intestine, with liberation of a *heat-labile enterotoxin* which acts mainly on the membrane permeability of the small intestine.

Diagnosis: strains that cause food poisoning also form part of the normal flora in 5–30% of the population, so that laboratory diagnosis of an individual case is difficult. However, there are many different serotypes of *C. perfringens*, and isolation of the same serotype in large numbers from the victims of an outbreak of food poisoning and from the suspect food (when available) is strong presumptive evidence that it is the cause.

Isolation: *culture* faeces or suspected food on *aminoglycoside blood agar, anaerobically*.

Observe for typical colonies, β-haemolytic or non-haemolytic. Identify by Nagler reaction; serotype in a specialist reference laboratory for epidemiology.

Detection of enterotoxin: Examine stools, by latex agglutination test.

Treatment: sometimes, rehydration. Antibiotic therapy is unnecessary.

Epidemiology: *C. perfringens* is often present in large numbers as a commensal in the animal and human intestine; it is also ubiquitous in the environment.

Control: *food hygiene*: adequate cooking of meat and meat products, with prompt refrigeration if stored before consumption.

LESS COMMON BACTERIAL CAUSES OF DIARRHOEA

BACILLUS SPECIES

Diarrhoea caused by these relatively non-pathogenic organisms is typically associated with Chinese restaurants, because of their frequent use of rice.

Bacillus species are aerobic, spore-forming Gram-positive bacilli, often found in soil and the air and dust of the environment. *B. cereus* is the principal cause of this form of food poisoning, but members of the *subtilis* group (e.g. *B. subtilis*, *B. pumilus* and *B. licheniformis*) are increasingly implicated.

Clinical features

Two distinct types of illness:

- *Short incubation period*: 1–2 h, with nausea and vomiting, often followed by diarrhoea: associated with bulk-prepared rice. This is by far the more common type.

• *Longer incubation period*: 6–16 h, with sudden onset of abdominal pain and diarrhoea: associated with soups and sauces.

Pathogenesis: the disease is due to an enterotoxin produced by *Bacillus* species.

Diagnosis: culture suspected food, vomit, faeces on ordinary media. Observe for significant numbers of the typical 'curled hair' colonies.

Treatment: disease is self-limiting.

Epidemiology: *Bacillus* species and their spores are widespread in soil, and cereals are commonly contaminated with them. Some spores survive cooking – if storage is at a warm temperature, there is germination into vegetative bacilli, which multiply and produce toxin.

Control: correct storage of cooked food; reheating should be rapid.

CLOSTRIDIUM DIFFICILE

Diarrhoea is a common side-effect of oral antibiotic therapy, probably as a result of disturbance of the normal intestinal flora owing to the antibacterial action of the drug. This diarrhoea is usually mild and self-limiting. However, antibiotic therapy – particularly in the elderly in hospitals and nursing homes – can cause severe diarrhoea, which is occasionally fatal: due to *Clostridium difficile*.

C. difficile is acquired as part of the intestinal flora, most often as a result of cross-infection, either from other patients who are excretors, or from contamination in the environment. Antibiotic or other therapy suppresses other bacteria and allows *C. difficile* to proliferate and produce toxins. In severe cases the disease may take the form of fulminant pseudomembranous colitis (Fig. 7.4).

Clindamycin is particularly associated with this form of diarrhoea, but other antibiotics, notably ampicillin and cephalosporins, can also cause it.

C. difficile can also cause diarrhoea in the absence of antibiotic therapy, and is carried by 3–5% of healthy people.

Clinical features

Varies from mild diarrhoea to the life-threatening disease pseudomembranous colitis; the diarrhoea can be very profuse (up to 20 stools per day); abdominal discomfort, fever and leukocytosis are often present. Sometimes fatal, especially in the vulnerable elderly.

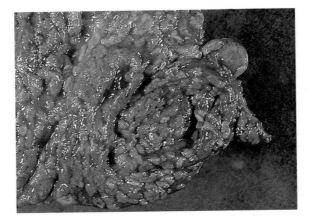

Fig. 7.4 Pseudomembranous colitis. Segment of large bowel with typical pseudomembranous plaques. The plaques consist of fibrin and polymorphs and are the characteristic gross and microscopic lesions in the condition. (Photograph courtesy of Dr Hugh Gilmour, Pathology Department, University of Edinburgh.)

Pathogenesis: toxin production within the colon. *C. difficile* produces two toxins:

- *Toxin A*: *an enterotoxin*: responsible for the gut symptoms
- *Toxin B*: *a cytotoxin*: has a cytopathic effect in cell cultures; a useful marker for identification, as it is always associated with toxin A.

Diagnosis: *clinically*, a high index of suspicion is necessary. *Proctosigmoidoscopy* may show the characteristic membrane, or isolated areas of white or yellow material adhering to the colonic mucosa: these areas should be biopsied for histological examination; the rectum is sometimes unaffected.

Laboratory diagnosis: *demonstration* of toxin in *faecal filtrate*, by testing for cytotoxic effect on cells in tissue culture (e.g. Vero or human embryo lung cells). The toxic effect is neutralized by antiserum to *Clostridium sordellii*, which cross-neutralizes *C. difficile* cytotoxin in tissue culture.

Isolation of *C. difficile* from faeces on selective media, with subsequent demonstration of toxigenicity.

Treatment: oral vancomycin or metronidazole.

Epidemiology: *outbreaks* of infection have been reported in elderly patients in long-stay wards, and are often associated with contamination of the ward environment by *C. difficile*. Many cases in hospital patients are sporadic.

CLOSTRIDIUM SEPTICUM

C. septicum can cause *neutropenic enterocolitis*, a rare disease seen in neutropenic patients (e.g. associated with cytotoxic therapy for leukaemia): it is sometimes associated with septicaemia. *Neonatal necrotizing enterocolitis*, an important and life-threatening complication in preterm babies, is not antibiotic associated and no bacterial cause has been established.

YERSINIA

Yersinia are not a common cause of diarrhoea in Britain, but have been reported as important enteric pathogens in Europe (especially Belgium and Scandinavia) and North America (particularly Canada). The most common causal organism is *Y. enterocolitica*.

Clinical features

Acute gastroenteritis, with abdominal pain and fever; as a rule, resolves without treatment in 1–3 weeks. Yersiniosis may mimic appendicitis, and the disease can cause acute terminal ileitis and mesenteric lymphadenitis. Infection may progress to septicaemia – usually in debilitated patients. Reactive polyarthritis is a recognized complication (see Chapter 15).

Diagnosis: culture of faeces, blood cultures or mesenteric lymph nodes (if specimens of these are available). *Serology*: demonstration of a rising antibody titre.

Treatment: tetracycline, aminoglycosides, co-trimoxazole or chloramphenicol. Treatment is of doubtful value as the disease is usually self-limiting; however, systemic yersiniosis carries a high mortality despite antibiotic therapy.

Epidemiology: *reservoir of infection*: pigs. Infection spread: probably via the faecal–oral route, directly person-to-person, or from animals by contaminated food and water. However, most cases are sporadic and their epidemiology is uncertain.

Note: *Y. pseudotuberculosis* is a zoonosis: infection in humans takes the form most often of mesenteric adenitis, causing abdominal pain that can mimic appendicitis. It rarely' causes diarrhoea. The organism is widespread in birds and wild animals, especially rodents and other small mammals.

VIBRIO PARAHAEMOLYTICUS

This organism, acquired from shellfish, is a rare cause of infective diarrhoea. *V. parahaemolyticus* is a marine bacterium found in warm coastal waters and in fish and shellfish.

Clinical features

Acute onset of vomiting and diarrhoea, usually 8–24 h after eating raw seafood, especially imported shellfish.

Epidemiology: more prevalent in warmer months. Most common in the Far East, where raw fish is a delicacy and large outbreaks have been reported; cases in Britain have been due to imported seafood, although the organism exists in British sea waters.

LISTERIA MONOCYTOGENES

Outbreaks of gastroenteritis due to this organism have been described, mainly in the USA (see Chapters 16 and 38).

CHOLERA

Cholera is caused by *Vibrio cholerae* O1, and also by non-O1 type 139.

In 1961 the world experienced the start of the seventh pandemic of cholera, which has persisted and spread over the succeeding 40 years: the six previous pandemics were during the 19th and early 20th centuries. Glasgow Royal Infirmary is built on the site of mass cholera graves from the epidemic of 1849. The factors that determine the onset of epidemic spread are unknown. In 1991, cholera broke out in an epidemic in Peru, later to spread to neighbouring countries in South America and to Mexico. *Late in 1992* a new epidemic of cholera appeared in Bengal, caused by non-O1 type O139, and spread causing many deaths in the Indian subcontinent.

Clinical features

Acute onset, after an incubation period of from 6 h to 5 days, of abdominal pain and diarrhoea – the diarrhoea being typically of exceptional severity, progressing to the continuous passage of 'rice-water' stools. Vomiting, dehydration, acidosis and collapse may follow. Some cases are much less severe, with only mild diarrhoea.

Two forms of disease are recognized:

- *Severe classic cholera*
- *Milder cholera, associated with the O1 El Tor biotype.*

Pathogenesis: *V. cholerae* produces a potent *exotoxin – cholera toxin (CT)*, very similar to the LT enterotoxin of ETEC, which is plasmid coded. The toxin stimulates the activity of the enzyme adenyl cyclase, which raises the concentration of cyclic AMP in cells; this causes an increase in the flow of water and electrolytes into the bowel lumen. The fluid lost has relatively high concentrations of bicarbonate and potassium.

V. cholerae is not invasive and does not penetrate the gut mucous membrane, although adhesion to gut epithelium plays a part in its pathogenicity.

Diagnosis: *culture* faeces on alkaline selective medium. *Observe* for typical colonies, which can be identified by slide agglutination, with polyvalent antiserum.

Treatment: correction of dehydration by intravenous administration of fluid and electrolytes, to restore the acid–base balance: mortality can be reduced from more than 50% to nil with fluid replacement treatment. Tetracycline, given orally or intravenously, may help to limit the duration of diarrhoea and reduce fluid loss.

Epidemiology: *reservoir of infection* is the human gut, and also the coastal marine environment.

Spread is faecal–oral, usually via contamination of the water supply with sewage, but sometimes via food contaminated by flies or unclean hands.

Symptomless carriers are common in epidemics – for example, the case:carrier ratio may reach 1:100 – and they form an important source of infection.

Pandemic: since 1961, the milder (El Tor) form of cholera has gradually spread through the Far East to reach Africa and beyond: air travel has probably increased the risk of importation of the disease into cholera-free areas. Poorly cooked seafood from contaminated estuarine waters probably played a role in its spread.

Control: *good sanitation*, with a clean water supply and adequate sewage disposal, together with personal hygiene (i.e. handwashing after defecation) are effective methods of controlling the spread of cholera. Unfortunately, in many areas of the world these methods are simply not practicable. Carriers and cases should, if possible, be isolated.

Vaccination: *A vaccine*, containing heat-inactivated organisms, is available (see Chapter 39). A live attenuated vaccine has also been developed, and has been shown to be effective in early trials. There is no protection against the non-O1 strain 139.

WHIPPLE'S DISEASE

A rare multisystem disorder, usually affecting middle-aged Caucasian males.

Pathology: many organs – but especially the small intestine, heart and CNS – are infiltrated with macrophages.

Causal organism: an actinomycete, *Tropherema whippelii*: not yet cultured, but demonstrated within macrophages and numerous other cell types.

Clinical features

Usually gradual in onset, with low-grade fever.

Symptoms include chronic diarrhoea, progressing to malabsorption with steatorrhoea, abdominal pain, weight loss and arthralgia. Anaemia is common, and there may be neurological signs and symptoms.

Diagnosis: microscopy of small bowel biopsy.

Treatment: co-trimoxazole, for 1 year.

NON-BACTERIAL INFECTIVE DIARRHOEA

It must never be forgotten that diarrhoea is often due to infection with non-bacterial agents. The more important of these are listed, with some of their characteristics, in Table 7.2.

BOTULISM

A rare but severe foodborne disease caused by ingestion of a bacterial toxin preformed in food; diarrhoea is not a symptom. Often fatal, with death being due to respiratory failure.

Causal organism: *Clostridium botulinum*, types A, B and E (rarely, types C, F and G).

Clinical features

Signs and symptoms are neurological, such as oculomotor and pharyngeal paralysis, vomiting, constipation, thirst, dryness of mouth, vertigo; sometimes difficulty in speaking. Seen 12–36 h after ingestion of the toxin, which acts by inhibiting acetylcholine release at neuromuscular junctions.

Table 7.2 Non-bacterial causes of diarrhoea

Agent	Disease	Diagnosis	Treatment
Viruses			
Rotavirus	Diarrhoea	Electron microscopy of stools; ELISA for antigen in stools	Symptomatic
Adenovirus	Diarrhoea	⎫	Symptomatic
Astrovirus	Diarrhoea	⎬ Electron microscopy of stools	Symptomatic
Norwalk-like viruses*	Diarrhoea	⎭	Symptomatic
Protozoa			
Entamoeba histolytica	Amoebic dysentery	Microscopy of stools; serology	Metronidazole
Giardia lamblia	Giardiasis	Microscopy of duodenal aspirate and stools	Metronidazole
Cryptosporidium	Diarrhoea	Microscopy of stools	Symptomatic
Cyclospora	Diarrhoea	Microscopy of stools	Symptomatic

*Also diagnosed by PCR

Pathogenesis: *C. botulinum* is a spore-forming anaerobe which forms an exceedingly powerful exotoxin. It is found in soil, water and sludge. If spores contaminate food in anaerobic conditions, germination follows and the vegetative bacilli multiply, with production of toxin during storage at room temperature. Spore germination and toxin formation are inhibited by a low pH, so are not usually a problem in acid fruits. It is important to note that the toxin is sensitive to heat and is destroyed by cooking.

Diagnosis: *demonstration of toxin* in suspected food, patient's serum or faeces by inoculation of mice. Observe for paralysis and death.

Test mice protected by antitoxins to toxin types A, B and E: protection by the corresponding antitoxin identifies the toxin present.

Isolation: from suspected food or patient's faeces.

Culture: after pasteurization of the food to destroy non-sporing bacteria, anaerobic culture at 35°C and identify suspect colonies.

Treatment: antibiotics are of no value. Treatment is supportive, with artificial ventilation etc. and the administration of antitoxin to neutralize absorbed toxin.

Epidemiology: Table 7.3 shows the habitat, geography and the kind of food associated with the three types of *C. botulinum* that cause human disease. The disease is extremely rare in Britain, but there was a small outbreak in Birmingham in 1978 caused by tinned Alaskan salmon contaminated with type E toxin.

Table 7.3   Main medically important types of *Clostridium botulinum*

Type	Habitat	Geography	Usual source of infection
A	Soil	USA Former USSR	Home-preserved vegetables, meat, fish
B	Soil	Europe USA	Meat, especially pork
E	Soil, sea water, sludge	Japan Canada Alaska	Raw or tinned fish

In 1989, a sizeable outbreak of botulism in Britain was caused by the contamination of hazelnut purée with *C. botulinum* type B: the toxin was ingested in hazelnut yoghurt.

Person-to-person spread does not occur.

Control: home canning and preservation of food should be avoided. Commercial canning and pickling processes should be carefully controlled: a temperature that will kill the heat-resistant spores of *C. botulinum* is essential, e.g. 120°C for 20 min.

INFANT BOTULISM

Rare in this country, but not uncommon in the USA. It is caused by the ingestion of *C. botulinum* spores, not preformed toxin.

Causal organism: *C. botulinum*, usually type A or B. The spores are sometimes found in contaminated honey.

Clinical features: affects infants, often when mixed feeding starts, causing constipation, failure to thrive, cranial palsies and even sudden death.

Pathogenesis: after colonization of the gut, spores germinate and the bacteria multiply and produce toxin; the subsequent absorption of toxin leads to symptoms.

Diagnosis: *isolation* of *C. botulinum* from stools. Toxin may be demonstrated in stools or serum.

WOUND BOTULISM

A complication of injecting drug abuse.

GASTRITIS AND PEPTIC ULCER

Although spiral bacteria were observed in the human stomach a century ago, it was not until 1982 that the organism now known as *Helicobacter pylori* was isolated from a gastric biopsy. Infection with *H. pylori* is an important causal factor in peptic ulceration.

Clinical associations

Infection results in a chronic gastritis (type B or non-autoimmune gastritis), which is often lifelong. Although the gastritis is usually asymptomatic, it is strongly associated with duodenal ulcer (present in 90% of cases), and less markedly with gastric ulcer (present in 65% of cases).

Long-term gastritis is a recognized risk factor in gastric carcinoma, and is implicated in about 60% of cancers involving the antrum and body of the stomach. It is even more closely associated with the much rarer tumour, primary malignant lymphoma.

Epidemiology: *H. pylori* has been demonstrated in saliva, dental plaque and faeces.

There is no evidence that the infection is a zoonosis – it is probably spread from person to person by the oral–oral and/or faecal–oral routes.

This common worldwide infection affects both males and females. Infection is commoner in developing countries and in lower socioeconomic groups in developed countries, indicating that poor living conditions are a predisposing factor. Infection may be acquired in childhood; in developed countries the prevalence increases with increasing age. Serological studies indicate an infection rate of 20% at 20 years of age, rising to 50% at age 50.

The majority of those infected do *not* develop peptic ulcers, and remain symptom free.

Pathogenesis: *H. pylori* is found associated with, but not invading, gastric-type epithelium in the stomach (particularly the antrum). It is also sometimes found in the duodenum, but only if there is ectopic gastric epithelium, a common finding in patients with duodenal ulceration.

The organism survives under a layer of mucus. Its intense urease activity produces ammonia from the urea in gastric juice, which neutralizes the bactericidal action of gastric acid. The organism induces an acute, then a chronic, inflammatory cell infiltrate within the mucosa, which later atrophies. Gastritis results in a dramatic increase in the release of gastrin, which in turn causes excess acid secretion. The reason for this is uncertain: gastrin production may be stimulated by a rise in mucosal pH, due to ammonia formed by bacterial urease activity, or by cytokines released in the inflammatory response. With the development of gastric atrophy there is progressive reduction in the secretion of acid, and eventually complete achlorhydria.

Although gastritis caused by *H. pylori* is associated with peptic ulcers, the mechanism linking the pathologies is uncertain and *H. pylori* infection must not be considered the *only* causal factor in peptic ulceration. However, gastritis does reduce the resistance of the epithelium to ulceration, and the longer-term atrophic changes, with metaplasia, predispose to cancer.

Infection provokes an antibody response, but this is not protective.

Diagnosis: three main methods, each having a diagnostic accuracy greater than 90%:

1. *Endoscopy and biopsy*: the samples removed are examined by:
   - histology
   - culture: isolation of *H. pylori* enables the antibiotic sensitivity of the infecting strain to be determined
   - direct urease test: a positive result makes an immediate diagnosis.

This method is invasive and expensive.

2. *Serology*: usually an ELISA test, to detect IgG antibody. This method allows large numbers of samples to be screened at low cost, but antibody levels take many months to fall after successful treatment.

3. *Breath test*: patient swallows ^{13}C- or ^{14}C-radiolabelled urea, which is split by *H. pylori* urease into ammonia and CO_2: detection of radiolabelled carbon in expired air (blown into a bag by the patient) makes the diagnosis. The test rapidly becomes negative after successful treatment.

Treatment: the indication for treatment is a peptic ulcer with evidence of infection. Eradication of infection allows healing of the ulcer, and this greatly reduces recurrence, which is usually due to relapse rather than reinfection.

All regimens use a combination of drugs: the complexity of treatment may result in poor patient compliance. Give *two antimicrobial agents for 2 weeks* – choose from tetracycline, metronidazole, amoxycillin, clarithromycin, bismuth compounds, along with *a gastric antisecretory drug for a longer period* – choose either an H_2-receptor antagonist (e.g. cimetidine, ranitidine) or a proton pump inhibitor (e.g. omeprazole). Resistance to metronidazole and clarithromycin has been reported, and this has resulted in some treatment failures.

Success rates of around 90% have been reported.

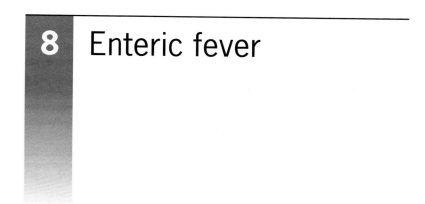

8 Enteric fever

Enteric fever includes typhoid and paratyphoid fevers. Both are caused by salmonellae which are markedly more pathogenic and invasive than those that cause food poisoning. Paratyphoid fever is generally a milder disease than typhoid fever.

The causal organism of typhoid fever is *Salmonella enterica* serotype typhi (*S.* Typhi). *S.* Paratyphi A, B and C cause paratyphoid fever. *S.* Paratyphi B is still sometimes seen in Britain; *S.* Paratyphi A and C are found in tropical countries.

Note: This chapter refers to both typhoid and paratyphoid fevers, except where otherwise indicated.

TYPHOID FEVER

Clinical features

Causal organism: S. Typhi

Incubation period: 14–21 days; sometimes longer.

Symptoms: a septicaemic febrile illness with headache, toxaemia, dullness and apathy. Rose-coloured spots (which contain the infecting organism) are often seen as a sparse rash on the trunk. Splenomegaly is sometimes present, together with some soft abdominal swelling and discomfort generally. Leukopenia is common. Diarrhoea is a late symptom, usually in the third week of illness.

Duration: untreated, about 4 weeks: symptoms clear up in about 3–4 days with antibiotic therapy.

Complications: relapse, intestinal perforation and haemorrhage are the most serious; rarely, periostitis, myocarditis, pneumonia.

Relapse is common, with recrudescence of symptoms about a week after the end of the primary illness.

Carriers: around 2–5% of patients with typhoid fever become chronic carriers, owing to persistent infection of the gall bladder: this results in *S.* Typhi being discharged into the gut and excreted in the faeces.

Pathogenesis

S. Typhi invades first the alimentary tract by ingestion, then via the lymphatic system and the thoracic duct into the bloodstream. This first septicaemic phase leads to infection of the reticuloendothelial system and the gall bladder. Infection of the gall bladder causes the discharge of organisms into the intestine, with heavy infection of the *Peyer's patches* and septicaemia – and the onset of symptoms.

PARATYPHOID FEVER

Causal organisms: *S.* Paratyphi A, B and C.

Clinically, a milder febrile illness than typhoid fever, with a shorter duration and incubation period. Transient diarrhoea and symptomless infection are common.

Carriers: patients become carriers less frequently than after typhoid fever.

Diagnosis

Best made by isolation of the infecting organism from faeces, blood and urine. Blood culture is positive in over 80% of patients in the first week of illness. *Blood and urine*: MacConkey medium (enrichment and selective media are not necessary). *Faeces*: use indicator medium (for non-lactose-fermenting colonies), and selective and enrichment media.

Identification:

- *Biochemical reactions (API test)*: *Note:* *S.* Typhi, unlike other salmonellae (including *S.* Paratyphi) produces no gas on fermentation of sugars.
- *Serological*: preliminary identification with salmonella polyvalent H and O antisera; final identification: send to Reference Typing Laboratory.
- *Phage typing*: useful in identifying different strains of *S.* Typhi (and also of *S.* Paratyphi B) for epidemiological investigation into the source of outbreaks.

Serology

The classic test is the *Widal test*: agglutination test for antibodies to flagellar H antigens and somatic O antigens of *S*. Typhi and *S*. Paratyphi A and B, but the results are difficult to interpret, especially if the patient has been immunized with typhoid vaccine. This test is no longer used in routine diagnostic laboratories.

Treatment

- *Ciprofloxacin*: is the drug of choice, especially with the emergence of multiresistance involving other antibiotics – but care is needed with children. The emergence of strains with decreased susceptibility has been reported and treatment failures noted. *Ceftriaxone* is a useful alternative in such cases.
- *Chloramphenicol*: effective, but resistance is now a problem; can rarely have serious side-effects.
- *Co-trimoxazole*: less good than chloramphenicol, but has less serious side-effects.

Carriers

It is notoriously difficult to eradicate *S*. Typhi from the gall bladder. Antibiotic therapy is effective in curing some carriers, but in a proportion the infection persists and they become long-term permanent carriers.

Epidemiology

Source of infection: carriers or cases who excrete the organism: excretion in faeces – less commonly in the urine – continues for about 2 months after the acute illness.

Route of infection: ingestion of water or food, contaminated by sewage or via the hands of a carrier. Direct case-to-case spread is rare.

Infecting dose: small numbers of *S*. Typhi can cause typhoid fever – hence waterborne infection is common, despite the dilution of organisms. Larger doses are required to infect in paratyphoid fever.

Sporadic cases are now rare in Britain, but infection is endemic in many tropical areas, e.g. Africa, Asia, Latin America.

Outbreaks are often explosive – sometimes involving large numbers of people. There are two main types:

- *Waterborne*: in which sewage containing organisms from a carrier pollutes drinking water, e.g. the outbreaks in Croydon in 1937 and in Zermatt in 1963.
- *Foodborne*: in which food becomes contaminated via polluted water or via the hands of carriers. 'Typhoid Mary', possibly the most famous carrier, worked as a cook in the USA and caused numerous outbreaks there in the early years of this century. Typhoid and paratyphoid bacilli multiply readily in most types of food.

Tinned food may become contaminated during canning – the large outbreak in Aberdeen in 1964 was due to a tin of corned beef which had been cooled in sewage-contaminated water; bacteria entered the can through tiny holes in the metal casing.

Shellfish often grow in estuaries, where the water may be polluted by sewage: if eaten uncooked, they may cause infection – in the past, a significant source of typhoid, but not paratyphoid, fever.

Milk or cream products, contaminated through handling by carriers, have caused outbreaks of both typhoid and paratyphoid fever.

Other foods, e.g. meat products, dried or frozen eggs, dried coconut, have been responsible for infection as a result of contamination by handlers who were carriers.

Animals: S. Paratyphi B, unlike S. Typhi, occasionally infects cattle; this has caused some outbreaks among humans, but much less commonly than infection from human sources.

Control

Public health. The most effective way of controlling typhoid and paratyphoid fevers is the provision of a clean water supply, adequate arrangements for sewage disposal, and supervision of food processing and handling.

Carriers are refractory to treatment and must not be employed in food preparation. When instructed in personal hygiene (i.e. washing hands after defecation), carriers are rarely a danger to family and close contacts.

Vaccination

Two effective typhoid vaccines are available: the oral live vaccine (Ty 21a) and the injectable Vi capsular polysaccharide vaccine (see Chapter 39).

9 Urinary tract infections

Urinary tract infections are the most common of all bacterial infections. Many consultations in general practice are because of urinary infections.

Infections of the urinary tract may involve:

- Bladder: *cystitis*
- Kidney: pelvis – *pyelitis*; parenchyma – *pyelonephritis*
- Urethra: *urethritis*.

It is difficult to distinguish between pyelitis and pyelonephritis, and it is probably better to refer to both as pyelonephritis. Urethritis is considered in Chapter 13.

Definitions

- *Urinary infection* is defined as *bacteriuria*, i.e. the multiplication of bacteria in urine within the renal tract.
- *Significant bacteriuria*: a concentration of more than 10^5 organisms/mL (10^8/L) in 'clean-voided' urine.
- *Pyuria*: presence of pus cells (polymorphs) in the urine; it usually (but not always) accompanies bacteriuria.
- *Asymptomatic bacteriuria* or 'covert bacteriuria' is the presence of significant bacteriuria in the absence of clinical symptoms.
- *Symptomatic abacteriuria*: presence of clinical symptoms of cystitis but without significant bacteriuria, although pyuria may be present. The symptoms may be recurrent, and this condition is also referred to as the '*acute urethral*' or '*dysuria–pyuria*' syndrome.

Clinical features

Cystitis: the classic symptoms are dysuria, frequency, urgency, suprapubic pain, and sometimes haematuria. Episodes of cystitis greatly outnumber those that involve the kidney.

Pyelonephritis: the signs are loin pain and tenderness, rigors and fever.

Chronic pyelonephritis: causes general ill-health and malaise, with nocturia.

Urinary infection is predominantly a disease of women of all ages (sex ratio 10:1); males are affected at the extremes of life.

Children: symptoms are often non-specific, e.g. failure to thrive in infants, febrile convulsions in toddlers, unexplained fever in older children.

Neonates: prevalence of 1%, greater incidence in males owing to urogenital congenital abnormalities, and in premature infants, half of whom have vesicoureteric incompetence.

Schoolgirls: prevalence of 1–2%, with a third symptomatic – 80% have reinfections after the initial episode, and 20% of girls with infection have vesicoureteric reflux.

Women: symptoms usually of cystitis, are surprisingly common.

Non-pregnant: 1–3% incidence in women aged 15–24, with an increase of 12% for each decade thereafter. Only a minority of women with symptoms consult their doctor, and of those who do only two-thirds have significant bacteriuria. The remainder have the '*acute urethral syndrome*'. It is found almost entirely in sexually active women, and aetiology is unclear.

Pregnant: twice the rate of non-pregnant women. Covert bacteriuria is present in over 60% of pregnant women. If untreated there is a high risk of developing pyelonephritis and subsequent premature onset of labour.

Screening to detect symptomless or covert bacteriuria has been advocated in schoolchildren and pregnant women.

Causal organisms

Escherichia coli is the cause of 60–90% of urinary infections. Certain serogroups of *E. coli* are particularly common in urinary infection (e.g. 01, 02, 04, 06, 07, 075, 0150): this is probably because they are often present in the colon, rather than because of inherently high pathogenicity for the urinary tract. However, some strains are reputed to be more invasive than others. *Factors associated with virulence* include: the possession of K (capsular) antigens, which inhibit phagocytosis and the bactericidal effect of normal human serum; and the ability to adhere to uroepithelium, owing to specialized fimbriae.

Staphylococcus saprophyticus is an important cause of infection, related to sexual activity in women under 25 years old. It is detected in 30% of such infections but, surprisingly, is seldom isolated from faeces and the anogenital region of young women. Also has a possible role in the aetiology of the acute urethral syndrome.

Proteus mirabilis: responsible for 10% of infections.

Klebsiella species: often multiply antibiotic resistant.

Enterococcus spp: often found accompanying infection with coliforms.

Fastidious Gram-positive bacteria (e.g. lactobacilli, streptococci, corynebacteria). Routine urine culture fails to grow these organisms but, when they have been detected by appropriate methods, it is claimed that they are associated with pyuria and symptoms of infection. Infection with them may be one cause of the acute urethral syndrome.

Pseudomonas aeruginosa
Staphylococcus aureus, including MRSA } (especially after catheterization or instrumentation.)
Candida albicans

Mycobacterium tuberculosis: renal tuberculosis is described in Chapter 14.

Acute uncomplicated urinary infection is usually due to one type of organism.

Chronic infection is often associated with more than one type of organism.

Source, route and factors influencing urinary infection

Source: the reservoir of urinary pathogens is the flora of the colon.

Route of infection is ascending via the urethra from the perineum.

Female preponderance is probably due to the shortness of the female urethra: the turbulence of urinary flow during micturition may result in bacteria entering the bladder.

Colonization of the periurethral area with potential pathogens is said to be a necessary prerequisite for infection: this may be prevented by the bactericidal activity of urethral and vaginal secretions.

Sterility of urine is maintained by 'flushing' (i.e. from the frequent and complete emptying of the bladder and the constant inflow of newly formed urine), by antibody and non-specific antibacterial substances in urogenital secretions, and by local defence mechanisms in the bladder wall.

Residual urine: after micturition the bladder should be empty – residual urine enables bacteria to multiply, and predisposes to infection.

Sexual intercourse, especially within the previous 48 h, is correlated with infection and the onset of symptoms in young women – possibly due to retrograde 'milking' of the urethra during coitus ('honeymoon cystitis').

Incompetence of the vesicoureteric valve, owing to congenital abnormality or inflammation of the bladder wall, causes reflux of urine into the kidney pelvis during micturition; this may lead to pyelitis and pyelonephritis.

The risk of infection is also greatly increased by abnormalities of the renal tract which cause *obstruction* and *stasis* in the tract, e.g. congenital structural abnormalities, urinary calculi, neurogenic bladder, prostatic enlargement.

Diagnosis

Specimen: a midstream specimen of urine (MSSU), collected to avoid contamination from perineum or vagina; in babies, use a strategically placed self-adhesive plastic bag, but suprapubic needle aspiration of the full bladder may be necessary. A catheter specimen of urine (CSU) is useful, but catheterization to obtain urine for laboratory examination cannot be justified because of the risk of introducing infection.

Transport: bacteria multiply in urine, so specimens must be submitted to the laboratory within 2–4 h of collection. If this is not possible, do one of the following:

- Refrigerate the specimen at 4°C.
- Use a container with boric acid, a bacteriostatic preservative, to give a final concentration in urine of 1.8%.
- Use a dip-slide coated on both sides with culture medium and inoculated by dipping into the freshly voided urine: can be read even after several days' delay.

Direct examination:

- *Wet film*: for the presence of pus cells and bacteria: erythrocytes and casts should be noted.

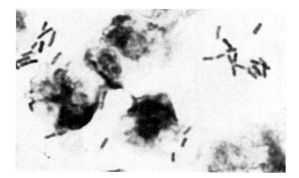

Fig. 9.1 Urinary deposit: coliform infection (× 1000).

- *Gram film*: not often required; sometimes useful for immediate presumptive identification of causal bacteria (Fig. 9.1)

   Culture: semiquantitative culture on appropriate media to prevent swarming of proteus.

   Observe and count the number of colonies obtained (Fig. 9.2).

- More than 10^5 bacteria/mL: evidence of urinary infection: carry out sensitivity tests with appropriate antibiotics.
- Between 10^4 and 10^5 bacteria/mL: significance uncertain: further specimens should be obtained except in infections with *S. saprophyticus* and *C. albicans*, where this level is significant.
- Less than 10^4 bacteria/mL: regard as contaminants (unless the patient is on treatment for a known urinary infection).

   Note: One cause of pyuria without bacteriuria is *renal tuberculosis*. When there is no obvious cause for pyuria without bacteriuria (e.g. recent urinary infection), three entire early-morning specimens should be examined for *M. tuberculosis*.

Treatment

Acute uncomplicated infections: numerous suitable oral antibiotics are available; all are excreted in the urine in high concentration:

- Trimethoprim
- Fluoroquinolones, e.g. ciprofloxacin
- Nitrofurantoin
- β-lactam antibiotics.

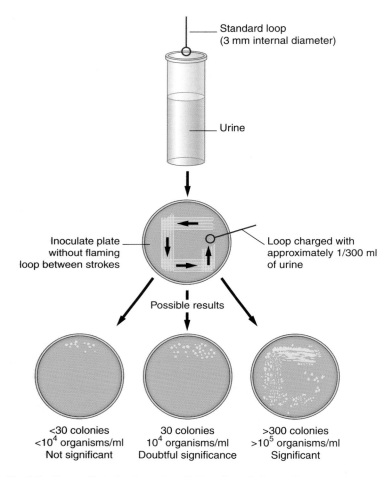

Standard loop
(3 mm internal diameter)

Urine

Inoculate plate
without flaming
loop between strokes

Loop charged with
approximately 1/300 ml
of urine

Possible results

<30 colonies
<10⁴ organisms/ml
Not significant

30 colonies
10⁴ organisms/ml
Doubtful significance

>300 colonies
>10⁵ organisms/ml
Significant

Fig. 9.2 Diagram illustrating the semiquantitative culture of urine specimens.

A short (3-day) course is usually adequate. A single dose is not as effective resulting in more recurrent infections.

β-lactam antibiotics (e.g. ampicillin, co-amoxiclav, cefalexin) are, in general, less effective.

Pyelonephritis or chronic recurrent infections: parenteral therapy with an aminoglycoside or β-lactam, e.g. cephalosporin, or fluoroquinolone. The efficacy of β-lactams given parenterally is not in doubt.

Cure rate of acute infections is around 90%, but 50% recur within a year and about 10% of patients have repeated recurrences, most likely if infection involves the kidney.

Recurrent infections: may be due to either:

- *Relapse*: recurrence within 1 month of stopping treatment, i.e. recrudescence of infection with the same organism: evidence of therapy failure, usually connotes significant parenchymal invasion. Underlying abnormality of the urinary tract (e.g. calculus, tumour) may be present and appropriate investigations should be considered. Often more difficult to treat, and long-term suppressive treatment with appropriate antibiotics is required.

or

- *Reinfection*: later recurrence is often a result of reinfection with a different organism. Normally implies superficial infection of the bladder mucosa, and requires shorter antibiotic treatment.

Prophylaxis: drinking cranberry – lingon berry juice twice daily can reduce recurrences.

Prognosis

In adults, bacteriuria, with or without symptoms, is a relatively benign condition and permanent or progressive renal damage is rare.

In children under 5 years of age the prognosis is much worse: bacteriuria with vesicoureteric reflux often results in progressive renal damage, with scar formation and impairment of kidney growth. Some of these children go on to develop chronic pyelonephritis, which accounts for 20% of end-stage renal failure. Reflux resolves spontaneously in most children as they grow older.

In children with chronic pyelonephritis renal scarring may be reduced by antibiotic treatment of acute episodes and prophylaxis against recurrence with long-term trimethoprim: this is essential if reflux is present.

HOSPITAL URINARY INFECTION

A particular problem in urological, renal and long-term geriatric patients.

Eighty per cent of hospital-acquired urinary tract infections are associated with urethral catheterization. Increasingly pathogens are multiresistant, e.g. MRSA and vancomycin-resistant enterococci.

Catheterization: the risk of infection after a single catheterization – even if carefully carried out – is about 5%: almost all patients with an indwelling catheter develop infection.

Septicaemia: one-quarter of septicaemias in hospital patients originate from urinary tract infection.

Source of infection

Endogenous: from contamination of the patient's urethra or perineum by bacteria from the colonic flora.

Exogenous: due to cross-infection with bacteria from the infected urinary tract of another patient: transmission is by instruments (e.g. cystoscopes, catheters) or by the hands of doctors and nurses (e.g. MRSA).

Prevention

Strict attention to aseptic technique: use of disposable plastic catheters; introduction of antiseptics into the urethra before instrumentation. Careful handwashing and drying between patients is *essential*.

Indwelling catheters should be attached to a closed drainage system, to prevent retrograde bacterial spread into the bladder from the collection bag.

Short-term antibiotic prophylaxis to reduce the risk of septicaemia may be given at the time of operations on, or the removal of catheters from, an infected urinary tract.

10 Bacterial meningitis

Bacterial meningitis (classically, 'pyogenic' or polymorphonuclear meningitis) is a much more severe disease than viral meningitis (classically 'aseptic' or lymphocytic) and, untreated, is almost always fatal. Even with antibiotic therapy bacterial meningitis remains a serious cause of morbidity and mortality, and is a bacteriological emergency requiring urgent diagnosis and treatment.

Clinical features

Symptoms: severe headache with malaise and fever – the onset is often abrupt. Vomiting, photophobia and convulsions are sometimes seen; patients often show irritability and are lethargic, with drowsiness progressing to unconsciousness.

Signs of meningeal irritation: neck and spinal stiffness; pain and resistance on extending the knee when the thigh is flexed (Kernig's sign). 'Meningism' (signs of meningeal irritation without meningitis) may be a feature of other types of severe infection: the diagnosis of meningitis has to be differentiated from meningism, subarachnoid haemorrhage and cerebral abscess.

Age: although meningitis is largely a disease of infancy and childhood, the disease is encountered throughout life.

Neonatal meningitis: the characteristic clinical features of meningitis are usually absent, the only presenting features being that the baby is obviously unwell, with failure to feed and, often, vomiting. The condition is much more common in premature than in full-term babies.

The elderly and the immunocompromised: typical clinical signs and symptoms of meningitis may again be absent; mental confusion is sometimes a prominent feature.

Sequelae

There are extensive pathological changes within the CNS (Fig. 10.1) and, despite appropriate antibiotic therapy, neurological sequelae can follow in survivors. The commonest sequela is deafness; other, rarer, neurological sequelae include encephalopathy, cranial nerve palsies and obstructive hydrocephalus.

CAUSAL ORGANISMS

The most common causal organisms are:

- *Neisseria meningitidis* (meningococcus)
- *Haemophilus influenzae*
- *Streptococcus pneumoniae* (pneumococcus)
- *Mycobacterium tuberculosis*.

Neisseria meningitidis (meningococcus)

The main cause of meningitis in Britain: affects all ages, but most common in infants, children and young adults. In the UK, group B strains are responsible for the majority of infections, but group

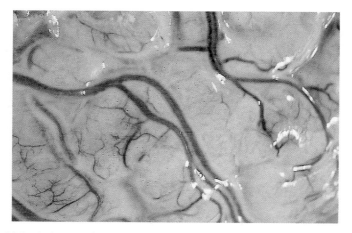

Fig. 10.1 Surface of brain in pneumococcal meningitis. *Note:* Congested meningeal vessels with purulent exudate, best seen within the sulci.

C strains have become more common in recent years. The other serogroups (see Chapter 4) are usually found in carriers rather than in cases. The disease is endemic, and sometimes epidemic.

Meningococcal septicaemia: is a dangerous early manifestation of meningococcal meningitis. It has a high mortality rate and is associated with adrenal haemorrhages, causing sudden collapse (Waterhouse–Friderichsen syndrome). During the meningococcaemia a characteristic petechial rash, rare in other types of meningitis, is common (Fig. 10.2).

Incubation period of meningitis: short: around 3 days.

Source: the reservoir is the human nasopharynx.

Spread: via infected respiratory secretions from carriers and cases (i.e. 'droplet spread'). Carriage rate in normal populations is about 10–25%: this may rise to 50% or more in household contacts of sporadic cases and during epidemics in closed communities, e.g. institutions, military camps.

Route of infection: from nasopharynx, probably via the bloodstream, to the meninges.

Treatment: penicillin is the drug of choice: cefotaxime or ceftriaxone are alternatives. Chloramphenicol can be used in penicillin-allergic patients.

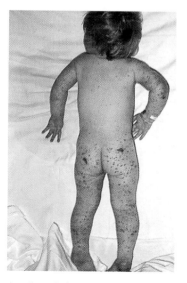

Fig. 10.2   Meningococcal septicaemia: haemorrhagic rash. (Photograph courtesy of Dr D. H. M. Kennedy.)

Chemoprophylaxis: use for *close* contacts of a patient, e.g. members of the same household, possibly contacts in school, to eradicate the organism from the nasopharynx. Ciprofloxacin (not for children or pregnant women) and rifampicin are the drugs of choice; an alternative is ceftriaxone (by injection only).

Vaccine: *N. meningitidis* type B is unfortunately non-immunogenic. Effective vaccines are available for types A and C. The introduction of *N. meningitidis* type C vaccine in 1999 in UK has reduced the number of cases by over 80%.

Haemophilus influenzae

A cause of meningitis in infants and preschool children aged 1 month to 4 years. The causal strains are capsulated and almost always of serological type b. Spread to the meninges is from the nasopharynx, probably via the bloodstream.

Treatment: Cefataxime or ceftriaxone are the drugs of choice. Chloramphenicol is an alternative.

Chemoprophylaxis of close contacts: rifampicin.

Vaccine: Hib vaccine has now been introduced for the immunization of infants (see Chapter 39) and has caused a dramatic fall in the incidence of the disease.

Streptococcus pneumoniae (pneumococcus)

Although not uncommon in children, this is the usual cause of meningitis in the middle-aged and elderly, especially in patients who are in poor general health. This type of meningitis is often the sequela to pneumococcal infection of the middle ear, sinuses or lungs; fracture of the base of the skull, communicating with the nasopharynx, is another risk factor.

Case fatality rate: is high, despite appropriate antibiotic therapy – around 20%.

Treatment: penicillin: but note that a small proportion of *S. pneumoniae* are now penicillin resistant: if so, use cefotaxime, ceftriaxone or vancomycin plus rifampicin.

Mycobacterium tuberculosis

Seen in people of all ages – but most common in children – and at any stage after the primary infection. Now rare in developed countries: about 100 cases per year in England and Wales. Typically lymphocytic (aseptic) meningitis, although polymorphs are present in the early stages.

Treatment: triple therapy with isoniazid, rifampicin and pyrazinamide: include ethambutol and streptomycin if resistance suspected. Continue isoniazid and rifampicin for 12 months, with pyrazinamide for the first 2 months. Steroids are given with the antibiotics to reduce the inflammatory response.

Rare causes of meningitis

- *Listeria monocytogenes*: mainly seen in infants, the elderly and immunocompromised patients; often, but not always, a lymphocytic meningitis.
- *Cryptococcus neoformans*: meningitis due to this yeast is rare in previously normal people, but is found in immunocompromised patients, e.g. those with leukaemia or lymphoma.
- *Leptospira* spp.: a lymphocytic meningitis.

Neonatal meningitis: a serious form of meningitis: mainly due to Gram-negative bacilli such as *Escherichia coli, Klebsiella* species and *Proteus* species, but also to *L. monocytogenes* and β-haemolytic streptococci of Lancefield group B (usually acquired from the mother's vagina). Premature (low birthweight) babies are at greatest risk, especially if there has been a prolonged interval between rupture of the membranes and delivery (see chapter 38).

Treatment of neonatal meningitis: if due to coliform bacilli: give cefotaxime or ceftriaxone. If due to listeria, give netilmicin with amoxycillin.

Group B β-haemolytic streptococcal meningitis in babies is best treated with penicillin and netilmicin in combination. Cefotaxime is an alternative.

Diagnosis

Laboratory diagnosis of bacterial meningitis depends on examination of the CSF. Table 10.1 lists the results of CSF examination in meningitis compared to those in the other two most important diseases in the differential diagnosis, subarachnoid haemorrhage and cerebral abscess.

Red blood cells may be present in a normal CSF owing to accidental damage to a blood vessel during lumbar puncture (universally known as a 'bloody tap'): in such cases the supernatant fluid after centrifugation is clear, whereas in subarachnoid haemorrhage it is stained yellow to orange (xanthochromic).

Table 10.1 Findings in cerebrospinal fluid

	Causal microorganisms	Appearance	Cells/mm³	Microbiology	Protein	Glucose
Normal	–	Clear, colourless	0–5 lymphocytes	Sterile	150–450 mg per litre	2.8–3.9 mmol per litre
Bacterial meningitis	Neisseria meningitidis Haemophilus influenzae Streptococcus pneumoniae	Turbid	500–20 000, mainly polymorphs, few lymphocytes	Bacteria in Gram-stained deposit. Growth on culture. PCR	Markedly raised	Reduced or absent
Viral (aseptic) meningitis	Enteroviruses Mumps virus	Clear or slightly turbid	10–500, mainly lymphocytes	Viruses rarely isolated from CSF. Diagnose by stool culture (enteroviruses) or serology (mumps). PCR	Normal or slightly raised	Normal
Tuberculous meningitis	Mycobacterium tuberculosis	Clear or slightly turbid	10–500, mainly lymphocytes, polymorphs in early stages	AAFB in ZN-stained deposit – often scanty. Growth on LJ culture. PCR	Moderately raised	Usually reduced
Cerebral abscess	Streptococcus milleri Bacteroides species, Staphylococcus aureus, Proteus species	Clear or slightly turbid	0–500, mainly polymorphs, some lymphocytes	Organisms often not present in CSF	Normal or raised	Normal
Subarachnoid haemorrhage	–	Turbid, often blood-stained; supernatant yellow–orange	Large numbers of red blood cells	Sterile	Markedly raised	Normal

AAFB: acid- and alcohol-fast bacilli; ZN: Ziehl–Neelsen; LJ: Löwenstein–Jensen.

Isolation: *specimens*: CSF obtained by lumbar puncture; blood.
Examination of CSF:

- In a counting chamber, for white blood cells and erythrocytes
- Gram film of centrifuged deposit, for bacteria and cells
- If indicated, Leishman film of centrifuged deposit, to differentiate polymorphonuclear leukocytes from lymphocytes
- If indicated, Ziehl–Neelsen film of centrifuged deposit, for tubercle bacilli.

Culture of CSF:

- centrifuged deposit on to blood agar and chocolate agar, and into glucose broth and cooked meat broth: incubate plates in air plus 5% CO_2
- if indicated, Löwenstein–Jensen medium, for culture for tubercle bacilli.

Blood culture: positive in over 40% of patients with meningitis due to *N. meningitidis*, *H. influenzae* or *S. pneumoniae*.

Demonstration of bacterial antigen or DNA

Of value when meningitis has been partially treated and no infecting organisms can be seen or cultured: detect immunologically by latex agglutination or Phadebact coagglutination for *N. meningitidis*, *H. influenzae* type b and pneumococci : detect DNA by PCR.

Antibiotic treatment: *before* the results of laboratory tests are available, if meningitis is suspected give high-dose intravenous penicillin immediately: this may be life-saving in the case of meningococcal septicaemia.

The treatment of meningitis of known cause is covered in the corresponding sections above.

Meningitis of unknown cause

When many polymorphs are present in the deposit of the CSF, but no bacteria have been detected and there is no growth on culture, treatment must be empirical. This state of affairs is usually the result of inadequate treatment, given outside hospital before the patient is admitted. Broth cultures may give a positive result after a few days' incubation when cultures on solid media remain negative.

On a '*best-guess*' basis, give either benzyl penicillin or cefotaxime or ceftriaxone. Add amoxycillin if *Listeria* spp. suspected. If history of anaphylaxis to β-lactams give chloramphenicol.

11 Sepsis

The term 'sepsis' covers numerous and diverse purulent infections, some trivial and others serious, which are among the most common encountered in medicine. They include:

- Superficial skin infections
- Cellulitis
- Necrotizing fasciitis
- Peritonitis
- Abscesses
- Septicaemia
- Wound infections.

SKIN INFECTION

The skin is an efficient barrier to infection, but nevertheless, skin infections are common but uncomfortable and unsightly rather than serious. The main forms of skin sepsis are shown in Table 11.1.

Clinical features

Boils, carbuncles, styes, sycosis barbae

Below are listed some characteristics of these infections:

1. Due to *Staphylococcus aureus*, mainly of phage groups I or II.
2. Tend to be recurrent, appearing in crops at the same site, often over weeks or months.
3. Infection is usually endogenous and due to a strain carried in the nose and on the skin.

Table 11.1 Skin infections

Infection	Site	Causal organism
Boil	Hair follicle	*Staphylococcus aureus*
Carbuncle	Multiple hair follicles	*Staphylococcus aureus*
Stye	Eyelash follicle	*Staphylococcus aureus*
Sycosis barbae	Shaving area	*Staphylococcus aureus*
Impetigo	Cheeks, around mouth	*Staphylococcus aureus* *Streptococcus pyogenes*
Erysipelas	Face, sometimes limbs	*Streptococcus pyogenes*
Pemphigus neonatorum	Infant's skin	*Staphylococcus aureus*
Toxic epidermal necrolysis	Infant's skin	*Staphylococcus aureus*
Acne vulgaris	Face and back	*Propionibacterium acnes*

4. Generally more common in males than females: seen in previously healthy young males surprisingly often. *Sycosis barbae*, seen only in males (Fig. 11.1), is a chronic septic pustular rash on the shaving area spread by the minor trauma inflicted on skin and hair follicles by a razor.

Carbuncles are rarely seen nowadays except in diabetics, who have a predisposition to develop septic lesions: they are associated with considerable malaise and systemic disturbance.

Treatment: boils and styes do not require antibiotic therapy, which in any event does not prevent recurrences. Severe infections such as carbuncles should be treated with penicillin or, if

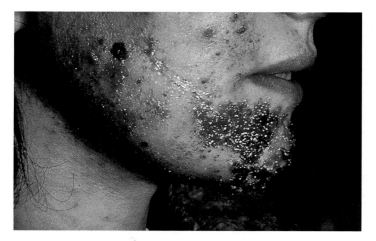

Fig. 11.1 Sycosis barbae. Staphylococcal infection of the skin of the shaving area. (Photograph courtesy of Dr A. Lyell.)

causal strain is resistant, flucloxacillin. Treat sycosis barbae topically with cream containing neomycin and bacitracin, fusidic acid or mupirocin (reserve for methicillin-resistant *S. aureus* – MRSA).

Carriage sites: difficult to clear: apply to the nostrils creams containing the topical antibiotics listed above. Regular use of hexachlorophane soap reduces overall skin carriage.

Impetigo

A disease of young children, with vesicles on the skin around the mouth that later become purulent, with characteristic honey-coloured crusts. Nowadays most often due to *S. aureus*, but *Streptococcus pyogenes* can also cause impetigo (Fig. 11.2).

Outbreaks are not uncommon in schools, where infection is spread by contact, shared towels and contaminated fomites.

Glomerulonephritis has been described following impetigo due to *S. pyogenes*, especially Griffith type 49.

Treatment: topical antibiotics, e.g. tetracycline, chloramphenicol, bacitracin, mupirocin (reserve for MRSA).

Erysipelas

Nowadays rare: caused by *S. pyogenes*; a spreading infection, with a red, indurated and sharply demarcated area of skin, often with

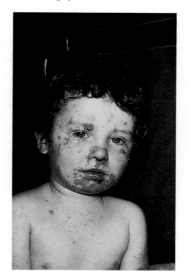

Fig. 11.2 Impetigo. (Photograph courtesy of Dr W. C. Love.)

oedema causing a characteristic 'orange-peel' texture to the skin; the patient may be acutely ill, with high fever and toxaemia.

Treatment: penicillin.

Neonatal skin sepsis

S. aureus can become epidemic in neonatal nurseries – with outbreaks of pustules, sticky eyes, boils and abscesses – where babies readily become carriers in the nose, skin and umbilical stump.

Two severe infections in neonates and infants are associated with skin splitting; caused by staphylococci of phage group II producing an epidermolytic toxin that causes skin splitting and desquamation:

- *Pemphigus neonatorum*: in which the skin splitting is focal or localized in large vesicles or bullae; a more serious disease than the neonatal infections above, but responds well to antibiotics.
- *Toxic epidermal necrolysis*, also called Ritter–Lyell's disease or, more descriptively, 'scalded skin syndrome': a more severe infection in which large areas of skin desquamate, leaving a red weeping surface resembling a scald (Fig. 11.3). Predominantly seen in neonates, but also in young children and occasionally in adults; usually responds to antibiotics, with full recovery.

Treatment: flucloxacillin.

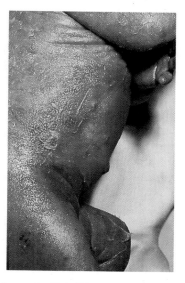

Fig. 11.3 Ritter–Lyell's disease: 'scalded skin' produced by epidermolytic toxin of *Staphylococcus aureus*. (Photograph courtesy of Dr W. C. Love.)

DIAGNOSIS OF SKIN INFECTIONS

Specimens: swabs from lesions: pus, exudate. *Direct Gram film*: observe for bacteria, especially typical forms of any Gram-positive cocci (see Figs 3.2 and 3.4). *Culture* aerobically.

Acne vulgaris

A common and disfiguring skin disease of adolescence that sometimes persists into adult life with residual pitting or scarring; not primarily an infectious disease, but bacteria play a cofactor role in its pathogenesis.

Propionibacterium acnes (and *P. granulosum*) can regularly be isolated from inflamed comedones (whiteheads). These bacteria may induce an inflammatory reaction in the skin by the production of lipase, which liberates irritant fatty acids from lipid in the sebum within sebaceous glands.

Treatment: topical erythromycin, tetracycline, clindamycin. In severe cases: tretinoin or other non-antibacterial drugs.

Note: Bacteriology plays no part in diagnosis.

CELLULITIS

An infection of subcutaneous tissue seen as two clinical syndromes:

1. *Acute pyogenic cellulitis*
Due to *Streptococcus pyogenes*: a red, painful swelling, usually of a limb, associated with lymphangitis and lymphadenitis, involving local draining lymph glands (Fig. 11.4).
Treatment: penicillin.

2. *Anaerobic cellulitis*
Rare – may be due to non-sporing anaerobes (e.g. 'bacteroides') or clostridia, but more usually a synergistic infection with both aerobic and anaerobic bacteria (the aerobes produce reducing or anaerobic conditions, enabling the anaerobes to multiply).
Causal organisms: a combination of aerobes (coliforms, *P. aeruginosa, S. aureus, S. pyogenes*) and anaerobes (most often 'bacteroides' or anaerobic cocci; rarely, clostridia).
Clinically: redness, swelling and oedema around a primary wound (which may be traumatic or surgical): usually on the abdomen, buttock or perineum, less commonly the leg.
Treatment: penicillin, metronidazole: other appropriate antibiotics.

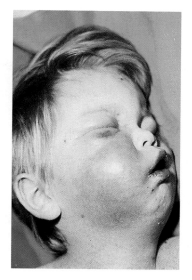

Fig. 11.4 Acute streptococcal cellulitis. (Photograph courtesy of Dr A. K. R. Chaudhuri.)

NECROTIZING FASCIITIS

A serious infection, most often due to *S. pyogenes* but sometimes to a mixture of organisms, such as streptococci, staphylococci, coliforms, 'bacteroides' and anaerobic fusiform bacilli. Two main syndromes are recognized, but their clinical features overlap.

1. *Necrotizing fasciitis*
Originally described as 'streptococcal gangrene': the external appearance of the skin is initially normal, while the infective–ischaemic process spreads along the fascial planes with extensive necrosis. Later the overlying skin, deprived of its blood supply, discolours, becoming painful and red, and finally numb and necrotic. The patient is severely ill, with fever, toxaemia and shock. Due to *S. pyogenes*.
Treatment: wide excision of the skin to expose the entire area of necrosis, with general supportive measures including appropriate antibiotics.

2. *Progressive bacterial synergistic gangrene*
Caused by mixed infection with aerobic and anaerobic organisms; often follows surgery. The overlying skin becomes purplish and there may be central necrosis (Fig. 11.5). When the infection involves the peno-scrotal area it is known as 'Fournier's gangrene'.
Treatment: surgery, with appropriate antibiotics.

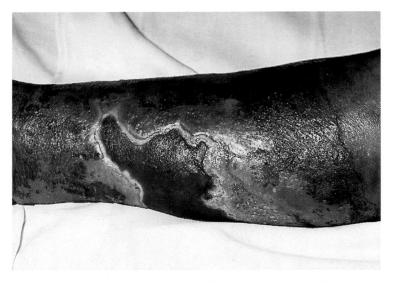

Fig. 11.5 Progressive bacterial gangrene due to *Streptococcus pyogenes* and *Bacteroides* species. (Photograph courtesy of Dr D. H. M. Kennedy.)

PERITONITIS

A serious complication of abdominal surgery and of diseases that cause perforation of the gastrointestinal tract, e.g. peptic ulcer, diverticulitis, acute appendicitis, Crohn's disease; perforated typhoid ulcer is still a cause of death in enteric fever.

Causal organisms: usually mixed infection with faecal flora, i.e. coliforms, enterococci, 'bacteroides'; sometimes *Clostridium perfringens*.

CAPD: peritonitis is a common and serious complication of continuous ambulatory peritoneal dialysis for renal failure. Most commonly caused by coagulase-negative staphylococci (from patient's skin) but Gram-negative organisms such as *E. coli* (from the peritoneal cavity) can also cause CAPD peritonitis.

Clinically: the patient's condition deteriorates, with fever, toxaemia and shock; there may be tenderness on palpation of the abdomen, and the absence of bowel sounds owing to paralytic ileus.

Diagnosis: a specimen of peritoneal exudate is examined in the same way as pus from a wound.

Treatment: start *appropriate antibiotics* (even before sensitivity results are available), e.g. a combination of amoxycillin, gentamicin and metronidazole. Alternatively: a cephalosporin such as cefotaxime; or ciprofloxacin; or imipenem with cilastatin. If coagulase-negative staphylococci, consider vancomycin; review therapy when results of sensitivity tests are known.

ABSCESSES

Abscesses, both obvious and cryptic, are an important part of the work of hospital bacteriology laboratories and can be very difficult to diagnose. A collection of pus within – often deeply within – the body, is walled off by a barrier of inflammatory reaction with fibrosis. This often makes it impossible to treat abscesses satisfactorily by antibiotics alone: surgery and drainage are also needed.

Abscesses can form in almost any tissue or organ of the body: the commonest sites are listed in Table 11.2.

Note that tuberculosis commonly causes abscesses but that these are 'cold', i.e. not accompanied by pain, redness or an acute inflammatory response (see Chapter 14).

Clinical features

Abscesses may be:

- *Clinically obvious*: includes those at sites such as the breast, axilla, peritonsillar (quinsy), perianal, ischiorectal and Bartholin's glands: there is painful swelling with local inflammation, fever, and often some degree of systemic upset. Brain abscess commonly presents with the signs of a space-occupying lesion, most often in the temporal lobe (Fig. 11.6).
- *Cryptic*: such abscesses can be exceedingly difficult to diagnose and, unfortunately, are relatively common. Many abdominal and pelvic abscesses are of this type: the patient presents with vague, progressive ill health and fever and, although obviously toxic, there are no definite localizing signs.

Investigations: clinical history; computerized tomography (CT) scan; X-ray – a subphrenic abscess may be detected; a positive blood culture confirms the diagnosis of sepsis and the type of organism may indicate the source; laparotomy if there is a high degree of clinical suspicion.

Pathogenesis: abscesses do not necessarily form at the site of primary infection: there may be tracking of pus, leading to a puru-

Table 11.2   Abscesses – some common sites

Site	Route of infection, predisposing factors	Bacteria usually responsible
Subcutaneous tissues, finger pulp, palmar space	Penetrating wounds	*Staphylococcus aureus*
Axilla	Extension of superficial infection via lymphatics to axillary lymph nodes with suppuration	*Staphylococcus aureus*
Breast	Breastfeeding – infected from infant	*Staphylococcus aureus*
Peritonsillar (quinsy)	Streptococcal sore throat	*Streptococcus pyogenes*
Intra-abdominal, e.g. appendix, subphrenic, paracolic	Appendicitis: abdominal sepsis; peritonitis due to any cause	Faecal flora *Streptococcus milleri*
Ischiorectal	Direct from rectum	Faecal flora
Perianal	Infected hair follicle round anus	*Staphylococcus aureus* Faecal flora
Pelvic	Abdominal or gynaecological sepsis	Faecal flora Genital flora
Tubo-ovarian (pyosalpinx)	Gynaecological sepsis; gonorrhoea	Genital flora *Neisseria gonorrhoeae*
Bartholin's glands	Local spread	Genital flora *Neisseria gonorrhoeae*
Perinephric	Extension of acute pyelonephritis	Coliforms
Cerebral	Otitis media; sinusitis Haematogenous	*Streptococcus milleri* 'Bacteroides' *Staphylococcus aureus,* *Proteus* species
Hepatic	Ascending cholangitis; portal pyaemia	Faecal flora *Streptococcus milleri*
Lung	Aspiration pneumonia; bronchial obstruction with collapse (e.g. tumour)	Oropharyngeal flora
	Staphylococcus aureus pneumonia	*Staphylococcus aureus*

Note: The anaerobic commensals ('bacteroides', anaerobic cocci etc.) also play a role in abscess production, usually in conjunction with other organisms.

lent collection at a site some distance from the original infection, e.g. subphrenic and pelvic abscesses.

Metastatic abscesses: occasionally, multiple abscesses form as a result of bloodborne or 'pyaemic' spread of infected thrombi: such abscesses are found in many sites. *Portal pyaemia*, in which

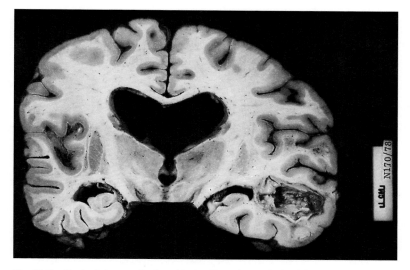

Fig. 11.6 Cerebral abscess. Section of brain with an abscess in the right temporal lobe, secondary to suppurative otitis media. (Photograph courtesy of Professor J. Hume Adams.)

the source is intra-abdominal sepsis (often the appendix), results in liver abscesses.

Diagnosis: *specimens*: pus (which may have to be collected at operation or by aspiration); blood. *Culture*: aerobically and anaerobically – incubation may have to be continued for some days.

Treatment: antibiotics are rarely sufficient on their own and surgical intervention and drainage may be necessary – under appropriate antibiotic cover, depending on the site of the abscess and the likely infecting bacteria (see Table 11.2).

SEPTICAEMIA

Literally, 'sepsis of the blood'. In the past, the terms *bacteraemia* and *septicaemia* have been used to describe the presence of organisms in the bloodstream. It is no longer considered useful to distinguish between them, and septicaemia is now preferred. Usually a complication of a localized infection, e.g. pyelonephritis, peritonitis, cholangitis, pneumonia, osteomyelitis, abscesses of internal organs, but also a basic feature of generalized infections such as enteric fever or brucellosis.

Causal organisms: the organisms that cause septicaemia and the underlying infections or associated clinical conditions are shown in Table 11.3. In about 95% of cases a single infecting organism is responsible for an episode of septicaemia.

Note: Infective endocarditis (also associated with septicaemia) is described in Chapter 12, infection in the immunocompromised in Chapter 37.

Table 11.3 Bacteria commonly causing septicaemia

Predisposing factor	Causal organisms
Abdominal sepsis (peritonitis, hepatobiliary infection, abscess etc.)	Coliforms 'Bacteroides' Enterococci *Streptococcus milleri*
Infected wounds, burns, pressure sores	*Staphylococcus aureus* *Streptococcus pyogenes* Coliforms 'Bacteroides'
Gynaecological sepsis (puerperal infection, pelvic abscess, salpingitis etc.)	Coliforms Enterococci 'Bacteroides' *Streptococcus pyogenes* Lancefield group B streptococci
Urinary tract infection	Coliforms Enterococci
Osteomyelitis Septic arthritis	*Staphylococcus aureus*
Pneumonia	*Streptococcus pneumoniae*
Meningitis	*Streptococcus pneumoniae* *Neisseria meningitidis* *Haemophilus influenzae*
Meningitis in neonates	Coliforms Lancefield group B streptococci
Food poisoning	*Salmonella* species (not *S.* Typhi or *S.* Paratyphi) *Campylobacter jejuni*
Drip sites, shunts, intravascular catheters	*Staphylococcus aureus* Coagulase-negative staphylococci Coliforms
Intravenous drug abuse	*Staphylococcus aureus*
Splenectomized patients	*Streptococcus pneumoniae*
Immunosuppressed patients	Coliforms *Staphylococcus aureus* *Pseudomonas aeruginosa* *Streptococcus pneumoniae*

Clinical features

Variable – sometimes minimal, sometimes severe and rapidly progressive: those of the underlying disease (e.g. pneumonia, peritonitis) may predominate. The presenting feature is usually a worsening of the patient's condition, with fever, rigors, tachycardia, tachypnoea, cyanosis, hypotension; in elderly patients there may be confusion, agitation or behavioural changes.

Septicaemia may develop into the very serious complications of sepsis syndrome or septic shock.

SEPSIS SYNDROME AND SEPTIC SHOCK

Sepsis syndrome: defined as evidence of infection with signs of a systemic response such as tachypnoea, tachycardia, fever (or hypothermia); results from microorganisms initiating a cascade of reactions, with the sequential release of endogenous mediators: these include cytokines – tumour necrosis factors and interleukins are of particular importance. A central mediator does not seem to exist.

Septic shock occurs when the sepsis syndrome progresses to severe hypotension and tissue anoxia, leading to multiple organ failure (e.g. heart, lungs, liver, kidneys) despite fluid resuscitation. This has a poor prognosis, despite antibiotics and supportive therapy, with case fatality rates often higher than 50%.

Septic shock is usually a complication of septicaemia, with Gram-negative and, much more rarely, Gram-positive bacteria. The main virulence factor of Gram-negative bacteria is bacterial endotoxin or lipopolysaccharide (LPS). Endotoxin is derived from the outer membrane of Gram-negative bacteria: it activates the complement system, causing intravascular coagulation and the release of vasoactive substances and various cytokines. Septic shock is sometimes called *endotoxic shock*.

Diagnosis: blood culture – more than one may be required. Take two or three separate sets of cultures from different veins at intervals of about 5 minutes before antibiotics are administered.

Treatment: bactericidal therapy is required, administered intravenously; surgical intervention may be required (e.g. to drain an abscess, resuture a ruptured viscus).

Septic shock: in addition to antibiotic therapy, special resuscitative measures, with fluid replacement, inotropic support and artificial ventilation, are necessary. Newer approaches to therapy, such as monoclonal antibodies to endotoxin and TNF, have proved disappointing.

TOXIC SHOCK SYNDROME

Seen mainly in menstruating women using tampons, which encourage the growth of *S. aureus*, present as a commensal in the vagina.

Clinically: fever, collapse, diarrhoea and vomiting, with a diffuse erythematous macular rash followed by skin desquamation. The patient may be severely ill and there is a significant mortality, with multisystem organ failure and shock.

Pathogenesis: due to toxin released by *S. aureus* – TSST-1 (toxic shock syndrome toxin).

Diagnosis: *culture*: tampon or swab from vagina for toxin-producing strain of *S. aureus*.

Treatment: flucloxacillin.

WOUND INFECTION

Minor wounds are commonplace in everyday life and, naturally, some become infected, most often with *S. aureus*; most heal without antibiotic treatment.

SURGICAL WOUND INFECTION

A more serious problem because the majority of surgical wounds involve not only skin and subcutaneous tissue but also muscle and deeper tissues, e.g. bone, peritoneum and viscera.

Clinical features

Starts with reddening of the wound edges, usually followed by pus formation – sometimes in the deeper layers of the wound to form a *wound abscess* (as a rule, this eventually discharges to the surface through the sutured incision); there may be fever, but systemic disturbance is often minimal. Infection delays healing and so prolongs hospitalization, with a considerable increase in the cost of treatment (see chapter 35).

Complications:

• *Dehiscence*: the wound may break down completely, sometimes with exposure of viscera, and needs to be resutured.
• *Spread of infection to local tissues*, e.g. the peritoneum in the case of abdominal wounds, or the blood, causing septicaemia.

Causes: the main bacterial causes of surgical wound infections are shown in Table 11.4.

Table 11.4 Main bacterial causes of surgical wound infection

Bacteria	Species	Most common site
Aerobic	Staphylococcus aureus	Any wound
	Escherichia coli	Any wound, but especially abdominal, urological and gynaecological
	Proteus species	
	Klebsiella species	
	Enterococci	
	Pseudomonas aeruginosa	Urological; burns
Anaerobic	'Bacteroides'	Abdominal and gynaecological
	Anaerobic cocci	
	Clostridium perfringens	

S. aureus: (including MRSA strains) usually present in pure culture.

Mixed infection: it is common to find more than one species of coliform, together with enterococci, 'bacteroides' or *C. perfringens* – i.e. faecal flora – the usual cause of abdominal wound sepsis. Note that the presence of *C. perfringens* does not imply the onset of gas gangrene.

Pseudomonas aeruginosa is not usually found in the human bowel but is a particular problem where there are breaches of mucosa, such as after prostatectomy or with skin ulcers such as bed sores; usually acquired exogenously from contaminated water, fluids, ventilators, humidifiers, even antiseptic solutions; often highly antibiotic resistant.

Sources

Endogenous infection: many wound infections are due to organisms carried on the patient's skin.

Exogenous infection: generally acquired during operation, from the surgeon, other theatre personnel, the theatre environment, or in the ward postoperatively.

Factors affecting surgical wound sepsis

The risk of wound infection is increased by:

• Operations involving opening of the bowel
• The presence of drains, catheters, venous lines or other foreign bodies
• Long operations

• Large wounds with considerable tissue trauma
• Obesity.

Incidence: the sepsis rate of surgical wounds therefore varies:

• *Low*: in clean elective surgery, e.g. hernia repairs, 'cold' orthopaedic operations: around 1%.
• *High*: in operations, and particularly emergency surgery, in a contaminated site (e.g. large bowel): around 15%.

DIAGNOSIS OF SURGICAL WOUND INFECTION

Specimens: swab of pus, exudate or tissue from wound. *Direct Gram film*: examine for organisms present. *Culture*: aerobically and anaerobically.

Treatment: appropriate antibiotic therapy – may not be necessary in the absence of generalized symptoms.

Prevention: difficult and complex: needs rigid observance of aseptic and antiseptic technique, both in theatres and wards, combined with appropriate antibiotic prophylaxis (see Chapter 19).

OTHER TYPES OF WOUND INFECTION BURNS

Burns have a large moist exposed surface, always heavily colonized with bacteria. Three organisms present particular problems in burns units:

• *S. pyogenes*: can cause life-threatening septicaemia and loss of skin grafts.
• *P. aeruginosa*: can be difficult to eradicate both from patients and the ward environment; of low invasive powers.
• *S. aureus*: including MRSA, often in outbreaks.

Complications: bacteria from the burn commonly invade the bloodstream: dangerous, but does not necessarily indicate septicaemia.

ORTHOPAEDICS

Wound infection is a particular problem in orthopaedic surgery, in which healing of bone by first intention is important for future weight-bearing and movement. *S. aureus* is the principal cause.

Joint replacement: about 1–5% of these operations fail as a result of low-grade chronic infection, which causes the prosthesis to work loose; most often due to coagulase-negative staphylococci.

INDWELLING CATHETERS

The usual route of infection is by colonization of the catheter with skin commensals and their subsequent shedding into the blood or other tissues or fluids, and infection is especially likely if the catheter is in situ for long periods (e.g. for total parenteral nutrition, or in the peritoneum for continuous ambulatory peritoneal dialysis) – or from urinary catheters.

Causes: coagulase-negative staphylococci; less often, coliforms, *S. aureus*, yeasts.

TRACHEOSTOMIES

Tracheostomies have a marked tendency to become colonized with coliforms – often multiply antibiotic resistant – from the resident hospital flora. Low-grade pathogens such as *Acinetobacter* and *Serratia* species can be particularly difficult to eradicate, although their presence and that of other coliforms in tracheal secretions may not actually harm the patient.

PUERPERAL SEPSIS (INCLUDING SEPTIC ABORTION)

Formerly due mainly to *Streptococcus pyogenes*, the important causes nowadays are streptococci of Lancefield group B, *Bacteroides* and anaerobic cocci; still a severe disease which requires prompt treatment.

Clostridium perfringens is a rare but dangerous cause of puerperal sepsis.

ANAEROBIC WOUND INFECTION

Two types of anaerobic infection of wounds can be conveniently considered here – although neither can be classified as sepsis: pus is not produced, and typically the wounds ooze a serous exudate.

The first, *gas gangrene*, is due to anaerobic clostridia of various species.

The second is *tetanus* due to one species of anaerobic clostridia, *Clostridium tetani*.

GAS GANGRENE

A rare disease in peacetime, but a scourge among wounded armies in the field, notably during the First World War.

Causal organisms:

- *Clostridium perfringens* (65% of cases)
- *Clostridium novyi* (20–40% of cases)
- *Clostridium septicum* (10–20% of cases).

Often more than one species is present.

Clinical features

A spreading gangrene of the muscles, with profound toxaemia and shock. There is oedema, with blackening of the tissues and a foul-smelling serous exudate, and crepitus (palpable crackling or bubbling) detected under the skin caused by gas production by the clostridia (Fig. 11.7).

Severity: a serious disease with a high case fatality rate, often requiring wide excision or amputation.

Pathogenesis: due to contamination of wounds by dirt and soil containing clostridia from animal faeces: risk is increased with extensive wounding and the presence of necrotic tissue, blood clot

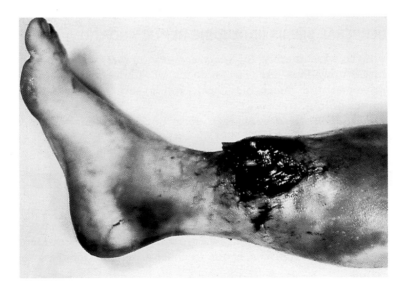

Fig. 11.7 Clostridial gas gangrene complicating a compound fracture. (Photograph courtesy of Professor J. G. Collee.)

and foreign bodies, all of which produce anaerobiosis. Vascular damage may also impair blood supply to the site.

Toxins: clostridia produce powerful toxins which cause tissue damage – and hence anaerobiosis – thereby enhancing spread of the infection.

Epidemiology: gas gangrene can follow major trauma and, occasionally, operations on the bowel (*C. perfringens* is a normal bowel inhabitant), and on ischaemic limbs. Recent reports of *C. novyi* infection in drug users who 'muscle pop'.

Diagnosis: *specimens*: exudate, tissue. *Direct Gram film*: observe for typical Gram-positive bacilli – spores may or may not be seen. In clinical material *C. perfringens* is usually capsulated but does not form spores. *Culture*: anaerobically (but also aerobically).

Treatment: *surgical*: by wide excision or amputation of affected tissue, with large doses of penicillin, often with metronidazole in addition.

Antitoxin: widely used in wartime; of doubtful value.

Hyperbaric oxygen, to reduce anaerobiasis in tissues, has been reported to be effective. This supportive treatment requires special apparatus.

TETANUS

Tetanus also follows contamination of wounds, and although a very rare disease in the UK (fewer than 10 notified cases each year), wounds from which it can develop are common and often trivial.

Clinical features

Incubation period: 5–15 days.

Symptoms: severe and painful muscle spasms: the masseter muscles are often affected, causing 'lockjaw' (the familiar name for tetanus) and 'risus sardonicus' the characteristic facial grimace produced by spasm of the facial muscles. The extensor muscles of the body are more powerful than the flexors so that, as the spasms progress, the body becomes arched in *opisthotonus* (Fig. 11.8).

Death is due to exhaustion, asphyxiation or intercurrent infection, and the case fatality rate is still high despite intensive therapy.

Pathogenesis: *C. tetani* produces a protein exotoxin (although this is mainly released by bacterial lysis). One of the most powerful toxins known, it has two components:

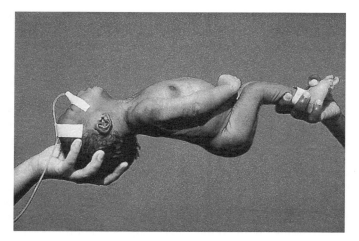

Fig. 11.8 Neonatal tetanus. Infant with opisthotonus due to extensor muscle spasm. (Reproduced with permission from Abbott Laboratories *Slide Atlas of Infectious Diseases*, 1982, Gower Medical Publishing, London. Photograph courtesy of Dr T. F. Sellers Jr.).

- *Tetanospasmin*: acts on synapses, to block the normal inhibitory mechanism that controls motor nerve impulses.
- *Tetanolysin*: lyses erythrocytes.

Spread: *C. tetani* does not spread beyond the wound but the toxin, absorbed at the motor nerve endings, travels via the nerves to the anterior horn cells in the spinal cord.

Site: wounds of the face, neck and upper extremities are more dangerous than those of the legs and feet: they are associated with more severe disease and a shorter incubation period.

Tetanus neonatorum, in which the umbilical stump is the portal of entry, is still common in some developing countries.

Diagnosis: often clinical: attempts at bacteriological confirmation often fail.

Specimen: swab or exudate from wound. *Direct Gram film*: examine for characteristic Gram-positive bacilli with round terminal spores – 'drumsticks' (see Fig. 3.8). *Culture*: anaerobically (and also aerobically).

Epidemiology

Source: faeces of animals, especially horses: wounds become contaminated with spores which, in anaerobic conditions, germinate to produce vegetative bacilli that produce toxin.

Worldwide in distribution, but the incidence is much higher in the Third World, where it is an important cause of death.

Classically, associated with severe wounds contaminated with soil or dust, today in countries with good medical services prophylactic measures prevent patients with such wounds developing the disease. Tetanus now often follows minor injuries disregarded by the patient: in a few reported cases in the UK no wound could be found.

Treatment: supportive, artificial ventilation, with muscle relaxants to control spasms; excision of wound. *Antitoxin*: give large doses intravenously, to neutralize toxin: metronidazole or tetracycline to prevent further toxin production.

Prophylaxis: thorough cleansing of the wound, with administration of antitoxin (see Chapter 39).

12 Infective endocarditis

Infective endocarditis is an infection of the endocardium that most commonly affects the heart valves and the endocardium around congenital defects. The infection was formerly known as bacterial endocarditis: the change in nomenclature recognizes that organisms other than bacteria can cause endocarditis.

Mortality: before antibiotics were available the disease was always fatal: progressive damage to the heart valves led to cardiac failure and death; even nowadays the case fatality rate is around 30%. Rapid diagnosis, careful antibiotic treatment and optimal surgery can reduce mortality associated with treatment to 10%.

Causal organisms

These have changed over the years. Viridans streptococci remain the most common, but staphylococci are now a major cause (see Table 12.1). *S. aureus* is the commonest cause of endocarditis in intraveneous drug users, in patients with diabetes and in the immunocompromised. Coagulase-negative staphylococci are the commonest cause of prosthetic valve endocarditis.

Clinical features

The disease used to be described as 'acute' or 'subacute', based on the progression of the untreated disease. This terminology is now no longer used: it is preferable to assess the disease in terms of the causative microorganism and the underlying pathology.

Signs and symptoms: classically fever, malaise, weight loss, cardiac murmur, anaemia, splinter haemorrhages (i.e. under the

Table 12.1   Causes of infective endocarditis

Organism		Percentage of cases
Bacteria		
Streptococcus sanguis		
Streptococcus bovis	Viridans or	
Streptococcus mutans	non-haemolytic	50–60
Streptococcus mitior	streptococci	
Enterococci		
Staphylococcus aureus		20–30
Coagulase-negative staphylococci		
Other bacteria		5–10
(e.g. corynebacteria,		
Haemophilus species, coliforms)		
Fungi		
Candida albicans		Rare
Aspergillus species		
Rickettsia, chlamydia		
Coxiella burnetii		Rare
Chlamydophila psittaci		

fingernails), haematuria, petechiae, splenomegaly. Nowadays these classic features are rarely seen fully developed: most patients who present with significant malaise and fever are diagnosed at an early stage.

Clinical course: unless adequately treated (and even in some patients apparently so treated) there is progressive damage to the heart valves, leading to cardiac failure and death.

Pathogenesis

Although most patients are known to have pre-existing cardiac disease, a substantial proportion – about one-third – have previously normal hearts or undiagnosed abnormalities.

Cardiac and other abnormalities that predispose to infective endocarditis are:

- *Rheumatic valvular disease*: e.g. stenosis or incompetence of the mitral and aortic valves following rheumatic fever (see Chapter 6)
- *Congenital defects*: e.g. bicuspid aortic valve, septal defects, patent ductus arteriosus, coarctation of the aorta
- *Intracardiac prostheses*: usually, replacement of diseased heart valves with prosthetic valves
- *Degenerative cardiac disease*: e.g. calcific aortic stenosis

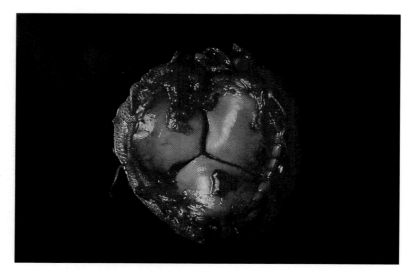

Fig. 12.1 Infective endocarditis. The ventricular surface of a Carpentier Edwards aortic valve, explanted 5 weeks postoperatively because of prosthetic valve endocarditis caused by *Staphylococcus epidermidis*. Vegetations are seen attached to all three cusps. (Reproduced with permission from *Current Medicine 4*, Churchill Livingstone.)

- *Drug use*: addicts who take drugs intravenously have a high risk of endocarditis, often with atypical clinical features.
  Involvement of the tricuspid valve is particularly common: usually due to *S. aureus*.

Formerly an infection of adolescence and young adult life, the mean age of patients in developed countries is now over 50 years, owing to the increasing importance of degenerative disease and the decreasing incidence of rheumatic heart disease.

Pathology

Infective endocarditis usually occurs at the site of a predisposing heart lesion or congenital defect, where the velocity of blood is such as to cause turbulence, resulting in damage to the surface of the endocardium. On such roughened surfaces, usually of the mitral or aortic valves, thrombi of fibrin and platelets form. Circulating microorganisms colonize the avascular thrombi and convert them into infected *vegetations*: the end result is destruction of the valve (Fig. 12.1). As a rule, only a single valve is affected.

Infection of endocardial thrombi results from:

- *Transient asymptomatic bacteraemia*: usually with organisms derived from the normal flora, particularly that of the mouth – which explains the frequency of viridans streptococci as a cause of infective endocarditis. Although this type of bacteraemia is common after dental surgery (e.g. extractions), a history of recent significant dental treatment is surprisingly uncommon. Other predisposing procedures include surgery on the gastrointestinal and genitourinary tracts, including even minor manipulations such as endoscopy or catheterization.
- *Septicaemia*: usually part of a generalized infection with more virulent organisms (such as *S. aureus, S. pneumoniae*).

Vegetations: organisms are shed from these into the blood-stream, often over long periods of time. Minute thrombi are also dislodged, to give rise to distant embolic manifestations of the disease: cerebral emboli are an important complication.

Immune complexes can also form, and may produce vasculitis and glomerulonephritis.

Prosthetic valve endocarditis

An important complication of cardiac surgery. *Early-onset* endo-carditis has a high mortality: the infection is acquired at opera-tion, when it is usually due to coagulase-negative staphylococci. *Late-onset* endocarditis may be acquired in the same way as that of natural valves, and although the infecting organisms reflect the normal microbiological pattern of the disease (Table 12.1), coagulase-negative staphylococci are a frequent cause. The dis-tinction between early-onset and late-onset endocarditis is becom-ing less clear-cut.

Diagnosis: close collaboration between the microbiologist and the clinician is essential: prompt diagnosis and early treatment are imperative.

Blood culture

The cornerstone of diagnosis and important for the subsequent treatment of the patient: repeated cultures may be necessary to isolate the causal organism, e.g. two to six, if possible taken over 48 h. Take blood cultures before the start of antibiotic treatment; however, in seriously ill patients therapy should not be delayed until blood culture results are available.

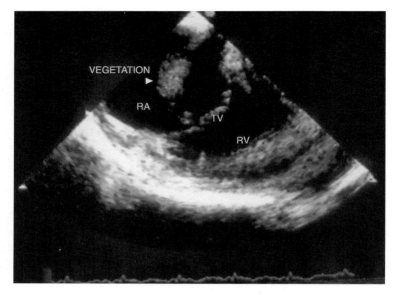

Fig. 12.2 A transoesophageal echocardiogram showing a large vegetation on the tricuspid valve. (Photograph courtesy of Dr S. D. Pringle.)

Observe: early signs of growth.
Subculture: to blood agar, aerobically and anaerobically.
Identification: as appropriate for the organism isolated.

Echocardiography

This is a useful investigative technique and complementary diagnostic aid: it can detect vegetations on heart valves. Diagnostic sensitivity varies and is dependent on the echocardiographic technique used, the size of the vegetations and the stage of the infection. The ability of echocardiography to detect the intracardiac manifestations of infective endocarditis has continued to improve, especially with the introduction of transoesophageal imaging (Fig. 12.2).

Antibiotic sensitivity tests

The usual disc diffusion method of testing is generally considered to be inadequate in infective endocarditis. The following tests should be carried out:

• *Minimum inhibitory concentration* of potentially useful drugs, both singly and in combination

- *Minimum bactericidal concentration* is now no longer recommended as a routine determination.

Culture-negative endocarditis

In 10% of cases no organisms can be grown from blood cultures. This may be due to:

- Infection with *Coxiella burneti* or *Chlamydia psittaci*: perform serological tests to confirm or exclude these diagnoses
- Recent antibiotic therapy: repeat blood cultures over a few days, in the absence of chemotherapy
- Infection with fastidious organisms, difficult to grow in ordinary media, e.g. the HACEK group (see Chapter 4), which are fastidious and may require 2–3 weeks for primary isolation; repeat blood cultures using special media if these are suspected.

Management and treatment

The modern management of infective endocarditis is very much a team effort involving cardiologists, microbiologists and cardiac surgeons.

Antimicrobial therapy

Depends on adequate – and this usually means high – dosage with an antimicrobial drug: two drugs in combination are recommended.

The antibiotic regimen selected must be:

- bactericidal
- parenteral (at least initially)
- continued for several weeks.

High doses of bactericidal drugs are necessary because the aim of therapy is to eliminate the organisms from their sites enmeshed in the relatively avascular vegetations. Some of the antibiotic regimens used are shown in Table 12.2.

Duration of treatment

The length of treatment depends on the causative microorganism, its antibiotic sensitivity pattern and the clinical response.

Table 12.2 Antibiotic regimens for infective endocarditis

Causal organism	Antimicrobial drugs
Viridans streptococci	Penicillin or cephalosporin, plus gentamicin
Enterococci	Penicillin or ampicillin plus gentamicin*
Staphylococcus aureus	Flucloxacillin plus gentamicin
Staphylococcus epidermidis	Vancomycin plus gentamicin and/or rifampicin
Fungi	Amphotericin B plus 5-fluorocytosine or fluconazole
Coxiella burnetii	
Chlamydophila psittaci	Tetracycline

* Although enterococci are not sensitive to either penicillin or gentamicin alone, this combination is usually bactericidal and, in practice, effective.
Note: Vancomycin is also a useful drug for infections due to streptococci and Staphylococcus aureus, especially in patients hypersensitive to the penicillins.

Uncomplicated infective endocarditis caused by viridans streptococci can be treated with penicillin and aminoglycoside for 2 weeks. Otherwise, 4 weeks of treatment is necessary, but the aminoglycoside component of treatment can be reduced to 2 weeks.

Laboratory monitoring of therapy

- *Estimation of the antibiotic level* in the patient's serum: rarely necessary if large doses are being given intravenously, but may be indicated when there is a switch to oral therapy. Also used to avoid overdosage with potentially toxic drugs (e.g. aminoglycosides).
- *Measurement of C-reactive protein* is useful in monitoring the response to treatment, and also in detecting intercurrent infections and complications.
- *Estimation of the bactericidal activity* of the patient's serum against the causal organism: although of little prognostic value, a poor result (e.g. no killing at a 1 in 8 dilution of a 'peak' serum sample) indicates that the antibiotics chosen, their dose and route of administration should be reconsidered.

Surgery

Replacement of damaged valves is now accepted as part of the management of cases of infective endocarditis; it is often life-saving.

Prophylaxis

Although not of proven value, 'at-risk' patients (e.g. those with valvular or congenital heart disease) should be given prophylactic antibiotics – oral amoxycillin or, if hypersensitive to penicillins, oral clindamycin or parenteral vancomycin – before dental procedures. Prior to surgery or instrumentation on the gastrointestinal or urinary tract, parenteral ampicillin with gentamicin is an appropriate prophylactic combination.

In addition, much more emphasis should be placed on improving oral hygiene, by encouraging all people to seek regular routine dental care.

13 Sexually transmitted diseases

Some infectious diseases are transmitted by sexual intercourse. The causal organisms are generally delicate and do not remain viable for long outside the body: their survival as pathogens therefore depends on transmission by direct contact between mucosal surfaces. They often (but not always) produce genital lesions; however, several give rise to severe, systemic disease.

After an increase in incidence during the 1970s and early 1980s, possibly because of changing social attitudes, there was a decline during the late 1980s and early 1990s, particularly in gonorrhoea. Since 1995 there has been a dramatic rise in diagnoses of acute sexually transmitted diseases in the UK: 55% increase in gonorrhoea, 54% in syphilis, 20% in genital warts and 76% in chlamydial infections. This is due to unsafe sexual behaviour, particularly in the young heterosexual and male homosexual populations.

Sexually transmitted diseases affect male homosexual partners as well as heterosexual relationships. In its early years in the USA and UK AIDS was primarily transmitted through homosexual (anal) intercourse. Variations in sexual behaviour can result in sexually transmitted diseases producing lesions in the rectum or oropharynx.

The main sexually transmitted diseases are listed in Table 13.1.

GONORRHOEA

A worldwide disease, with over 60 million cases per annum. In the UK cases have been rising each year since 1995, with a 25% rise in 1999. The majority of patients are aged 15–29.

Causal organism: Neisseria gonorrhoeae.

Table 13.1   Sexually transmitted diseases

Disease	Cause
Bacterial	
Gonorrhoea	*Neisseria gonorrhoeae* (the gonococcus)
Vaginitis	*Gardnerella vaginalis*, anaerobes
Chancroid	*Haemophilus ducreyi*
Granulmona inguinale (donovanosis)	*Calymmatobacterium granulomatosis*
Spirochaetes	
Syphilis	*Treponema pallidum*
Chlamydia	
Non-specific urethritis	*Chlamydia trachomatis* types D–K
Lymphogranuloma venereum	*Chlamydia trachomatis* types L1, 2, 3
Mycoplasma	
Pelvic inflammatory disease	*Mycoplasma hominis*
Non-specific urethritis	*Ureaplasma urealyticum* (T-strain mycoplasma)
Protozoa	
Trichomoniasis	*Trichomonas vaginalis*
Dysentery*	*Entamoeba histolytica*
Diarrhoea*	*Giardia lamblia*
Fungi	
Vaginal thrush*	*Candida albicans*
Ectoparasites	
Pubic lice	*Phthirius pubis*
Genital scabies	*Sarcoptes scabei*
Viruses	
AIDS	HIV-1
Genital herpes	Herpes simplex, type 2 (and 1)
Warts	Papilloma viruses types 6, 11, 16 and 18
Hepatitis*	Hepatitis B

* Not always sexually transmitted.
Note: This chapter deals only with gonorrhoea, non-specific urethritis, trichomoniasis, thrush, syphilis and *Gardnerella vaginalis*.

Clinical features

Purulent urethral or vaginal discharge of acute onset: often with dysuria and frequency in males; asymptomatic infection is common in females. The disease may involve the rectum or the oropharynx (usually asymptomatically).

Complications

Due to local spread:

• *Males*: prostatitis, epididymitis; rarely, urethral stricture in untreated cases.

- *Females*: pelvic inflammatory disease (salpingitis, endometritis, infertility).
- *Neonates*: ophthalmia neonatorum (gonococcal conjunctivitis) owing to infection during birth from maternal disease.

Occasionally: disseminated gonococcal infection (septicaemia, arthritis, meningitis, endocarditis) owing to haematogenous spread.

Gonococcal vulvovaginitis: a rare form of gonorrhoea in young girls, either following a sexual offence or sometimes acquired non-sexually by contact with infected exudates or fomites.

Diagnosis: *specimens*: urethral, cervical, rectal or throat smears and swabs – swabs directly plated or transported to the laboratory in transport medium (Amies' is best). *Direct Gram film*: examine for typical intracellular Gram-negative diplococci in smears: often convincingly positive in males (Fig. 13.1) but less useful in females because of difficulty in interpreting the microscopic appearances in the mixed normal flora.

Isolation

Culture: on gonococcal selective media (e.g. Thayer–Martin), because of contamination of sites such as vagina or rectum with other organisms.

Observe: typical translucent colonies, turning purple on addition of oxidase reagent.

Identify: by rapid carbohydrate utilization test for enzyme; alternatively, or in addition, by coagglutination with monoclonal antibody in a test kit.

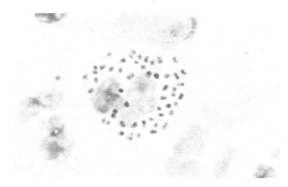

Fig. 13.1 Gonococcal pus (approx. × 1000).

Rapid diagnostic techniques: direct immunofluorescence test, ELISA and DNA probes all offer rapidity, but confer no significant benefit in terms of sensitivity and specificity over Gram film. They should not be substituted for culture, particularly in areas where resistant gonococci are common. Ligase chain reaction (LCR), a DNA probe amplification method, offers high sensitivity and specificity and may also be used in non-invasive specimens, e.g. urine.

Treatment

Patients tend to default, and whenever possible antibiotics should be given in one curative dose. Coexisting chlamydia infection occurs in 20–50% of patients and antibiotic regimens should include treatment for both organisms. All patients with gonorrhoea should be tested for syphilis. Empirical treatment for gonorrhoea has been complicated by the development of antibiotic-resistant strains.

Antibiotic resistance: normally *N. gonorrhoeae* is extremely sensitive to penicillin, but two types of penicillin resistance are now seen:

- Chromosomally mediated resistance: not due to β-lactamase production
- Penicillinase-producing *N. gonorrhoeae* (PPNG): due to a plasmid-coded β-lactamase. Increasing rapidly in the UK.

Resistance to other antibiotics exists:

- *Tetracycline resistance* (TRNG) can be both chromosomal and plasmid mediated. Incidence rising.
- *Spectinomycin resistance*: incidence remains low.
- *Quinolone resistance*: incidence in UK remains low (<5%). Most strains imported from Asia and Africa, where it is a major problem.

Standard treatment

Numerous different regimens have been proposed for uncomplicated disease. They include a large single (oral) dose of:

- *Quinolone, e.g. ciprofloxacin*: also provides treatment for chlamydia. Not for use in pregnancy.
- *Ceftriaxone* (intramuscular): safe in pregnancy.

- *Spectinomycin*: limited availability in UK. Recommended in pregnant women with β-lactam allergy; do *not* use in pharyngeal infection.
- *Amoxycillin*, with oral *probenecid* (to delay renal excretion) for penicillin-sensitive strains. Limited availability of probenecid in UK.
- *Macrolides* e.g. erythromycin for children and pregnant women. High-dose oral azithromycin effective but has significant side-effects.

CHANCROID

Chancroid, or *soft sore*, is a sexually transmitted disease common in the developing countries and strongly associated with HIV infection.
Causal organism: *Haemophilus ducreyi*.

Clinical features

Incubation period: 3–10 days.

A papule on the genital area erodes and forms a markedly painful, non-indurated ulcer with ragged edges and yellow exudate on the base; often accompanied by painful local lymphadenopathy.

Diagnosis: *direct Gram film*: slender Gram-negative bacilli, arranged *en masse,* giving a characteristic appearance of 'shoals of fish'.

Culture: on selective medium showing requirement for growth factor X.

Molecular: a sensitive PCR assay is available.

Treatment

Ceftriaxone, ciprofloxacin or macrolides, e.g. azithromycin, are effective. HIV patients may require prolonged treatment.

NON-SPECIFIC URETHRITIS OR CERVICITIS

Non-specific genital infection is now the commonest sexually transmitted disease in Britain. Seen predominantly in males – infection in females is often symptomless.

Cause: up to 50% of cases are due to *Chlamydia trachomatis* types D–K (see also Chapter 17). *Ureaplasma urealyticum* and possibly other species of mycoplasma are responsible for a proportion of cases.

Clinical features

Men: *acute purulent urethral discharge* with dysuria and urethral discomfort, indistinguishable clinically from gonorrhoea; pus cells are present in the first 10–15 mL of voided urine. A proportion of men are asymptomatic.

Complications: epididymitis, prostatitis, proctitis and Reiter's syndrome – a triad of urethritis, arthritis and conjunctivitis (with or without iritis); men who are HLA-B27 seem to have a genetic predisposition to develop Reiter's syndrome.

Women: *cervicitis*: most women have no symptoms, although some may show mucopurulent cervicitis on pelvic examination. The majority of infected women have male partners infected with *C. trachomatis*. May also be a cause of acute urethral syndrome in women (see Chapter 9).

Complications: pelvic inflammatory disease (PID), salpingitis – leading to infertility and risk of ectopic pregnancy; rarely, Curtis–Fitz-Hugh syndrome of perihepatitis with fever and abnormal liver function tests.

Diagnosis

Examine smears and swabs of urethral or cervical discharge for antigen by ELISA or immunofluorescence, but best by DNA probe or amplification. If a forensic case, attempt isolation by culture in specialized cell culture.

Screening: is now recommended annually for sexually active women, followed by appropriate treatment.

Isolation: now rarely done, but necessary for forensic cases.

Specimens: smears and swabs of urethral or cervical discharge: *culture*: in specialized tissue cultures and *observe* for intracytoplasmic inclusions by immunofluorescence.

Treatment

Tetracycline (doxycycline) for 7 days; alternatively, azithromycin in a single dose or erythromycin for 7 days.

LYMPHOGRANULOMA VENEREUM

A sexually transmitted disease endemic in Asia, Africa and South America. Virtually unknown in temperate climates.

Cause: *C. trachomatis* serotypes L1, 2 and 3 (see also Chapter 17).

Clinical features

Males: the primary lesion is a painless ulcer on the penis, often unnoticed, followed by spread with painful enlargement of the inguinal and femoral lymph nodes and later suppuration to form buboes, sometimes fluctuant, and leading to sinus formation. Proctitis is a common complication in homosexual men.

Females: the genitoanorectal syndrome is the most common disease with involvement of the pelvic rather than the inguinal lymph glands and extension to the rectum and rectovaginal septum causing proctitis, with rectal stricture, fistulae, bleeding and purulent discharge from the anus.

Diagnosis: serology – by CFT or microimmunofluorescence.

Treatment: tetracycline or doxycycline for 3 weeks; alternatively, 3 weeks' erythromycin.

TRICHOMONIASIS

A common disease in women: mainly, if not entirely, transmitted as a result of sexual intercourse with males who have a symptomless infection. See also Chapter 41.

Causal organism: a pear-shaped protozoon, *Trichomonas vaginalis*: motile by means of four flagella (Fig. 13.2).

Clinical features

Vaginal discharge – typically frothy, offensive and greenish-yellow. There may also be urethral discharge and excoriation of the vulva and perineum; the mucosa of the vagina and cervix is reddened and inflamed. The bladder may be involved, with dysuria and frequency. Infection is usually symptomatic, but varies from an acute severe vaginitis to a mild, low-grade or even symptomless infection. Infection in pregnancy has been associated with premature labour.

Diagnosis: *specimen*: swab of vaginal discharge in Amies' transport medium.

Direct: observe wet film for motile protozoa.

Culture: in special medium for trichomonas, for 5 days: examine for motile protozoa at 2 and 5 days.

Treatment

Metronidazole: orally for 7 days, or a large single dose. It is also recommended for use in pregnancy. Increased resistance to metronidazole is being reported.

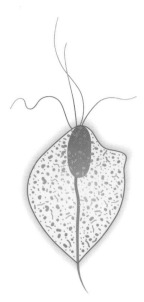

Fig. 13.2 *Trichomonas vaginalis*. This common protozoon is pear-shaped, with four flagella.

THRUSH (CANDIDIASIS)

Vaginal thrush is seen in females; genital candidiasis is rare in men.

Causal organism: *Candida albicans*, a normal commensal of mucous membranes, including those of the vagina and bowel. Infection may be endogenous and precipitated by systemic disease (e.g. diabetes) or drug treatment (e.g. broad-spectrum antibiotics), but some cases are sexually transmitted.

Clinical features

White membranous patches with itching and irritation of the vulva or vagina; white, thick or sometimes watery discharge may be present; many cases are virtually symptomless.

Diagnosis: can usually be made clinically, but best with laboratory confirmation.

Specimen: swab.

Direct Gram film: look for characteristic Gram-positive yeast cells, with budding pseudohyphae (see Fig. 6.1).

Culture: on appropriate medium.

Treatment: imidazole, e.g. clotrimazole or miconazole, applied locally for 3–14 days. Single-dose oral fluconazole is also effective.

SYPHILIS

Now a relatively rare disease, at least in the UK, but important because of its severity and long-term effects if inadequately treated or missed; may be associated with concomitant HIV infection. Increasing incidence both worldwide and UK in last 5 years.

Causal organism: the spirochaete *Treponema pallidum*.

Clinical features

Incubation period: 3–90 days (average 3 weeks).

There are four clinical stages: primary, secondary, tertiary, and late or quaternary.

Primary syphilis

A papule, usually on the genital area, which ulcerates to form the classic *chancre* of primary syphilis: a flat, dull, red indurated ulcer which exudes serous fluid (Fig. 13.3). This heals spontaneously in 3–8 weeks. There is painless enlargement of local lymph nodes.

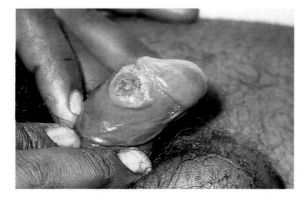

Fig. 13.3 Primary chancre, showing indurated ulcer on penis. (Reproduced with permission from Abbott Laboratories *Slide Atlas of Infectious Diseases*, 1982, Gower Medical Publishing, London. Photograph courtesy of Dr R. D. Caterall.)

Secondary syphilis

Two to 8 weeks after the primary lesion has healed the infection becomes generalized, with a rash, most often papular, of mucous membranes as well as of the skin. The lesions are highly infectious and contain many treponemes; they may coalesce in intertriginous areas (especially the perianal region) to form wart-like *condylomata lata*. There is generalized lymphadenopathy in half the patients at this stage, and there are snail-track mucosal ulcers in the mouth in about a third of patients.

Rarer manifestations include periostitis, arthritis, hepatitis, glomerulonephritis and, occasionally, iridocyclitis and choroidoretinitis.

Tertiary syphilis

Three to 10 years after the primary lesion: *gummata* or granulomatous nodules in skin, mucous membrane or bones; gummata commonly break down to form shallow punched-out ulcers.

Late or quaternary syphilis

Ten to 20 years after primary syphilis; there are two main clinical forms:

1. *Cardiovascular:* aortitis, aneurysm (classically of the aorta), aortic incompetence, coronary ostial stenosis (i.e. narrowing of the origins of the coronary arteries in the aortic sinus).
2. *Neurosyphilis:* may take the following forms:
   - *Tabes dorsalis,* with characteristic ataxic gait and trophic changes in joints (Charcot's joints); often associated with optic atrophy
   - *General paralysis of the insane,* with dementia, tremor, spastic paralysis
   - *Meningovascular syphilis,* with headache, cranial nerve palsies, pupillary loss of reaction to light (Argyll Robertson pupil).

Latent syphilis

The disease can lie dormant for many years with no clinical symptoms (but with positive serology). Latent syphilis can eventually develop into cardiovascular syphilis or neurosyphilis.

Congenital syphilis

Syphilis is one of the infections – rare among bacteria – capable of crossing the placental barrier to infect the fetus.

Transmission can take place early (10th week) until late in pregnancy; fetal infection is usually seen only with primary or secondary syphilis in the mother.

Clinically: congenital syphilis is seen clinically as:

1. *Latent infection*: more than half the infected infants have no symptoms but are serologically positive.
2. *Early*: up to the end of the second year of life. Most infants appear healthy at birth; symptoms develop in the first few weeks, starting with failure to thrive, then generalized infection with skin rash, snuffles, nasal deformity (saddle nose), hepatitis, bone lesions, meningitis, anaemia.
3. *Late*: manifestations appear after the second year of life: interstitial keratitis, bone sclerosis, joint effusions and arthritis, juvenile general paralysis of the insane and tabes, notching of incisor teeth (Hutchinson's incisors), deafness.

Diagnosis

Direct demonstration: but spirochaetes can be demonstrated in fluid or scrapings from chancre or ulcerated secondary lesions (except oral lesions), by dark-ground microscopy.

Serology

The most effective laboratory diagnostic methods are serological. Two types of tests are used:

1. *Non-treponemal*: detect IgG and IgM antibodies (reagin) directed against cardiolipin–lecithin–cholesterol antigen (not derived from spirochaetes). Tests can be quantified, but biological false-positive reactions are common; 13–40% of tests are false-negative in primary syphilis.
   Tests:
   • *VDRL* (Venereal Disease Reference Laboratory)
   • RPR (rapid plasma reagin)
   • ART (automated reagin test).
2. *Treponemal*: using *T. pallidum* as antigen. Tests using specific antigen involve fewer false-positive reactions than those using non-specific antigens, and they remain positive after treatment.

Tests:

- *TPHA* (*T. pallidum* haemagglutination test): detects IgG antibody.
- *FTA-ABS* (fluorescent treponemal antibody-absorption test): detects IgG and IgM antibody. Subjective and difficult to standardize.
- *ELISA*: detects IgG and IgM antibody. Easy to automate, but some false positives.

Important principles in syphilis serology testing are:

- Use either TPHA and VDRL combination, or ELISA for screening.
- A different treponemal test from that used in screening should be used to confirm a reactive result.
- Reserve FTA-ABS test for testing specimens that yield discrepant results.
- Other treponemal diseases, such as yaws, also give positive reaction in all serological tests for syphilis.
- Always test a patient with a positive syphilis test for HIV infection (with consent).

Table 13.2 lists the typical serological reactions in the different stages of syphilis.

Treatment

Penicillin: large doses continued for 10–21 days.

Table 13.2	Serological tests for syphilis			
Stage of disease	VDRL	TPHA	FTA-ABS	ELISA (IgG + IgM)
Primary	+ or −	−	+	+
Late primary	+	+ or −	+	+
Secondary and tertiary	+[†]	+	+[†]	+
Late (quaternary)	+	+	+	+
Latent	+ or −	+	+	+
Treated syphilis	−	+	+	+
Congenital syphilis	+	+	+[*]	+[*]

[*] IgM and IgG positive: detection of IgG only might represent passively transferred maternal antibody.
[†] May be negative in HIV-positive patients, particularly if CD4 count <200.
Note: The success of treatment can be monitored by the VDRL test, which becomes negative on successful treatment. The other tests remain positive.

Late or latent syphilis: large doses of penicillin for 21 days, usually followed by 10 injections at weekly intervals.

Tetracycline (doxycycline) or chloramphenicol can be used if patient is hypersensitive to penicillin.

BACTERIAL VAGINOSIS

Many episodes of vaginosis remain unexplained. Numerous organisms have been implicated. Infection is probably transmitted sexually, but infectivity appears to be low.

Possible causal organisms: *Gardnerella vaginalis*, *Mycoplasma hominis*, mobiluncus species, non-fragilis 'bacteroides', various anaerobes.

Clinical features

Thin, grey-white watery offensive vaginal discharge. Complications in pregnant women: chorioamnionitis, premature rupture of membranes and preterm delivery.

Diagnosis

Based on the presence of three of the following criteria:

1. Thin watery discharge
2. Vaginal pH fluid of ≥4.5
3. Presence of fishy or amine odour, intensified by the addition of potassium hydroxide – the *amine* or *whiff* test
4. Demonstration of '*clue cells*', i.e. squamous epithelial cells with many Gram-variable adherent bacilli in wet or stained films. Few polymorphs present.

Isolation: of little value in diagnosis.
Treatment: metronidazole or clindamycin.

CONTROL OF SEXUALLY TRANSMITTED DISEASES

'Sexually transmitted diseases are now second only to respiratory tract infections as a cause of morbidity due to communicable diseases in Europe' (WHO, 1992): prompt diagnosis and treatment are essential.

Whatever the disease, determined attempts should be made to persuade patients to name consorts, and for the consorts to submit themselves to examination and treatment. The tracing of partners' contacts, although difficult and time-consuming, is of great importance in the control of sexually transmitted diseases.

14 Tuberculosis and leprosy

TUBERCULOSIS

A chronic debilitating disease, once the scourge of Victorian Britain ('consumption', 'phthisis'), which remains a major health problem in much of the world today: 30–50% of the world population is infected, with 10 million new cases per year accounting for 3 million deaths a year. It is a particular problem in HIV-infected patients.

Causal organisms: *Mycobacterium tuberculosis* and *M. africanum*, both human tubercle bacilli; less often, *M. bovis*, the bovine tubercle bacillus.

Clinical features

Tuberculosis is a slowly progressive, chronic granulomatous infection which most often affects the lungs; other organs and tissues may also be involved. Clinically, tuberculosis is seen in three forms:

- *Primary*: generally the more invasive, with marked lymph node involvement. Mainly in children, but increasingly in adults
- *Latent*: asymptomatic dormant phase
- *Post-primary*: in which the development of delayed-type hypersensitivity modifies the infection, with limitation of spread and considerable fibrotic reaction.

Primary infection

Usually involves the lung.

Symptoms: clinically, many cases are symptomless. Symptoms, if present, are vague and non-specific – malaise, anorexia, weight loss, fever, sweats, tachycardia; cough may not be prominent.

Site of primary complex: the commonest form is a local lesion (Ghon focus), with marked enlargement of the regional hilar lymph nodes. The Ghon focus develops at the lung periphery, usually just below the pleura in the midzone, and is a small lesion. In most cases it heals with fibrosis.

A primary focus with enlargement of the draining lymph nodes can alternatively involve other sites, e.g. the tonsils, with cervical adenitis; the intestine, with mesenteric adenitis, peritonitis.

Progressive primary infection

Primary infection may progress to:

- *Tuberculous bronchopneumonia*: an acute diffuse extension of the infection throughout the lung, owing to discharge into the bronchial tree of caseous material from an expanding Ghon focus or, more often, from caseous hilar lymph nodes (Fig. 14.1). A serious and often fatal complication if untreated.

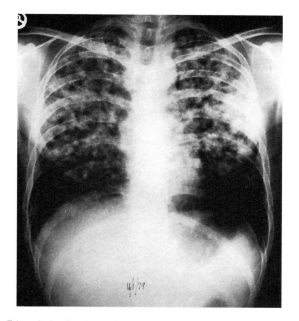

Fig. 14.1 Tuberculosis: chest X-ray of a patient with tuberculous bronchopneumonia. (Courtesy of Dr R. S. Kennedy.)

Caseation – the production of thick cheesy material consisting of pus cells and necrotic tissue – is characteristic of tuberculous inflammatory lesions.

- *Miliary tuberculosis*: small tuberculous foci (tubercles) disseminated widely throughout the body, as a result of haematogenous (bloodborne) spread of infection.
- *Tuberculous meningitis*: bloodborne spread of infection to penetrate the blood–brain barrier and involve the meninges; a serious disease, with considerable mortality and disabling sequelae in some survivors.
- *Bone and joint tuberculosis*: affects different sites: a common form is spinal tuberculosis, in which there may be collapse of the vertebrae, causing kyphosis and the formation of a 'cold' *psoas abscess* in the groin, owing to tracking of pus down the psoas muscle from the infective process in the spine.
- *Genitourinary tuberculosis*:
  - (a) *Renal tuberculosis* presents with frequency and painless haematuria: the urine shows a 'sterile' pyuria – numerous pus cells on microscopy, but no growth of pathogens when cultured on standard media.
  - (b) *Endometrial tuberculosis* in females.
  - (c) *Tuberculous epididymitis* in males.

Cold abscess: tuberculosis also causes 'cold' abscesses, i.e. without an acute inflammatory reaction. Neck abscesses, now rare and formerly associated with *M. bovis* infection, originate in an enlarged cervical lymph gland, with discharge of caseous pus and the formation of draining sinuses. Psoas abscess is another example.

Latent infection: during which the tubercle bacilli remain dormant before initiating active disease 10–80 years after the primary infection.

Post-primary: generally involves the lungs, with lesions in the apices: if untreated, progressive chronic disease develops, with areas of local exudation and caseation surrounded by dense fibrosis. Caseous lesions enlarge to coalesce and cavitate: cavities, sometimes large and containing fluid, can then be seen on radiography. Lymph node enlargement is much less marked than in the primary form.

Presenting symptoms: non-specific ill health, with fever, night sweats, weight loss; respiratory symptoms include cough, haemoptysis and a pneumonic illness that fails to respond to conventional antibiotics.

Source of post-primary infection can be:

- *Endogenous*: reactivation of latent foci formed at the time of primary infection
- *Exogenous*: reinfection, by inhalation of infected respiratory secretions from a case of 'open' tuberculosis (i.e. with tubercle bacilli in the sputum). Up to 30–40% of cases are reinfection, higher in cases with multidrug strains, highlighting the importance of continuing public health measures.

Dissemination: post-primary infection may disseminate and cause the manifestations listed above as progressive primary infections.

Delayed hypersensitivity in tuberculosis

Tubercle bacilli are readily phagocytosed, but can then multiply within mononuclear cells and resist digestion. This *intracellular parasitism* is associated with the development of *delayed hypersensitivity* (cell-mediated immunity), and of activated macrophages with increased ability to kill ingested bacilli.

Delayed hypersensitivity modifies the host response to a second challenge from tubercle bacilli, and differentiates primary from post-primary lesions. *Koch* recognized the phenomenon a century ago. He demonstrated that inoculation of tubercle bacilli into a guinea pig already suffering from a primary lesion, with caseating lymph nodes and disseminated infection, resulted in only a small superficial lesion at the site of the second inoculation – which healed rapidly without lymph node enlargement.

Skin tests in human infection: delayed hypersensitivity can be demonstrated by the *tuberculin test*. This is the intradermal inoculation of purified protein derivative (a purified filtrate from cultures of *M. tuberculosis*), either by multiple puncture (*Heaf test*) or by intradermal injection by syringe (*Mantoux test*). Result:

- Positive test (indicating delayed hypersensitivity) produces induration, followed by papule formation after 24–28 h.
- Negative test: no reaction.

Diagnosis

Specimens:

- *Respiratory*: *sputum* – if none available, laryngeal swab, bronchial washings or from gastric lavage
- *Meningitis*: CSF

- *Bone and joint*: samples removed at operation or by aspiration
- *Renal*: early morning urine (i.e. the 'overnight' urine voided on waking)
- *Repeated specimens*: three are usually necessary, especially with suspected respiratory and renal tuberculosis.

Laboratory diagnosis

During the last decade new techniques have been developed for rapid diagnosis which allow culture and identification of *M. tuberculosis* within 14–21 days, and antibiotic sensitivity within 1 month of receipt of specimen.

The following methods are used:

- *Direct microscopy*: detection of typical bacilli in a smear stained with Ziehl–Neelsen (Fig. 14.2) or auramine confirms a diagnosis of tuberculosis in most cases. Care is necessary with urinary deposits, however, as these may contain other types of acid-fast bacilli (smegma bacilli).
- *Culture*: a more sensitive method of detecting *M. tuberculosis* than microscopy which, even if positive, should always be followed by culture for antibiotic sensitivity test. Culture specimens on suitable solid media, e.g. Löwenstein–Jensen and liquid media. New rapid liquid culture isolation systems which are automated detect growth at an earlier stage and can also perform rapid antibiotic sensitivity tests.
- *Molecular methods*: increasingly being introduced for:
  (a) *direct detection* of tubercle bacilli in clinical specimens by PCR assay

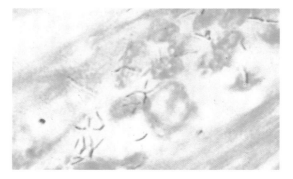

Fig. 14.2 *Mycobacterium tuberculosis* in sputum, stained with Ziehl–Neelsen stain (approx. × 1000)

(b) *typing*, e.g. PCR restriction enzyme assay
(c) *drug resistance*: by amplification of resistance genes.

Treatment

The discovery of streptomycin in 1944 revolutionized the treatment of tuberculosis. However, resistant strains emerge readily, and combinations of two or more drugs are used to minimize this risk. Treatment is both a personal and a public health measure. Directly observed treatment should be used for patients with a high risk of non-compliance and/or multidrug resistant (MDR) strains: resistance to isoniazid and rifampicin. Several national and local guidelines are available.

Recommended therapy for pulmonary infection

A combination of:

- Isoniazid ⎫
- Rifampicin ⎬ for 2 months
- Pyrazinamide ⎭

(Add ethambutol or streptomycin if high risk of MDR TB)

followed by:

- Isoniazid ⎫
- Rifampicin ⎬ for a further 4 months.

Treatment should be individualized with regard to the site and severity of disease and patient's immune status, e.g. prolonged treatment may be required for non-pulmonary infections (see Chapter 10).

Monitor:

- Side-effects due to drug toxicity
- Clinical, microbiological and radiological response. Failure to respond and positive cultures after 3 months may be due to: non-compliance, MDR strain or non-absorption. If MDR strain is suspected add two or more second-line drugs, e.g. ciprofloxacin, cycloserine, capreomycin or ethionamide.

Epidemiology

Route of infection: inhalation of infected respiratory secretions.
Reservoirs of infection: patients with 'open phthisis': tubercle bacilli are coughed up in the sputum.

Bovine tuberculosis: formerly common in cattle in Britain, and transmissible to humans through drinking infected milk. Now rare in the UK following the eradication of tuberculin-positive herds and *pasteurization* of milk.

Occupation: increased risk of tuberculosis in workers exposed to inhalation of stone or metal dust, such as quarrymen, blasters and tin miners, especially if there is contamination with silica, and healthcare workers.

Age incidence: formerly largely a disease of childhood, tuberculosis is now not uncommon in the elderly.

Race: Black people and Native Americans are more susceptible to tuberculosis than Caucasians; in the UK, the disease is especially common in Asian immigrants.

Immunocompromised patients, especially those infected with HIV.

Tuberculosis in HIV patients

Of the estimated 20 million people in the world infected with HIV, up to a half are coinfected with *M. tuberculosis*, often MDR strains. In 1987 the AIDS Case Definition was modified to include extrapulmonary tuberculosis in any HIV-seropositive patient.

Most cases are: *reactivation* – usually earlier than other opportunistic infections

Primary: not uncommon, patients are extremely susceptible to tuberculosis, and infection can be rapid and overwhelming: these highly infectious patients may be sources of infection to others, leading to further cases of *reinfection* and sometimes to institutional outbreaks.

Treatment

Often difficult, owing to:

• Higher rate of relapse: may require prolonged treatment
• MDR strains
• Interaction with antiretroviral agents
• Malabsorption
• Poor compliance.

Prevention and control

BCG (Bacille Calmette–Guérin) vaccine: see Chapter 39.

Control measures: to reduce the risk of person-to-person transmission should include:

- Nursing of hospitalized patients with open tuberculosis in respiratory isolation units until non-infectious
- Prompt notification of all cases to public health authority
- Consider HIV testing (with consent) for patients with tuberculosis.

LEPROSY (HANSEN'S DISEASE)

The scourge of the ancient world, and still afflicting millions of patients, mainly in Asia and Africa. Now, the outlook has been revolutionized by the introduction of effective treatment.

Clinical features

Leprosy is a slow, chronic and progressive infection affecting mainly the skin, where lesions present as nodules or thickened patches, sometimes with loss of pigmentation. Thickening of the peripheral nerves, with anaesthesia, is common: this leads to trophic changes in the tissues of the extremities (owing to repeated trauma as a result of loss of sensation) and so to the distressing mutilation characteristic of the disease (Fig. 14.3). Lesions affect mainly the skin and exposed, cooler extremities, such as the nose and ears.

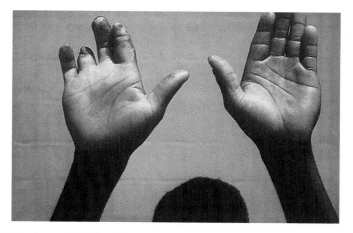

Fig. 14.3 Leprosy. Mutilation of fingers owing to trophic changes associated with anaesthesia caused by infection of peripheral nerves.

Causal organism: *Mycobacterium leprae*.
Incubation period: long, usually 3–5 years.
Three main forms of leprosy, depending on the patient's immunity, are recognized:

1. **Lepromatous (multibacillary)** leprosy: numerous bacilli are present in the lesions; sensory skin nerves are affected, causing 'glove and stocking' anaesthesia, with skin lesions causing nodules and diffuse thickening, and the characteristic 'leonine facies'. This form of leprosy is a systemic disease, with *M. leprae* spreading via the bloodstream: amyloidosis is a common complication.
2. **Tuberculoid (paucibacillary)** leprosy: the lesions are localized to the skin and peripheral nerves, with anaesthesia. There are only scanty *M. leprae* in the lesions, which tend to be benign, and the disease is often self-healing.
3. **Borderline leprosy**: the majority of patients have clinical features in between lepromatous and tuberculoid forms.

Delayed hypersensitivity mainly determines the clinical type of disease produced: patients with a high degree of hypersensitivity develop the tuberculoid form; in those with no, or only a low degree of, cell-mediated immunity the disease tends to be lepromatous.

Diagnosis

Specimens: skin biopsy or scrapings from lesions in the nasal mucosa.

Direct demonstration of acid-fast bacilli in smears or sections from lesions.

Propagation in the laboratory: *M. leprae* does not grow on artificial media in the laboratory; it can be cultivated in vivo by inoculation of armadillos, and into the footpads of mice. Culture is not used for diagnosis.

Treatment

- Dapsone
- Rifampicin
- Clofazimine

Triple therapy is required for lepromatous (multibacillary leprosy): duration at least 1 year.

Tuberculoid (paucibacillary) leprosy: give rifampicin and dapsone for 6 months.

There is controversy with regard to these WHO-recommended shorter regimens. Longer-duration treatment may result in more successful outcomes.

Minocycline, clarithromycin and ofloxacin are also useful alternatives.

Epidemiology

Spread in the community is slow.

Leprosy is often subclinical, and although patients with lepromatous leprosy shed numerous organisms from the nose, the incidence of disease in contacts is low. Leprosy is potentially quite infectious, but has a low expression of disease in infected people: the route of infection is probably mainly inhalation. Inoculation from soil may also be a possible transmission route. The incubation period is long – often years.

Geographic distribution is widespread (10 million cases worldwide), especially in tropical climates. The disease is also found in the southern United States and in Mediterranean Europe.

Control

The traditional horror of the disease may prevent early cases getting treatment. Hospitalization may be indicated at the start of treatment, but thereafter patients regarded as non-infectious can resume their normal activities.

Vaccine: BCG vaccine may offer a degree of protection.

DISEASES DUE TO ATYPICAL MYCOBACTERIA

Atypical mycobacteria, or MOTT (mycobacteria other than tubercle bacilli), form an ill-defined group of mycobacteria usually found as saprophytes in soil or water. Their laboratory characteristics differ from those of *M. tuberculosis*: for example, many produce pigment on culture, and grow at lower or sometimes higher temperatures. Also, their pathogenicity and infectivity are much lower.

Diseases

- *Pulmonary*:
  1. *Patients with AIDS*: most frequent opportunistic infections were due to *M. avium* complex (MAC), i.e. *M. avium* and

M. intracellulare (and possibly *M. scrofulaceum*). Infections occurred in up to 43% of patients and were often disseminated (see Fig. 31.1). Recently marked reduction in MAC infections owing to potent antiretroviral therapy.

2. *Non-AIDS patients*: infections due to MAC, *M. malmoense* and *M. kansasii*. Species prevalence varies with different geographical areas.

• *Cervical adenitis*: usually seen in children; can be due to *M. tuberculosis*, but also to MOTT such as *M. scrofulaceum*.
• *Skin ulcers*: e.g. 'fish-tank granuloma' and 'swimming-pool granuloma': due to *M. marinum*; occur in tropical countries. Progressive ulcers may be due to *M. ulcerans*.
• *Catheter-related infections*: associated with long-term catheters or shunts.

Treatment

Initial therapy: standard antituberculous drugs, but resistance is common. Clarythromycin is effective against *M. avium* complex; rifabutin is used for prophylaxis in AIDS patients.

The choice of drug combinations depends on the results of laboratory sensitivity tests. The identity of the isolate may indicate appropriate treatment, because some species have a predictable sensitivity pattern.

Epidemiology

Little is known. Infections due to MAC in AIDS patients may have been acquired from potable water or food. There is no evidence of person-to-person transmission.

15 Infections of bone and joint

Infections of both children and adults. Delay in diagnosis and inadequate treatment can result in protracted illness, with permanent disability.

The four main diseases are:

- Osteomyelitis
- Septic arthritis
- Infection of prosthetic joints
- Reactive arthritis.

OSTEOMYELITIS

Infection of bone and medullary cavity; may recur after treatment, which is therefore said to *arrest* rather than *cure* the infection.

Classification: can be based either *anatomically* or on *pathogenesis*:

- Haematogenous
- Contiguous-focus: *with* or *without vascular insufficiency*.

Infection can be *acute* or may progress to *chronic* disease.

Haematogenous osteomyelitis

Clinical features

Children: usually under 10 years old, present with *acute* metaphyseal disease. The metaphyseal region presents an ideal bacterial 'seeding' area: unusual end-artery capillary system forming venous sinusoids of slow-moving blood lacking in phagocytes.

The classic sites are the distal femur, proximal tibia and proximal humerus (Fig. 15.1).

Presentation: bone pain, with fever and local tenderness: the child is reluctant to move the affected limb. There may be a history of preceding mild trauma to the involved bone. Neonates may have no localizing features.

Causal organisms: *Staphylococcus aureus* (most common in all ages), *Streptococcus pyogenes*, *Haemophilus influenzae* (decreasing incidence since the introduction of vaccine); coliforms and group B streptococci in neonates.

Source: not always apparent; sometimes a septic focus elsewhere, e.g. a boil.

Adults: infection usually secondary to a distant focus elsewhere, e.g. infected injection site in intravenous drug user (IVDU). The diaphysis is involved in infection of the long bones, but more commonly the infection involves the vertebral and, in IVDU, the pubic and clavicular bones, often extending into the joint cavity.

Presentation: often non-specific pain and vague symptoms, but can also present with acute site-specific symptoms.

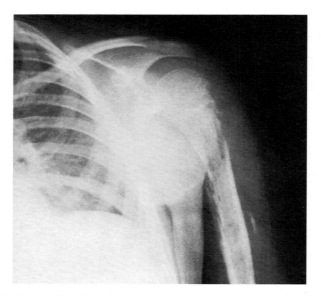

Fig. 15.1 Osteomyelitis of the upper humerus, showing bone destruction. (Reproduced with permission from Abbott Laboratories *Slide Atlas of Infectious Diseases*, 1982, Gower Medical Publishing, London. Photograph courtesy of Professor H. Lambert.)

Causal organisms: *S. aureus* (most common); *Pseudomonas aeruginosa*, coliforms, anaerobes, *S. pyogenes*, *Candida* spp.; *Salmonella* spp., and pneumococcus in patients with sickle cell anaemia.

Contiguous-focus osteomyelitis

Infection at any age may follow *direct contamination* of exposed bone:

Without vascular insufficiency, e.g.:

• After major trauma (compound fracture)
• Animal and human bites ('clenched-fist' injury)
• Puncture wound to calcaneum through soft 'training shoes'
• Extension of septic arthritis
• Orthopaedic surgical infections: may be device related, e.g. fixator sites.

Causal organism: *S. aureus* (including MRSA) is most common. *P. aeruginosa* (training shoes), *Pasteurella multocida* (bites), streptococci, anaerobes, coliforms. Infections are often polymicrobial.

With vascular insufficiency: predisposing conditions include peripheral vascular disease and diabetes. Small bones of the feet usually affected. Difficult to diagnose and treat.

Causal organisms: usually polymicrobial: *S. aureus* (including MRSA), coliforms, streptococci and anaerobes.

Chronic osteomyelitis

All forms of osteomyelitis can progress to chronic disease.

Presentation: pain; bone destruction, with the formation of sequestrum and discharging sinuses or enclosement by new bone formation: involucrum. May also present as Brodie's abscess (late, localized abscess) or progress to involve adjacent joint or distant spread, e.g. endocarditis.

Causal organisms: as above, but also other uncommon causes: *Mycobacterium tuberculosis*, *Brucella* spp. and actinomycosis (usually involving dental infections).

Laboratory diagnosis

Isolation of the causal organism, with antibiotic sensitivity tests, confirms the clinical diagnosis and directs treatment, but not always possible.

Culture:

- *Blood*: positive in many haematogenous cases; several cultures may be necessary.
- *Pus*: collected from the diseased bone, either by needle aspiration or by bone biopsy at open operation, particularly in cases of chronic contiguous-focus osteomyelitis. Culture of sinus tract is unreliable.

Haematology: in acute cases: a polymorphonuclear leukocytosis, raised ESR and C-reactive protein (CRP). Useful for monitoring treatment progress.

Radiology: imaging techniques: radionuclide, CT, magnetic resonance can help identify complex infections, e.g. diabetic foot.

Treatment

General: *Antibiotic treatment* is normally effective, and should be started early. Initial empirical treatment should be parenteral, high dose and targeted against *S. aureus*: flucloxacillin (with the addition of gentamicin if Gram-negative bacilli suspected). Later the choice will depend on culture and sensitivity.

Surgery: is essential to drain pus, remove sequestra, obliterate any dead space and restore vascular supply. A variety of orthopaedic procedures, e.g. bone grafting, stabilization of fractures, have an important role in management.

Specific: antibiotic choice should take into consideration bactericidal activity, bone penetration and route of administration (initially parenteral; later switch to oral).

- *S. aureus*: flucloxacillin; plus either gentamicin, clindamycin, fusidic acid or rifampicin (the latter three have excellent bone penetration): combination therapy preferred. MRSA strains: vancomycin; plus either fusidic acid or rifampicin
- Streptococci (group A, B, pneumococci): penicillin or clindamycin
- *H. influenzae*: ampicillin or ceftriaxone or ciprofloxacin
- Coliforms, *Salmonella*: ciprofloxacin or ceftriaxone
- *P. aeruginosa*: ciprofloxacin and gentamicin: combination preferred
- Anaerobes: metronidazole or clindamycin
- Tuberculous, Brucella, actinomycosis osteomyelitis: see relevant chapters.

Note: Treatment must be continued for up to 6 weeks.

SEPTIC ARTHRITIS

Infection of the joint space, usually seen as:

1. A complication of septicaemia, especially if there is pre-existing joint disease – particularly rheumatoid arthritis
2. An extension of osteomyelitis, or other infection near to the joint
3. Infection following intra-articular injection, arthroscopy or orthopaedic surgery, especially insertion of joint prostheses.

Clinical features

The most striking feature is severe pain, which limits movement of the affected joint: in general only one joint is involved, the most common being the knee. The onset may be sudden, with fever, swelling and redness over the joint. Crippling sequelae are common, despite antibiotic therapy.

Causal organisms: similar to those responsible for osteomyelitis, *S. aureus* being the most common, but in addition *Neisseria gonorrhoeae* (an important cause in sexually active adults, especially women), *Neisseria meningitidis*, *Mycoplasma hominis*, *Ureaplasma urealyticum* and *Borrelia burgdorferi*.

Laboratory diagnosis

Examination of fluid aspirated from the joint. *Direct Gram film*: observe for polymorphs and bacteria; the appearance may allow a presumptive diagnosis and advice regarding immediate chemotherapy. *Culture*: on a variety of media to isolate the causal pathogen.

Blood culture: positive in 30–60% of cases.

Culture of specimens from any other infected site, e.g. throat, genital tract, meninges. If tuberculosis is suspected, examine sputum and urine.

Serological tests for brucellosis and Lyme disease.

Molecular methods: detection of bacterial DNA in synovial fluid, e.g. *B. burgdorferi*, *M. hominis*, *N. gonorrhoeae*.

Treatment

Antibiotic therapy on a 'best-guess' basis should be started as soon as diagnostic specimens have been taken. When a causal organism has been isolated, the drug of choice is the same as for osteomyelitis. For treatment of specific pathogens, e.g. Lyme borreliosis, *N. gonorrhoeae*, refer to the relevant chapters.

INFECTION IN PROSTHETIC JOINTS

The insertion of artificial joints, usually hip or knee, has a high long-term success rate (over 90%): failure is due to either mechanical loosening or infection. Infection causes considerable morbidity and a major financial burden on healthcare systems. The introduction of inert material predisposes to infection, often with organisms of low pathogenicity. Major risk factors are rheumatoid arthritis, diabetes, malnutrition and obesity.

Clinical features

Infections may present as:

- *Early* fulminant, with haematoma or wound sepsis, usually within a month of operation: difficult to distinguish between superficial and deep involvement.
- *Delayed* indolent low-grade painful infection, within first year after surgery. Symptoms similar to those of aseptic loosening.

Source of infections: contamination of the site at the time of operation, with bacteria from the patient's skin or from the surgical team, by contact or via the theatre air.

- *Late-onset* septic arthritis (usually after 2 years): owing to organisms settling in the implant from a transient asymptomatic bacteraemia.

Causal organisms: *S. aureus* and coagulase-negative staphylococci are the most common. Occasionally anaerobes; 'coliforms' are usually colonizers from sinuses.

Laboratory diagnosis

Often impossible because of difficulty in accessing the joint. A combination of investigations is required:

Culture: perioperative surgical tissue (and surgical macroscopic opinion) are the most useful. Culture of sinus tract or superficial wound is *not* recommended

Haematology: ESR and CRP are usually elevated

Radiology: imaging studies may provide additional information.

Treatment

A complex issue consisting of antibiotic treatment, often a blind combination of vancomycin or cephalosporin and rifampicin; *and* replacement of the prosthesis as a one- or two-stage revision.

Prevention: a *key* issue: careful preparation of the skin site and scrupulous surgical technique: surgeons may wear special gowns and masks and operate in a laminar-flow ventilated theatre, which provides ultraclean air.

Antibiotic prophylaxis: perioperative, usually with a cephalosporin, often cefuroxime; probably the single most effective procedure. Prophylaxis for patients with prosthetic joints undergoing dental or other procedures is *not* recommended.

Infection rate with adequate precautions should be 1% or less.

REACTIVE ARTHRITIS

Acute arthritis of varying severity, affecting one or more joints, which develops 1–4 weeks after infection of either the genital or gastrointestinal tracts.

Due to an immunological mechanism: it is not the result of infection in the joint: culture of joint exudate is sterile.

Two forms of reactive arthritis are recognized:

1. **Post-sexual reactive arthritis**, in which the arthritis, usually accompanied by ocular inflammation (conjunctivitis, sometimes also iritis), presents after non-gonococcal urethritis – often caused by *Chlamydia trachomatis*. Almost all patients are males; the condition is common in the UK.

2. **Post-dysenteric reactive arthritis**, in which the arthritis presents after gastrointestinal infection with Gram-negative bacilli, such as shigella, salmonella, campylobacter or yersinia. Affects both men and women; patients may also develop urethritis or conjunctivitis. The condition is common in continental Europe, and is now being diagnosed more often in the UK.

Reiter's syndrome is a term used to describe patients who develop the triad of symptoms of arthritis, urethritis and conjunctivitis: much more common in post-sexual reactive arthritis.

Predisposing factor may be the antigen HLA-B27, present in 7% of the population but found in more than half of patients with reactive arthritis. Numerous hypotheses have been proposed to explain this apparent genetic predisposition, but the pathogenic mechanisms that link it with infection and arthritis remain speculative.

16 Bacterial zoonoses

Zoonoses are infections between vertebrate animals and humans. Many of those acquired by humans affect agricultural workers and veterinary surgeons, but the general public are also at risk, for example through contaminated meat and milk.

Table 16.1 lists the main bacterial zoonoses. Other zoonoses are caused by rickettsiae, chlamydiae, viruses, protozoa and fungi; animal ringworm is perhaps the commonest infection worldwide.

Domestic animals are more likely to be sources of infection than wild animals, owing to their closer contact with people. Table 16.2 shows the principal sources and routes of infection acquired from domestic animals.

Bacterial food poisoning caused by salmonella, campylobacter or *Escherichia coli* is by far the most common zoonosis in Britain. These infections, and tuberculosis due to *Mycobacterium bovis*, are described in Chapters 7 and 14, respectively. Although zoonoses such as brucellosis, anthrax and plague are very uncommon in the UK, they pose a public health challenge and are potential lethal agents of biological warfare.

BRUCELLOSIS

Although brucellosis is now a rare disease in the UK, it remains prevalent worldwide and is particularly common in the Mediterranean and Middle Eastern countries, and in parts of Africa and South America. In the UK there are 10–20 cases reported annually, mainly contracted abroad or acquired from imported dairy products.

Table 16.1   Bacterial zoonoses

Disease	Causal organism	Main animal host
Food poisoning	*Salmonella*	Cattle, poultry
Food poisoning	*Campylobacter* species	Poultry, other domestic animals
Food poisoning	*Escherichia coli* (VTEC)	Cattle
Tuberculosis	*Mycobacterium bovis*	Cattle
Brucellosis	*Brucella abortus*	Cattle
	Brucella melitensis	Goats, sheep
	Brucella suis	Pigs
	Brucella canis	Dogs
Anthrax	*Bacillus anthracis*	Cattle
Plague	*Yersinia pestis*	Rats
Mesenteric adenitis, enteritis	{ *Yersinia pseudotuberculosis* *Yersinia enterocolitica*	Various animals
Septic animal bite	*Pasteurella multocida*	Dogs, cats
Tularaemia	*Francisella tularensis*	Squirrels, other rodents
Leptospirosis	*Leptospira interrogans*	Rats, pigs, dogs, cattle
Lyme disease	*Borrelia burgdorferi*	Small mammals, deer
Listeriosis	*Listeria monocytogenes*	Various domestic and wild animals
Erysipeloid	*Erysipelothrix rhusiopathiae*	Pigs, fish, other animals
Rat-bite fever	*Streptobacillus moniliformis* *Spirillum minus*	Rats, mice
Cat-scratch disease	*Bartonella henselae*	Cats

Table 16.2   Domestic animals: sources and routes of infection

Source	Route	At risk
Infected animals	Contact, inoculation	Farm workers, veterinary surgeons, slaughtermen: may be associated with injury, animal and insect bites
Contaminated pastures, straw, dust, soil	Inhalation, contact	Farm workers, veterinary surgeons
Food: dairy products*, meat	Ingestion	General public
Hides, bones, other animal products	Contact inhalation	Industrial workers handling animal products; occasionally, general public

* Almost all milk retailed in the UK is heat treated. The sale of raw milk is no longer permitted in Scotland but, although discouraged, is not yet prohibited in England and Wales.

Brucellosis is a zoonosis primarily of domestic animals, causing a chronic, debilitating septicaemic disease leading to abortion. The causal *Brucella* species are named after Sir David Bruce, who discovered the cause of one form of the disease while serving in Malta.

Causal organisms: brucellae are small Gram-negative coccobacilli: the main species are listed in Table 16.1. Infection with *B. suis* and *B. canis* is less common than that due to *B. abortus* or *B. melitensis*.

Clinical features

Incubation period: 1–3 weeks, occasionally several months.

Signs and symptoms: *undulant fever*, a prolonged debilitating febrile illness with remissions and relapses, often persisting for months or even years. Symptoms are non-specific: sweating, anorexia, constipation, rigors, weakness and lassitude. 'Psychiatric morbidity' (usually depression) may overshadow physical symptoms. Brucellosis is a *septicaemic* illness: abortion is not a feature of human brucellosis. The spleen and lymph nodes are often enlarged, and there may be arthritis, orchitis and neuralgia.

Classification: into '*acute*' and '*chronic*' stages is arbitrary. Chronic brucellosis (symptoms for >1 year) is usually associated with persisting deep foci of infection.

Severity: brucellosis due to *B. melitensis* and *B. suis* tends to be a more severe disease than that due to *B. abortus*. Even before antibiotics, brucellosis had a low case fatality rate – around 2% – mostly due to infective endocarditis.

Pathogenesis

Route of infection: most infections acquired by:

- *Ingestion*: of unpasteurized contaminated dairy produce
- *Inhalation*: ⎫ of placental or uterine discharges
- *Inoculation*: ⎭ from infected animals.

NB: Animal tissues and products, such as placenta, uterus and milk, that are rich in *erythritol* (a growth factor for brucellae) can be heavily contaminated and highly infectious.

Spread in the body is analogous to that of *typhoid fever*: via lymphatics, replication within lymph nodes, and then wide haematogenous spread to organs and tissues.

Intracellular parasitism: brucellae have a particular tendency to persist intracellularly, notably in the reticuloendothelial system: this is the reason for the well-known difficulty in eradicating the infection by antibiotic therapy.

Diagnosis

Isolation: *culture* of blood, bone marrow and tissue fluids. Alert laboratory because of infection risk and need to maintain cultures for 6 weeks.

Positive blood cultures make certain the diagnosis of acute brucellosis, but numerous sets should be taken because the organism is difficult to isolate: *B. melitensis* is much more readily cultured than *B. abortus*.

Identification: by morphology, biochemical, serological and bacteriophage lysis.

Serology: diagnosis based on demonstration of high or rising titres of specific antibodies. Interpretation of results is often difficult. The most widely used test is:

Direct (standard) agglutination test: detects non-species specific Brucella antibodies, mainly IgM. Although no single antibody titre is absolutely diagnostic, a titre above 1:160 in patients from non-endemic areas, and above 1:640 from endemic areas, are regarded as positive. Lower titres (1:80), especially with relevant clinical symptoms from non-endemic areas, may be indicative of infection: serology should be repeated to demonstrate rising titres and further confirmatory tests (see below) performed.

False-negative: reactions due to *prozones* (i.e. absence of agglutination in low dilutions of serum which contain high levels of antibodies) are common.

False-positive: reactions may be due to cross-reactivity with antibodies to *Y. enterocolitica*, *F. tularensis* and *V. cholerae*. *Avoid* false reactions by diluting serum beyond 1:320.

Confirmatory tests:

- *Complement fixation test*: detects mainly IgG; a titre of 16 or more is significant.
- *ELISA* and *immunoradiometric assay* are also available.

Acute brucellosis: antibody levels are almost always high. IgM antibody levels rise within a week after infection and persist for years. IgG titres fall rapidly after successful treatment.

Chronic brucellosis: levels of IgG (but not IgM) are elevated: the complement fixation test may be positive and the direct agglutination test negative.

Treatment

Acute brucellosis should be cured if appropriate treatment is given promptly and continued for an adequate period. Monotherapy is ineffective. Give *doxycycline*, a tetracycline, for 6 weeks, with either *rifampicin* for the duration of treatment or *streptomycin* for the first 3 weeks of the course. In children co-trimoxazole and rifampicin should be used.

Control

Eradication: brucellosis was eradicated in cattle in the UK in 1981 by a policy of identifying affected herds and slaughtering infected animals.

Vaccination: effective vaccination of calves with a live attenuated *B. abortus* (RB51) and *B. melitensis* (strain Rev-1) is available. There is an urgent need for a safe vaccine for humans owing to the potential use of *Brucella* spp. for biological warfare.

ANTHRAX

Anthrax is a disease of animals which occasionally infects humans. Although a wide variety of animals are susceptible, anthrax is mainly a disease of herbivores, especially cattle and sheep.

Causal organism: *Bacillus anthracis*: a large, sporing, capsulated Gram-positive bacillus (Fig. 3.1).

Clinical features

Cutaneous anthrax, or malignant pustule, is due to direct inoculation of the skin from infected animals or animal products: an inflamed but painless lesion with surrounding oedema and a characteristic black eschar. Local lymph nodes are usually enlarged. If untreated it may progress to septicaemia, with death from overwhelming infection. In the UK almost all cases are of this type: about 11 per year were reported in the 1960s, but this has dwindled to an average of less than one annually.

Acquired in two ways:

- *Occupational*: the majority of cases, most often in those associated with the meat trade, but also in workers handling leather or wool, tanners, workers in bonemeal factories and in agriculture. Malignant pustule of the neck and shoulders was an occupational hazard of hide porters, caused by rubbing of infected hides carried on their backs.
- *Non-occupational*: occasionally affects the general public: formerly due to contact with infected shaving brushes, leather goods and clothes; now sometimes seen in amateur gardeners who use bonemeal.

Pulmonary anthrax – also called woolsorter's disease, a name indicating its mode of spread, via inhalation of spores by workers handling contaminated wool; now a rarity – a disease of the 19th century. A severe disease with high mortality.

Gastrointestinal anthrax – also a lethal disease: caused by ingestion of *B. anthracis* or its spores; fortunately very rare.

Pathogenesis

Long regarded as a classic example of a disease due purely to the invasive properties of the causal organism; however, *B. anthracis* is now known to produce three important toxins:

1. Oedema factor
2. Protective factor (antibody to this is responsible for immunity to the disease)
3. Lethal factor.

Diagnosis

Specimens: swab or sample of exudate from malignant pustule; sputum from suspected pulmonary anthrax.

Direct film: Gram-stained: observe typical large Gram-positive bacilli.

Culture: on ordinary media: observe growth of typical 'curled hair lock' colonies.

Treatment

Penicillin, erythromycin in patients hypersensitive to penicillin. Ciprofloxacin can be used as prophylaxis in those exposed to anthrax spores.

Animal anthrax

Animal anthrax is a rapidly fatal, septicaemic infection in which huge numbers of organisms are present in the blood and are shed in discharges from the body orifices. *Pastures* used by infected animals become contaminated with anthrax spores and may remain infective for many years.

Control

The decline in incidence of anthrax in occupational 'at-risk' groups is probably due to the introduction in 1965 of vaccination with an alum-precipitated toxoid, prepared from the protective factor – and to the wearing of protective clothing.

Animals suspected of being infected must be notified to the authorities. Dead animals must be disposed of by burning or, if this is not possible, by burying in quicklime; a careful check must be kept on the rest of the herd.

Animal products imported from countries where anthrax is a problem are subject to inspection and disinfection.

PLAGUE

Plague is a natural disease of rats which occasionally spreads to humans via the bite of infected fleas: one of the great epidemic diseases, it was the Black Death (which killed one-quarter of Europe's population in the 14th century) and the Great Plague of London and elsewhere in Britain during the mid-17th century. Plague still exists in endemic foci in Africa, India and the Far East.

Causal organism: *Yersinia pestis*, a small Gram-negative bacillus.

Clinical features

There are three forms of plague: bubonic, pneumonic and septicaemic.

1. *Bubonic plague*: the most common form: characterized by fever, prostration, mental confusion and enlargement, with profuse pus formation, of the inguinal glands to produce *buboes*. High mortality rate: about 50% in untreated cases. Not contagious – acquired by the bite of fleas.
2. *Pneumonic plague*: a rare but highly infectious form of plague, affecting the lungs. The route of infection is by inhalation of infected respiratory secretions: virtually always fatal.

3. *Septicaemic plague*: either bubonic or pneumonic plague may progress to an invariably fatal septicaemia characterized by haemorrhages: the Black Death was septicaemic plague.

Diagnosis

Isolation: *specimens*: needle aspirate of lymph node (bubo pus); sputum; blood culture.

Gram film: examine for Gram-negative bacilli, stained darker at the ends than in the middle (bipolar staining).

Culture: ordinary media.

Identification: biochemical and serological reactions.

Serology: demonstrate a fourfold rise in antibody titre against *Y. pestis*.

Treatment

Streptomycin; tetracycline or chloramphenicol are other effective drugs.

Epidemiology

Reservoir is mainly *urban* rats or *sylvatic* (wild) rats and other wild mammals; most human epidemics have been due to spread of the disease to urban rats.

Vector: the rat flea, *Xenopsylla cheopis*: plague spreads among rats via infected fleas, which transmit the disease during biting; the bacilli multiply in the flea, and are injected from its proventriculus when it bites and sucks blood again.

Spread: to humans by:

• bites from infected rat fleas
• rarely, person-to-person spread by inhalation of respiratory secretions.

Control

Urban plague: by quarantine, rat control and use of insecticides.

Sylvatic plague: difficult, owing to wild rodent reservoirs.

INFECTIONS WITH OTHER *YERSINIA* SPECIES

Gastrointestinal infection with *Yersinia enterocolitica* and *Yersinia pseudotuberculosis* is considered in Chapter 7.

PASTEURELLA INFECTIONS

Pasteurella multocida, also known as *P. septica*, is a commensal of the mouths of dogs and cats: it is a not uncommon cause of sepsis, which is sometimes severe, after bites by domestic animals.

TULARAEMIA

A plague-like disease spread from rodents, e.g. squirrels, in the USA and elsewhere – but not yet in the UK; due to *Francisella tularensis*, a small Gram-negative bacillus.

LEPTOSPIROSIS

Leptospires infect many different wild and domestic animals, rodents, cattle, dogs and pigs, which usually remain well. Leptospires are transmitted to humans by direct or indirect contact with animal urine. Entry of the pathogen is through skin cuts and abrasions, or via the nasopharynx or conjunctiva following bathing or accidental immersion in infected water – usually stagnant ponds or canals.

Human disease, often due to occupational contact, predominantly affects males and is most common in late summer and autumn. In an average year about 50 cases are diagnosed in the UK, with three deaths. Occupations most at risk are farmers, veterinary surgeons, abattoir workers and water sports enthusiasts. Formerly a disease of sewage workers and miners, but in recent years they have been protected by pest control and protective clothing.

Causal organism: *Leptospira* spp.: the species is traditionally divided into more than 200 serovars (see p. 96).

Clinical features

Incubation period: about 5–14 days.

Many infections are asymptomatic and detected only by serology. Three main clinical syndromes are recognized. All have an initial *septicaemic phase* lasting 3–7 days, presenting as an *influenzal illness* with notable features of myalgia and conjunctival suffusion. The majority of cases are self-limiting and diagnosis is rarely established.

There follows an *immune phase*, when leptospires have disappeared from the blood and antibodies begin to appear: characterized by signs of an acute *aseptic (lymphocytic) meningitis* (headache, vomiting and conjunctival suffusion).

The third syndrome of severe leptospirosis (*Weil's disease*), associated with hepatorenal failure and haemorrhages, is rare but potentially fatal and usually due to icterohaemorrhagiac infections.

Diagnosis

Isolation: difficult, and rarely accomplished.

Specimens: blood, CSF and urine during the first week of illness; urine (the sample *must* be fresh) during the second and third weeks of illness.

Inoculate and observe: a suitable serum-enriched liquid medium; for growth of leptospires.

Serology: the usual method of diagnosis: antibodies are not present in the first week of illness, but as a rule can be detected in the second and third weeks; initially of the IgM class, but IgG is developed later and may persist for years. Detection of IgG antibody can be taken as evidence of previous exposure.

1. *Screening tests using a genus-specific antigen*:
   • ELISA tests, which can be used to detect IgM or IgG
   • IHA: indirect haemagglutinin assay.
2. *Confirmation tests using serovar-specific antigens* – live suspensions of leptospires representative of those serovars prevalent in the area – in a *microscopic agglutination test*.

Demonstrate a rising titre to the infecting serovar in serial samples. Cross-reactions may be found in early tests; results from later samples are more specific and diagnostic.

Molecular methods: rapid detection of leptospiral DNA in serum, urine and CSF using PCR is highly sensitive.

Treatment

Penicillin for the treatment of moderate to severe infections. Ampicillin or doxycycline for mild cases.

Control

Prevention of occupational exposure by protective clothing and pest control.

Vaccination of livestock and dogs has reduced transmission.
Prophylaxis with doxycycline for those at risk is effective.

LYME DISEASE

A bacterial zoonosis with widespread clinical manifestations which usually follows an initial skin eruption, erythema migrans (EM). Although in 1909 EM was attributed to a tick bite, the bacterial cause was only established in the early 1980s.

Causal organism: a spirochaete, *Borrelia burgdorferi* and related European genospecies: *B. afzelii*, *B. garinii* and *B. japonica*. Geographic variability of clinical symptoms (*see below*) may be related to different genospecies.

Clinical features

EM starts as a red macule at the site of the tick bite: often associated with fever and malaise. It spreads to become an annular erythema with central clearing. Weeks or months later, in a proportion of patients there are early and late disseminated manifestations:

- *Nervous system*, e.g. chronic meningoencephalitis, peripheral neuritis; more common in Europe
- *Joints* – arthritis of large joints, often recurrent; common in USA, less so in UK
- *Heart* – myocarditis, pericarditis, conduction defects
- Skin, e.g. acrodermatitis chronica atrophicans, lymphocytoma; mainly in Europe.

Diagnosis

Often difficult: no single reliable test available.
  Serology: tests available:

- *ELISA*: screening test used for detection of IgM and IgG antibody in serum and CSF. Titres dependent on stage and treatment of disease. False-negative and -positive results often make interpretation difficult.
- *Western blot*: confirms positive ELISA test. Geographic strain variation may affect result.

Culture: unreliable, slow, and special media required.
  Molecular methods: DNA amplification by PCR, variable results possibly due to geographic strain variation.

Treatment

For EM: doxycycline, amoxycillin or azithromycin.

For later stages: cefotaxime or ceftriaxone are more effective.

Epidemiology

Reservoir of infection: field mice, voles and larger mammals, e.g. deer.

Route of infection: transmission by the bite of a hard tick, in Europe usually *Ixodes ricinus* and *I. persulcatus*.

Geographical distribution: hard body ticks live in temperate zones below an altitude of 1500 m: in UK, disease most common in the New Forest, Exmoor, East Anglia and the Scottish highlands.

At risk: farmers, forestry workers, walkers.

Control

Prevent: tick bites by protective clothing and insecticide.

Vaccine: offer to those at high risk. Works by inactivation of bacteria in the tick midgut by preformed antibody ingested from the victim's blood.

LISTERIOSIS

Formerly a rare disease: a tenfold increase in incidence in 10 years resulted in over 300 cases being recorded in the UK in 1988, but the incidence has declined sharply, by almost two-thirds, since then. The increase was thought to be real and not due to better diagnosis.

Causal organism: *Listeria monocytogenes*, a diphtheroid-like Gram-positive bacillus.

Clinical features

Mild or inapparent infection – as a non-specific febrile illness – is probably not uncommon in the general population.

Non-pregnancy associated listeriosis is rare in the healthy: usually found in the immunocompromised or elderly, who develop either a septicaemia or a meningoencephalitis.

Pregnancy-associated listeriosis affects the fetus: in early pregnancy results in abortion; later, causes stillbirth or neonatal septicaemia/meningitis. Maternal infection often asymptomatic (see Chapter 38).

Mortality of fully developed disease at any age is high – about 30%.

Diagnosis

Isolation: *specimens*: blood cultures, CSF, swabs from genital tract.

Culture: on to blood agar. *Observe*: small colonies surrounded by a narrow zone of β-haemolysis.

Identification: small Gram-positive bacilli, like corynebacteria but actively motile when grown in broth at 25°C. Use biochemical tests to distinguish from other listeria.

Treatment

Ampicillin, or ampicillin and gentamicin.

Epidemiology

Source: *L. monocytogenes* is widely distributed in nature: in soil, silage, water and a wide range of animal hosts (cattle, pigs, rodents, birds, fish); asymptomatic human faecal carriage is not uncommon.

Infection is probably foodborne: often sporadic, but food-associated outbreaks incriminating coleslaw, milk, pâté and several types of soft cheese have been reported. Listeria can multiply slowly at 6°C and is therefore able to grow in refrigerated foods.

Reduction in incidence since 1988 is probably due to 'at-risk' groups following advice to avoid pâtés, soft cheeses and cook–chill foods; also to increased vigilance by the food industry.

ERYSIPELOID

An inflammatory lesion of the skin, usually of the fingers, hand and forearm, resembling erysipelas but due to a Gram-positive bacillus, *Erysipelothrix rhusiopathiae* – the cause of swine erysipelas, but also found in other animals, birds and fish.

Occupational hazard of meat and fish handlers, veterinary surgeons.

Treatment

Penicillin or tetracycline.

RAT-BITE FEVER

Includes two separate, rare diseases transmitted to humans through rat bites: sometimes seen in laboratory workers handling experimental rats.

Causal organism: either *Streptobacillus moniliformis*, or *Spirillum minus*, a spiral organism.

Treatment

Penicillin or tetracycline (for both organisms).

BARTONELLA INFECTIONS (see also Chapter 18)

Cat-scratch disease

Clinically, a benign granulomatous disease of skin and sometimes internal organs, with regional lymph node involvement. Lesions may progress to abscess formation. Children and adolescents are usually affected. The condition is well recognized in the USA, but rarely diagnosed in the UK.

Cause: *Bartonella henselae*, a rickettsia-like organism. Acquired after close contact with apparently healthy cats, often kittens; normally, a history of scratch or bite.

Diagnosis: *serology*: by immunofluorescence test for antibodies to *B. henselae*.

Culture: on enriched blood agar or in Vero cell cultures.

Histology: still often diagnosed by histological examination of biopsied lymph node.

Bacillary angiomatosis

A rare complication of AIDS and some other immunosuppressed states, usually due to infection with *B. henselae*. The purplish lesions can be confused clinically with those due to Kaposi's sarcoma.

Bacillary angiomatosis can also be caused by *B. quintana*, which was responsible for trench fever in both World Wars. This epidemic infection, transmitted by the body louse, was characterized by relapsing fever and crops of erythematous maculopapules on the trunk.

17 Chlamydial diseases

Chlamydiae are small Gram-negative bacteria that, like viruses, grow only within living cells. In the human body they invade and replicate in cells of columnar epithelium. They are not restricted to human populations, being widespread in nature and in different species of animal.

There are four main species of chlamydia that are pathogenic for humans:

1. *Chlamydia trachomatis*
2. *Chlamydophila* * *pneumoniae*
3. *Chlamydophila* * *psittaci*
4. *Chlamydophila* * *abortus*.

* These three species have recently been placed in a separate genus, *Chlamydophila*.

Although distinguishable by immunofluorescence, all chlamydiae share a common group antigen in complement fixation test. Table 17.1 lists their serotypes and associated diseases.

CHLAMYDIA TRACHOMATIS

The most important human chlamydia and the cause of a variety of oculogenital syndromes.

Genital infection

The most common sexually transmitted infection (see also Chapter 13), causing non-specific urethritis in males and, although usually asymptomatic on primary infection in women,

254

Table 17.1 Chlamydia

Species	Hosts	Main diseases	Serotypes
Chlamydia trachomatis	Humans	Oculogenital	D, E, F, G, H, I, J, K
		Trachoma	A, B, Ba, C
		Lymphogranuloma venereum	L1, 2, 3
Chlamydophila pneumoniae	Humans	Pneumonia	–
Chlamydophila psittaci	Birds	Psittacosis, ornithosis	–
Chlamydophila abortus	Sheep, goats	Abortion, stillbirth, severe generalized infection in pregnancy	–

responsible in the longer term for pelvic inflammatory disease, with consequent problems of infertility and risk of ectopic pregnancy.

Caused by *C. trachomatis* serotypes D–K.

Clinical features

1. *Males*: acute urethritis with epididymitis, prostatitis and risk of proctitis in homosexual males; rarely, followed by arthritis and Reiter's syndrome (a triad of urethritis, arthritis and conjunctivitis) in under 1% of cases.
2. *Females*: infection commonly involves the cervix but can later spread, with the development of salpingitis, endometritis and, rarely, perihepatitis (Curtis–Fitz-Hugh syndrome).

Treatment: tetracycline, azithromycin, erythromycin.

Ocular infection

C. trachomatis causes two types of eye infection:

- Inclusion conjunctivitis
- Trachoma.

Inclusion conjunctivitis

1. *Neonatal*: acquired during birth by passage through the mother's infected birth canal; acute follicular conjunctivitis with

profuse mucopurulent discharge appears some 5–12 days after birth.

2. *In older children and adults*: subacute follicular conjunctivitis with discharge and ipsilateral preauricular lymphadenopathy; older children often acquire infection at swimming pools, probably due to indirect contact from genital infection: also seen in sexually active adults as a result of spread from infected genital areas.

Cause: *C. trachomatis* types D–K.

Treatment: in infants, erythromycin or sulphamethoxazole; in adults, tetracycline or doxycycline.

Trachoma

A major cause of blindness in the world and a scourge of tropical countries; tragically, a cause of needless suffering because it responds well to treatment. Spread is from case to case by contact, contaminated fomites and flies.

Clinical features: a severe follicular conjunctivitis (Fig. 17.1) with pannus (i.e. invasion of the cornea by blood vessels): corneal scarring, which results in blindness, is a common sequela.

Cause: *C. trachomatis* serotypes A, B, Ba and C.

Treatment: topical or oral tetracycline, erythromycin, azithromycin.

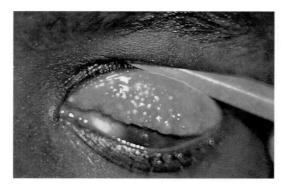

Fig. 17.1   Trachoma, showing severe follicular hyperplasia and papillary hyperplasia in the conjunctiva. (Photograph courtesy of the late Josef Sowa, reproduced, with the permission of the Stationery Office, from MRC Special Research Series Report No. 308.)

Pneumonia

C. trachomatis (serotypes D–K) also causes pneumonia in neonates, often (but not always) following chlamydial conjunctivitis.

Clinical features: affected infants develop symptoms usually some weeks after birth, often preceded by upper respiratory symptoms; the pneumonia is relatively mild, with dry spasmodic cough and rapid breathing: the infant is not usually febrile. Chest X-rays show diffuse infiltration of the lungs.

Treatment: erythromycin.

LYMPHOGRANULOMA VENEREUM (see also Chapter 13)

A sexually transmitted disease, common in tropical countries but almost unknown in temperate climates.

Clinical features

In both males and females: after primary infection with a papule or ulcer on the genitalia, there is swelling and inflammation of the local lymph glands leading to suppuration; complications include strictures and fistulas.

Cause: *C. trachomatis* types L1, 2 and 3.

Treatment: tetracycline, doxycycline, erythromycin: possibly also sulphamethoxazole.

Diagnosis of *C. trachomatis* infections

Chlamydia detection: in swabs, smears, scrapings, by immuno-fluorescence or ELISA using monoclonal antibody: DNA technology is now increasingly being used for this.

Isolation: in specialized tissue cultures with detection of chlamydial inclusions using monoclonal antibody.

Note: In cases of suspected child abuse it is essential to try and isolate chlamydiae.

Serology (less useful for diagnosis but important for epidemiological investigation): by immunofluorescence, but this is type specific so that sera must be tested against the appropriate range of serotypes (i.e. D, E, F, G, H, I, J and K); can also detect the presence of IgM antibody as an indicator of recent infection.

Complement fixation tests: genus specific, i.e. only detect antibody to chlamydiae in general, but often useful, especially in lymphogranuloma venereum.

CHLAMYDOPHILA PNEUMONIAE

A cause of acute respiratory disease worldwide.

Clinical features

Many infections are symptomless and reinfection appears to be common.

Respiratory disease: most often mild atypical pneumonia, with sore throat and hoarseness, cough and fever. Chest X-ray shows bilateral infiltrates.

A possible association with coronary artery disease has been described – still under investigation.

Epidemiology

Adults show a variable but quite high prevalence of antibody to *C. pneumoniae* – around 20–70% – showing that infection is common in the community. Children under 5 years old rarely have antibody.

Outbreaks of pneumonia due to *C. pneumoniae* have been reported.

Diagnosis

Serology: immunofluorescence test.

Treatment: tetracycline, erythromycin.

CHLAMYDOPHILA PSITTACI

C. psittaci infects a variety of birds – not only psittacine birds – from which infection can be transmitted to humans. Infected birds often, but not always, show signs of disease called *ornithosis* – if in psittacine birds (e.g. budgerigars and parrots) the disease is known as *psittacosis*. Most human cases are acquired from budgerigars or parrots, but other birds, such as pigeons, ducks and other domestic flocks, can also be a source of infection.

In Britain, psittacosis is relatively rare. Outbreaks of infection involving veterinary surgeons and workers in processing plants have been traced to infected flocks of ducks.

Clinical features

Incubation period: 7–10 days.

Signs and symptoms: most often a primary atypical pneumonia, with fever, cough and dyspnoea, and extensive opacities in the lung fields on chest X-ray; headache is common. Severity ranges from a mild influenza-like illness to a severe disease with generalized systemic features; rarely, infective endocarditis, as well as myocarditis and pericarditis; renal involvement and disseminated intravascular coagulation are occasional complications. Males are affected more often than females.

Case fatality rate: low (probably less than 1%).

Treatment: tetracycline, erythromycin.

Diagnosis

Serology: immunofluorescence or complement fixation test – look for rising titre against chlamydial common group antigen: less sensitive, but still widely used in diagnosis.

CHLAMYDOPHILA ABORTUS

A natural infection of sheep and goats (and other domestic animals) which affects pregnant animals, causing abortion. Occasionally transmitted to pregnant farmers' wives, causing severe generalized infection with abortion in the first trimester – or stillbirth when infection is at a later stage. Can be life-threatening. Pregnant farm workers must avoid helping at lambing or handling lambs; contaminated clothing of other farm workers is another possible source of infection (see Chapter 38).

Treatment: erythromycin intravenously; possibly add chloramphenicol if response slow.

18 Rickettsial diseases, bartonellosis

Rickettsiae are not viruses but are atypical bacteria that replicate only intracellularly: like chlamydiae, they are traditionally diagnosed in virus laboratories. The most notorious rickettsial disease is typhus – an epidemic scourge in conditions of poverty and malnutrition (e.g. the German concentration camps of the Second World War) and of armies in the field. Typhus played a major part in the disintegration of Napoleon's army in the retreat from Moscow.

There are three genera within the family of rickettsiaceae:

1. *Rickettsia*
2. *Coxiella*
3. *Ehrlichia.*

RICKETTSIAE

Diseases due to *Rickettsia* are transmitted by arthropod vectors, which are often also the reservoirs of infection. Their distribution is worldwide (although not found in the UK). The main diseases, together with their reservoirs, vectors and geographical distribution, are shown in Table 18.1.

Clinical features

Incubation period: 1–2 weeks.

Signs and symptoms: acute febrile illness, with rash a common feature; malaise, which may be severe, progressing to prostration; chills, myalgia, headache; haemorrhage and petechiae are common with the spotted fevers. Lymphadenopathy is seen in boutonneuse fever and scrub typhus.

Table 18.1 Diseases due to *Rickettsia* species

Disease	Causal organism	Reservoir	Vector*	Geographical distribution
Typhus group				
Typhus	*R.⁺ prowazekii*	Humans Flying squirrels	Lice	Americas, Africa Asia
Murine typhus	*R. typhi*	Rats, mice	Fleas	Worldwide
Scrub typhus	*O.# tsutsugamushi*	Mites, rodents	Mites	Far East
Spotted fever group				
Rocky Mountain spotted fever	*R. rickettsii*	Rodents, dogs	Ticks	Americas
Boutonneuse fever	*R. conorii*	Rodents, dogs	Ticks	Mediterranean, Africa
African tick-bite fever	*R. africae*	Rodents	Ticks	Sub-Saharan Africa
Queensland tick typhus	*R. australis*	Rodents, marsupials	Ticks	Australia
North Asian tick fever	*R. sibirica*	Rodents	Ticks	Asian part of former Soviet Union, China, Mongolia
Rickettsial pox	*R. akari*	Mice	Mites	USA, former Soviet Union

* Ticks also act as reservoirs, maintaining the infectious cycle in nature.
Note: *R.⁺* = *Rickettsia* species; *O.#* = *Orientia* species.

Rash: a common, but not invariable, feature – usually maculopapular, except with rickettsial pox, in which the lesions are vesicular.

Eschar: a skin ulcer with blackened centre, at the site of the infected bite, is a particular feature of boutonneuse and African tickborne fevers and scrub typhus.

Recurrent infection (Brill–Zinsser disease) is a recurrent form of typhus: recurrences may be years after the primary illness and are usually mild.

Fatality: varies, but rickettsial diseases are often severe. Case fatality rate in untreated typhus is from 10 to 40%, and in untreated Rocky Mountain spotted fever around 13–25%: most of the other rickettsial diseases have lower fatality rates.

Pathology: the principal site of infection is the vascular endothelium, causing rash, inflammatory lesions, thrombosis in small blood vessels.

Epidemiology

Geographical distribution: rickettsial diseases exist as endemic foci in the areas listed in Table 18.1.

Transmission: via an infected vector, either by a bite or by scratching faeces from an infected vector into skin abrasions.

Epidemics: rare nowadays; the most important – at least historically – is typhus, classically a disease of war and famine.

Vector control: has been effective in cutting short epidemics of typhus.

Bacteriology

Coccobacilli, just visible by light microscopy: replicate intracellularly by binary fission: grow in the yolk sac of the chick embryo and in some specialized cell cultures.

Diagnosis

Serology: by immunofluorescence, ELISA test, sometimes complement fixation.

Treatment

Tetracycline (doxycycline) or chloramphenicol if tetracycline not possible.

COXIELLA BURNETII

Coxiella burnetii, the only member of the genus *Coxiella*, is the cause of Q (or 'query') fever. A sporadic disease in Britain, it was first described in an outbreak of respiratory disease among meat workers in Queensland, Australia.

ACUTE Q FEVER

Clinical features

Incubation period: 2–3 weeks.

Signs and symptoms: pyrexia, headache (a prominent symptom), with generalized aches, anorexia and slow pulse; some cases have enlargement of the liver and abnormal liver function tests; more rarely, splenomegaly. Q fever is a generalized septicaemic infection.

Pneumonia: about half the patients have the signs and symptoms of primary atypical pneumonia, with patchy consolidation of the lungs on chest X-ray.

Duration: about 2 weeks, but sometimes prolonged for 4 or more weeks, especially in older patients.

Pathology: not a disease of vascular endothelium; infection first involves the lungs, then spreads via blood to become a systemic infection.

Prognosis: is good and complete recovery is usual.

CHRONIC Q FEVER

Infective endocarditis: the most serious form of chronic infection when Q fever is followed by infection of the heart valves with the formation of vegetations. The signs and symptoms are similar to those of bacterial infective endocarditis, i.e. fever, finger clubbing, anaemia, heart murmurs and splenomegaly; liver enlargement is common. The disease is usually (but not always) seen in patients with damaged heart valves; a much more serious disease than Q fever, and generally fatal if untreated.

Other forms of chronic Q fever: include hepatitis, meningoencephalitis and interstitial pulmonary fibrosis, in addition to prolonged fever and purpura.

Epidemiology

Animal reservoirs: sheep, cattle, other domestic and some wild animals; ticks are also infected and probably play a role in spreading *C. burnetii* among animals, although generally transmission is via inhalation or ingestion of infected dust, straw, pasture etc. At parturition, very large numbers of organisms are shed in the placenta, fluids and discharges.

Geographical distribution: worldwide.

Route of human infection: mainly by inhalation of contaminated dust or via placentas, fluids etc. at parturition: infection has been known to spread downwind some considerable distance from the primary source: sometimes by handling infected animals; infection can also be acquired by drinking unpasteurized, contaminated milk from infected cows, although this seems to be an unusual route.

Occupational hazard: animal workers have an increased risk of Q fever.

Sex: the majority of patients are male, probably reflecting the occupational hazard.

Seasonal incidence: Q fever is more common in spring and the early summer months.

Bacteriology

A typical rickettsia, but *C. burnetii* is resistant to drying.

Diagnosis

Serology: complement fixation test with two different antigenic phases of *C. burnetii* differentiates acute from chronic Q fever.

Phase 1: freshly isolated strains of *C. burnetii* give no reaction with sera of acute cases, but react well with sera from patients with chronic infection (e.g. endocarditis).

Phase 2: after repeated passage in eggs, *C. burnetii* reacts well with sera from both acute and chronic infection.

Isolation: by inoculation of guinea-pigs with material from valvular vegetations and spleen: after an interval test the guinea-pig sera for antibodies to *C. burnetii*; now rarely attempted.

Treatment

Tetracycline (doxycycline): but endocarditis requires long-term treatment and doxycycline should be combined with ciprofloxacin or rifampicin; this tends to suppress rather than eradicate the organism, and careful follow-up is necessary. Removal of the diseased heart valves and replacement with valve prostheses has greatly improved the prognosis, and long-term survival can now be achieved.

EHRLICHIAE

Ehrlichiae are tickborne rickettsiae that infect a variety of animals and of which some species are pathogenic for humans:

- *E. sennutsu*: found in Japan
- *E. chaffeensis*: the cause of human monocytic ehrlichiosis in the USA
- *E. equi*, *E. phagocytophilia* and 'the HGE agent': cause human granulocytic ehrlichiosis also in the USA
- *Other species*: *E. ewingi*, associated with dogs, also a cause of granulocytic ehrlichiosis; *E. canis* infects macrophages and is also a dog pathogen.

Clinically: ehrlichiosis is a febrile disease of variable severity; clinically, Sennutsu fever resembles infectious mononucleosis and is generally mild; the American diseases, which can be severe – even life-threatening – are fevers, with headache, myalgia, malaise, but with leukopenia: both forms cause thrombocytopaenia, anaemia and raised serum transaminases: *E.chaffeensis* primarily attacks monocytes, whereas in the granulocytic disease neutrophils are the targets of infection, and clumps of the organisms (morulae) can be demonstrated within neutrophils in peripheral blood films. Granulocytic ehrlichiosis may cause a degree of T-cell dysfunction with a propensity to develop opportunistic infections.

Reservoirs: humans, deer and dogs (*E. chaffeensis*); humans, mice, dogs, deer, other animals (*E. phagocytophila*).

Vector: ticks are the vectors of the American disease; none has been found for Sennutsu fever.

Diagnosis: *serology*: refer to reference laboratory.

Treatment: doxycycline – possibly with rifampicin, but this is not yet evaluated.

BARTONELLA

The three main species of *Bartonella* and the diseases they cause are shown in Table 18.2.

1. *B. bacilliformis*: found only in South America, where infection is transmitted to humans by sandfly vectors; the reservoirs are infected humans. Oroya fever is a febrile disease characterized by severe haemolytic anaemia due to massive infection of red cells and subsequent erythrophagocytosis, and generalized lymphadenopathy: untreated, the case fatality rate is from 10 to 90%. Verruga peruana is due to the same organism and is a benign skin eruption with haemangioma-like nodules in the skin and subcutaneous tissues: it may follow Oroya fever or an asymptomatic infection, sometimes after a long interval, and tends to recur.

Table 18.2 Species of *Bartonella* and the main diseases they cause

B. bacilliformis	Oroya fever
	Verruga peruana
B. henselae	Cat scratch fever
	Bacillary angiomatosis
B. quintana	Trench fever

2. *B. henselae*: now known to be the cause (perhaps not the only cause) of cat-scratch fever, a mild febrile illness with malaise and regional lymphadenopathy following a primary cutaneous papule at the site of a cat scratch or bite (cat fleas may be vectors). The organism also causes bacillary angiomatosis, a skin eruption of haemangiomatous (neovascular) nodules; sometimes seen in AIDS patients and liable to be misdiagnosed as Kaposi's sarcoma.

3. *B. quintana*: cause of trench fever, a louseborne disease which was the scourge of infantry troops in the First World War, but now found in many countries in association with poverty, deprivation and homelessness; clinically, fever with headache, severe pain in the shins and back, maculopapular rash and, commonly, splenomegaly, bacteraemia – sometimes with endocarditis. There is a marked tendency to recur; also causes bacillary angiomatosis, especially in AIDS patients, when it may be misdiagnosed as Kaposi's sarcoma.

Diagnosis: *isolation*: in specialized media; *serology*: refer to reference laboratory.

Treatment: for *B. bacilliformis* – chloramphenicol or doxycycline: antibiotic therapy is of uncertain value in cat-scratch disease – azithromycin appears to hasten resolution. Doxycycline for trench fever.

19 Antimicrobial therapy

Bacterial infections are among the few diseases in medicine for which specific therapy is available. Despite this, infections are still common and treatment may fail. Of increasing concern is the dramatic rise in antimicrobial resistance posing a constant challenge to medicine.

ANTIBIOTICS

More than a century ago, Pasteur observed that the growth of one microorganism could be inhibited by the products of another. However, most of these early products, or 'antibiotics', were toxic to mammalian as well as to bacterial cells, and were therefore of no therapeutic use. Penicillin, discovered in 1929 but not available for clinical trials until 1940, is the product of a mould, *Penicillium notatum*, and was the first antibiotic. Other antibiotics are the products of soil streptomycetes and bacteria of the genus *Bacillus*. The semisynthetic penicillins and cephalosporins have been prepared by the chemical manipulation of existing drugs. Trimethoprim, ciprofloxacin and linezolid are examples of synthetic chemotherapeutic agents.

Selective toxicity is the ability to kill or inhibit the growth of a microorganism without harming the cells of the host: an essential requirement for any successful antibiotic.

Antimicrobial therapy aims to treat infection with a drug to which the causal microorganism is sensitive. This can be achieved if a sound knowledge of microbiology indicates the most likely pathogen in a given patient and its usual antibiotic sensitivity, i.e. on a '*best-guess*' basis; it is better still if the infection is investigated bacteriologically by culture and in vitro sensitivity testing.

Antimicrobial drugs are often classified as *bactericidal* – when they kill the infecting bacteria – or *bacteriostatic* – when they prevent multiplication but do not kill the bacteria. This classification is not always clear-cut and may depend on the local concentration of the drug. In all but a few conditions, notably infective endocarditis, appropriate bacteriostatic drugs give excellent therapeutic results.

This chapter deals with the main antibiotics and antimicrobial agents in current use, from the point of view of a clinical bacteriologist. Pharmacokinetics are not considered. The tables summarize information about them, including their clinical use: inevitably oversimplified, use only as a guide to antibiotic therapy.

PENICILLINS (PENAMS)

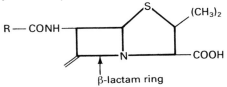

Mode of action: bactericidal: inhibit cell wall synthesis by combining with the transpeptidase responsible for cross-linking of the peptidoglycan; activity depends on an intact β-lactam ring.

Resistance: common: due to bacterial *β-lactamase*, which inactivates penicillin by acting on the β-lactam ring: often plasmid coded.

Antibacterial spectrum: varies with individual penicillins: activity determined by the side chain of the penicillin nucleus. The principal penicillins and their antibacterial spectra are shown in Table 19.1.

Toxicity: virtually non-toxic. Very large doses can cause neurotoxicity. Hypersensitivity can occur in the form of rashes (especially with ampicillin) and, rarely, anaphylaxis (with any penicillin given by injection). Broad-spectrum penicillins can cause antibiotic-associated colitis.

β-Lactamase inhibitors

Clavulanic acid, tazobactam and sulbactam are β-lactam compounds that have no intrinsic antibacterial activity but which are irreversible inhibitors of most plasmid-mediated (but generally not chromosomally mediated) β-lactamases. They do inhibit the chromosomal β-lactamase of most 'bacteroides'. Combined with a β-lactamase-susceptible penicillin, they enable the penicillin to resist degradation.

Table 19.1 The penicillins

Penicillin	Administration	Antibacterial spectrum	Clinical use
Penicillins			
Benzylpenicillin (penicillin G)	i.m., i.v.	Most Gram- positive bacteria and *Neisseria* species	Streptococcal (not enterococcal), clostridial infection, syphilis, leptospirosis, anthrax, actinomycosis. Sensitive staphylococcal and pneumococcal infections
Phenoxymethyl penicillin (penicillin V)	Oral		
Aminopenicillins			
Ampicillin	Oral, i.m., i.v.	Similar to penicillin, but in addition sensitive strains of enterococci, *Haemophilus influenzae* and coliforms	Community urinary and respiratory infections; listerosis. Use with caution in hospital-acquired infections owing to increased resistance
Amoxycillin (better oral absorption)			
Isoxazolyl penicillins			
Flucloxacillin	Oral, i.m., i.v.	Less active than penicillin but stable to staphylococcal β-lactamase. Ineffective against enterococci, neisseria and listeria	Staphylococcal infections; but note emergence of methicillin-resistant strains (MRSA)
Methicillin (now discontinued)			
Carboxypenicillins			
Ticarcillin (available only with potassium clavulanate)	i.v.	Similar to aminopenicillins but in addition *P. aeruginosa* and most *Proteus* spp. and 'bacteroides'	Principal use for infections due to *P. aeruginosa*
Acylureidopenicillins			
Piperacillin	i.m., i.v.	Similar to carboxypenicillins but in addition, infections due to *Klebsiella* species and greater activity against pseudomonads	Urinary, respiratory, burns and other infections due to sensitive bacteria, especially *P. aeruginosa*; severe sepsis, usually in combination with other drugs
Amidinopenicillins			
Mecillinam	Oral	Coliforms; low activity against Gram-positive bacteria and *P. aeruginosa*	Urinary infections

i.m.: intramuscular; i.v.: intravenous.
Note: in this book, reference to penicillin is taken to mean penicillin G or penicillin V.

Co-amoxiclav: combination of amoxycillin and potassium clavulanate.

Administration: oral; also intravenous.

Antibacterial spectrum: active against β-lactamase-producing coliforms, staphylococci, 'bacteroides' and *Haemophilus* spp.

Clinical use: urinary and respiratory tracts, skin and soft tissues, e.g. bites and dental infections.

Toxicity: The Committee on Safety of Medicines (CSM) has warned that the use of clavulanic acid is associated with cholestatic jaundice, most commonly in males and those aged over 65 years. *Duration* of treatment should not exceed 14 days.

Piperacillin with tazobactam

Administration: intravenous.

Clinical use: broad-spectrum antibiotic: lower respiratory, urinary, hepatobiliary tracts, intra-abdominal, skin and soft tissue infections. In neutropenic patients often combined with an aminoglycoside.

Ticarcillin with clavulanic acid

Administration: intravenous.

Clinical use: alternative to acylureidopenicillins.

Toxicity: as co-amoxiclav. Ticarcillin itself may cause a bleeding diathesis.

CARBAPENEMS

Semisynthetic β-lactam compounds.

Imipenem (with cilastatin) **and meropenem**

Imipenem (but not meropenem) is rapidly metabolized in the kidney by a dipeptidase: therefore administered with an enzyme inhibitor, cilastatin, which increases urinary and serum concentrations of the antibiotic and also reduces the potential for nephrotoxicity.

Administration: intravenous.

Mode of action: bactericidal: potent inhibitors of bacterial cell wall synthesis. Extremely stable to degradation by plasmid and chromosomal β-lactamases. Carbapenems are also β-lactamase inhibitors.

Resistance: uncommon; may develop in *P. aeruginosa* during treatment, when used as single agent: due to decreased permeability.

Antibacterial spectrum: extremely broad; active against Gram-positive and Gram-negative aerobes and anaerobes. Exceptions are *Stenotrophomonas maltophilia* (chromosomal carbapenemase), *Burkholderia cepacia*, *Enterococcus faecium* and MRSA.

Clinical use: reserve for serious infection, especially if hospital acquired and a polymicrobial cause is likely.

Toxicity: similar to other β-lactam antibiotics. Imepenem has been associated with central nervous system toxicity.

MONOBACTAMS

Monocyclic β-lactam antibiotics, e.g:

Aztreonam

First monobactam available for clinical use.

Administration: intramuscular, intravenous.

Mode of action: bactericidal: inhibits cell wall synthesis; β-lactamase stable.

Resistance: uncommon; may develop in *P. aeruginosa* during treatment.

Antibacterial spectrum: narrow: active against aerobic Gram-negative bacteria, but most *S. maltophilia* and *Acinetobacter* spp. are resistant; Gram-positive bacteria and anaerobes resistant.

Clinical use: infections with aerobic Gram-negative bacteria, e.g. urinary tract infections, gonorrhoea (but not chlamydia); mixed bacterial infections if given with another antibiotic.

Toxicity: as for other β-lactam antibiotics, but less likely to induce hypersensitivity; may be given *with caution* to patients known to be allergic to penicillins and cephalosporins, but not with ceftazidime allergy.

CEPHALOSPORINS

Chemically similar to the penicillins: most are semisynthetic derivatives of cephalosporin C, an antibacterial compound produced by the mould *Cephalasporium*. The cephamycin compounds (derived from *Streptomyces* spp.) and the oxa-β-lactams (synthetic compounds) are also regarded as members of the cephalosporin class. Antibacterial activity can be altered by variation in the side chains of the cephalosporin nucleus. In clinical practice cephalosporins are arbitrarily assigned to four generations. Table 19.2 lists the main cephalosporins and some of their properties: it is not exhaustive and some drugs are not available in the UK.

Administration: mostly parenteral, but a few oral drugs have been developed, e.g. oral cefuroxime axetil.

Mode of action: bactericidal: similar to penicillin. Stable to many bacterial β-lactamases, and this stability has been increased with the later generations, the inferior antistaphylococcal activity of the newer drugs is due to their less avid binding to the target site.

Clinical use: most cephalosporins are given parenterally, so are restricted to hospital patients: most useful in seriously ill patients infected with more than one susceptible organism. Often used as an alternative to an aminoglycoside, especially in patients with renal impairment. A major use is in short-term perioperative prophylaxis.

Toxicity: low: rashes, fever, blood disorders, diarrhoea and antibiotic-associated colitis. *Hypersensitivity*: about 10% of people hypersensitive to penicillin are also hypersensitive to cephalosporins.

AMINOGLYCOSIDES

Family of extremely useful antibiotics. Main aminoglycoside antibiotics are listed in Table 19.3.

Administration: intramuscular; intravenous for systemic infections: in divided doses or once daily regimen. No oral absorption.

Mode of action: bactericidal: inhibition of protein synthesis owing to action on bacterial ribosomes; all aminoglycosides misread messenger RNA to produce amino acid substitution in proteins.

Resistance: increasingly common in hospital-acquired strains; amikacin is least affected: due to acquisition of plasmid-coded inactivating enzymes or decreased transport of drug into the bacterial cell.

Antibacterial spectrum: coliforms, staphylococci, *P. aeruginosa* (tobramycin most active, and netilmicin least active); streptococci and strict anaerobes intrinsically resistant.

Toxicity: dose related: ototoxicity (vertigo or deafness) and nephrotoxicity are major problems, because toxic levels are close to therapeutic levels necessary for treatment. Netilmicin *may* be safer than other aminoglycosides. Serum levels *must* be monitored in all patients, including those on once-daily regimens, and dose adjusted accordingly.

Table 19.2 The cephalosporins*

Cephalosporin	Administration	Antibacterial spectrum	Clinical use
First generation Cefalothin (oldest) Cefalexin Cefradine	i.m., i.v. Oral Oral, i.m., i.v.	A wide range of Gram-positive and Gram-negative bacteria: *P. aeruginosa*, *H. influenzae*, *Neisseria* spp. and 'bacteroides' are resistant	Largely replaced by second generation drugs; oral drugs still used in urinary infections
Second generation Cefuroxime Cefamandole Cefoxitin	i.m., i.v., oral i.m., i.v. i.m., i.v.	Wide: with marked stability to β-lactamases of Gram-negative as well as Gram-positive bacteria; active against *H. influenzae* and (especially cefoxitin) 'bacteroides'; inferior antistaphylococcal activity cf. to first generation	Mild to moderate respiratory, skin and soft tissue and intra-abdominal infections; widely used in surgical prophylaxis
Third generation Cefotaxime Ceftriaxone	i.m., i.v. i.m., i.v.	Similar to second-generation drugs, but less anti-staphylococcal activity and more against *Neisseria* spp.	As second-generation drugs, but particularly in serious sepsis, gonorrhoea and meningitis
Ceftazidime	i.m., i.v.	Active also against *P. aeruginosa*, but little Gram-positive activity	Infections in patients with neutropenia, cystic fibrosis
Fourth generation Cefepime	i.v.	As third-generation drugs, including *P. aeruginosa*, and greater activity against certain coliforms	Not yet licensed in UK

i.m.: intramuscular; i.v.: intravenous.
* MRSA, enterococci and *Listeria* spp. are resistant to cephalosporins.

Table 19.3 The aminoglycosides

Aminoglycoside	Main clinical use
Gentamicin Tobramycin Netilmicin Amikacin	Severe infections in hospital due to coliforms; gentamicin most widely used: in certain infections, given in combination with a β-lactam antibiotic
Streptomycin	Little used: reserved for tuberculosis, and (rarely) gentamicin-resistant enterococcal endocarditis
Neomycin	Given orally in 'gut sterilization' regimens, e.g. in hepatic failure; topically for skin or mucous membrane infections

TETRACYCLINES

Broad-spectrum antibiotics that are remarkably free of serious side-effects. Decreased general use because of increasing bacterial resistance, but remain the antibiotics of choice for specific infections. The following are available:

- Tetracycline
- Demeclocycline hydrochloride
- Lymecycline
- Oxytetracycline
- Doxycycline ⎱ more effective: can be given in
- Minocycline ⎰ smaller dosage and in renal failure.

Administration: almost always oral.

Mode of action: bacteriostatic: inhibit protein synthesis by preventing the attachment of amino acids to ribosomes.

Resistance: fairly common: generally plasmid mediated.

Antibacterial spectrum: broad: both Gram-positive and Gram-negative bacteria: many strains of *Streptococcus pyogenes*, pneumococci and *H. influenzae* are now resistant; *P. aeruginosa* and *Proteus* spp. are intrinsically resistant. Active against brucellae, *Mycoplasma pneumoniae*, rickettsiae, *Coxiella burneti*, chlamydiae, *Borrelia burgdorferi* and leptospira.

Main clinical use: treatment of genital and respiratory infections caused by mycoplasma and chlamydia, rickettsial infections, Q fever, brucellosis, Lyme disease; and in syphilis and leptospirosis in patients with penicillin allergy. Commonly used for treatment of acne vulgaris, and now infrequently used for infective exacerbations of chronic bronchitis.

Toxicity: diarrhoea, usually mild and self-limiting. Avoid in renal and hepatic failure; contraindicated in pregnancy, and in children because the drug may be deposited in the developing teeth, with permanent yellow staining, and also interfere with bone development.

METRONIDAZOLE

Exceedingly effective against anaerobic bacteria.

Administration: oral, rectal (suppositories), intravenous and topical.

Mode of action: bactericidal: converted by anaerobic bacteria to active (reduced) metabolite with inhibitory action on DNA synthesis.

Resistance: uncommon.

Antibacterial spectrum: strictly anaerobic bacteria, e.g. 'bacteroides', anaerobic cocci, clostridia, and certain microaerophilic organisms, e.g. *Gardnerella vaginalis* and *Helicobacter pylori*. No effect on aerobic organisms; actinomyces are resistant. Active against anaerobic protozoa (e.g. *Trichomonas vaginalis, Entamoeba histolytica, Giardia lamblia*).

Clinical use: any anaerobic infection, e.g. abdominal and gynaecological wound sepsis, deep abscesses, peritoneal sepsis, Vincent's angina, dental infections, *Clostridium difficile*-associated colitis, tetanus and bacterial vaginosis; perioperative prophylaxis in abdominal and gynaecological surgery; anaerobic protozoal infections, and as a component of *H. pylori* eradication regimen.

Toxicity: low; side-effects: nausea, metallic taste in mouth, and disulfiram-like reaction with alcohol.

LINCOMYCINS

Clindamycin is active against Gram-positive bacteria (except enterococci) and some anaerobes: penetrates tissue well and acts particularly well on *S. pyogenes* (group A streptococci), *S. aureus* (not MRSA) and 'bacteroides'. Excellent oral agent for infections in intravenous drug users, where venous access is a problem, and for staphylococcal bone and joint infections, *but* use with caution because of a warning notice from the CSM that it is associated with antibiotic-associated colitis.

MACROLIDES

Erythromycin

The prototype of the macrolide group of antibiotics.

Administration: oral, intravenous.

Mode of action: bacteriostatic by inhibition of protein synthesis; may be bactericidal at higher concentrations.

Resistance: occurs in S. aureus, pneumococci and S. pyogenes.

Antibacterial spectrum: penicillin-like, but includes in addition *Corynebacterium diphtheriae*, *Bordetella pertussis*, 'bacteroides' *Campylobacter* species, *Legionella pneumophila*, *M. pneumoniae* and chlamydiae. Poor activity against *H. influenzae*.

Clinical use: staphylococcal infections; variety of respiratory infections (tonsillitis, sinusitis, bronchitis and pneumonia, diphtheria, whooping cough, atypical pneumonia, psittacosis, Legionnaires' disease); non-specific urethritis; campylobacter enteritis. Useful second-line drug in patients hypersensitive to penicillin.

Toxicity: safe antibiotic except for erythromycin estolate, which may be hepatotoxic. Main side-effects are gastrointestinal.

Azithromycin and clarithromycin

New drugs with similar spectra to that of erythromycin. Both achieve higher tissue concentrations, and have enhanced activity against *H. influenzae*, *Moraxella catarrhalis* and atypical mycobacteria. Clarithromycin is also a component of *H. pylori* eradication regimens, and azithromycin is useful for genital chlamydial infections.

GLYCOPEPTIDES

Vancomycin

Available for over 30 years but initially little used; nowadays, indications for its use are common.

Administration: intravenous, oral.

Mode of action: bactericidal: by inhibition of cell wall synthesis: mechanism different from that of β-lactams.

Resistance: occurs in coagulase-negative staphylococci, enterocci, and more recently 'intermediate resistance' in S. aureus.

Antibacterial spectrum: staphylococci (including strains resistant to methicillin and other drugs), streptococci (but less active against enterococci), clostridia.

Clinical use: *intravenous*: serious infections, e.g. endocarditis, septicaemia due to streptococci, *S. aureus* and coagulase-negative staphylococci, especially if multiresistant or if the patient is hypersensitive to penicillins; *oral*: antibiotic-associated colitis; *intraperitoneal*: CAPD peritonitis.

Toxicity: phlebitis, ototoxicity, nephrotoxicity if given intravenously: monitor serum levels to control dosage.

Teicoplanin

Chemically related to vancomycin, with similar activity and toxicity. Once-daily dosage and can be administered intramuscularly.

Note: Glycopeptides have no advantage over the penicillins in treating penicillin-sensitive strains.

LINEZOLID

First of the oxazolidinones – a new class of synthetic antimicrobial agents – available in the UK.

Administration: intravenous, and oral (100% bioavailability).

Mode of action: bacteriostatic: by inhibition of protein synthesis. *Novel* action by preventing formation of the initiation complex required for ribosomal function; no cross-resistance with other antibiotics acting at ribosomal sites.

Resistance: has been reported in enterococci and a recent report in *S. aureus*.

Antibacterial spectrum: all Gram-positive bacteria, including MRSA and glycopeptide-resistant strains.

Clinical use: serious infections caused by multiresistant Gram-positive organisms.

Toxicity: potential monoamine oxidase inhibition and reversible bone-marrow suppression with prolonged use.

STREPTOGRAMINS

Quinupristin and dalfopristin: available in a combination of 30%/70% ratio.

Administration: intravenous (both as mesilate salts).

Mode of action: bactericidal: act in synergy by binding to 50 S ribosome and inhibition of protein synthesis.

Resistance: plasmid-mediated methylation of ribosome: confers resistance to quinupristin, macrolides and lincosamides. The combination is still active, but only bacteriostatic.

Antibacterial spectrum: all Gram-positive bacteria except *Enterococcus faecalis*.

Clinical use: serious Gram-positive infections; where conventional treatment has failed, and especially for infections caused by vancomycin-resistant *Enterococcus faecium*.

Toxicity: reversible athralgia/myalgia, cardiac arrhythmias.

QUINOLONES

Ciprofloxacin

First of the fluoroquinolones – synthetic antibacterial agents developed from nalidixic acid – available in the UK.

Administration: oral; also intravenous.

Mode of action: bactericidal: inhibits DNA-gyrase and topoisomerase activity by binding to chromosomal DNA strands. Interferes with DNA replication and prevents supercoiling within the chromosome.

Resistance: gradually increasing: result of chromosomal mutation: most likely to develop when used as monotherapy and for prolonged duration. Mechanisms: decreased drug permeation and altered target enzyme, resulting in cross-resistance between different quinolones. Resistance most often seen in *S. aureus*, particularly most strains of MRSA; *P. aeruginosa*, *Klebsiella pneumoniae* and gonococci strains in the Far East. Plasmid-mediated resistance has been recently reported in *K. pneumoniae*.

Antibacterial spectrum: broad: active against aerobic Gram-negative bacteria, including *P. aeruginosa* and staphylococci, but streptococci less sensitive. Anaerobes are resistant.

Clinical use: respiratory infections, including those due to *P. aeruginosa*, e.g. cystic fibrosis, but not pneumococcal pneumonia; Legionnaires' disease (combined with rifampicin); mycobacterial infections; uncomplicated and complicated urinary infections; gonorrhoea; prostatitis; wide range of gastrointestinal infections, including enteric fever; useful in travellers' diarrhoea; skin and soft tissue infections due to *P. aeruginosa*. Often used for prophylaxis in neutropenic patients. *Avoid* use in MRSA infections.

Toxicity: severe systemic adverse reactions rare: most important CSM warnings are: CNS stimulation to produce anxiety, nervousness, insomnia, even convulsions; and tendon damage: discontinue antibiotic immediately. Avoid administration to children because of potential to damage juvenile cartilage, although can be prescribed for pseudomonal infections in cystic fibrosis for children over

5 years. Decreases metabolism of theophylline, caffeine and warfarin – so toxic effects of these drugs encountered if administered with ciprofloxacin.

Levofloxacin and moxifloxacin

More recently introduced quinolones that are more active against pneumococci, but not as active against *P. aeruginosa*. Useful agents for respiratory infections, including pneumococcal and atypical pneumonias.

Numerous other compounds have been under development but have not been successful due to toxicity.

SULPHONAMIDES AND TRIMETHOPRIM

Both drugs act sequentially in the synthesis of tetrahydrofolate. Available in combination as co-trimoxazole or as separate components.

Co-trimoxazole

Contains: sulphamethoxazole and trimethoprim in 5:1 ratio.

Administration: oral, intramuscular, intravenous.

Mode of action: bacteriostatic: sulphonamide and trimethoprim block sequential steps in DNA synthesis: evidence of synergism in vitro.

Resistance: common: mainly due to production of resistant enzymes; gene for trimethoprim resistance often present on a transposon.

Antibacterial spectrum: broad: active against both Gram-positive and Gram-negative bacteria (*P. aeruginosa* is resistant) and also *Pneumocystis carinii*, *Toxoplasma gondii* and *Nocardia* spp.

Clinical use: because of possible serious toxicity, the CSM now recommends restricting the use of co-trimoxazole for pneumocystis pneumonia, toxoplasmosis and nocardiasis.

Toxicity: nausea and vomiting; numerous allergic reactions, rashes; occasionally serious side-effects: Stevens–Johnson syndrome; blood dyscrasias, including bone marrow depression – the antibiotic should be discontinued immediately.

Sulphonamides

Rarely used on their own because of increasing bacterial resistance and toxicity.

The most widely used preparation is topical silver sulfadiazine for the prophylaxis and treatment of infections in burn wounds.

Trimethoprim

Mainly used for urinary and respiratory tract infections, including mild to moderate MRSA infections: used in an oral combination with fusidic acid or rifampicin. Many MRSA strains in the UK remain sensitive to trimethoprim.

Toxicity: reduced incidence of side-effects compared with co-trimoxazole, but long-term use can result in serious blood disorders.

OTHER ANTIBIOTICS AND ANTIMICROBIAL DRUGS

Some other less commonly used antibiotics and antimicrobial drugs are listed in Table 19.4.

ANTITUBERCULOUS CHEMOTHERAPY

A *combination of antimicrobial drugs* is essential in tuberculosis, to prevent the emergence of resistant bacteria. Standard regimen for sensitive strains is 2 months of at least three of the following: isoniazid, rifampicin, ethambutol, pyrazinamide; followed by 4 months of isoniazid and rifampicin.

Isoniazid

Administration: oral; intramuscular and intravenous.

Mode of action: bacteriostatic: penetrates well into tissues and fluids, and acts on intracellular organisms.

Resistance: develops readily.

Toxicity: uncommon: peripheral neuritis, psychotic and epileptic episodes.

Rifampicin

Administration: oral or intravenous.

Mode of action: inhibits by combining with bacterial DNA-dependent RNA polymerase.

Resistance: develops rapidly unless other drugs used in combination.

Table 19.4 Some other antimicrobial drugs

Drug	Administration	Mode of action	Antibacterial spectrum	Clinical use	Other features
Fusidic acid	Oral, i.v.	Bacteriostatic	S. aureus	Abscesses, osteomyelitis, septicaemia	Good tissue penetration; resistance may emerge rapidly; give in combination
Chloramphenicol	Oral, i.m., i.v., topical	Bacteriostatic: arrests protein synthesis	Broad spectrum	Typhoid fever Eyedrops for conjunctivitis	Rarely causes fatal aplastic anaemia; this has restricted its use
Nalidixic acid*	Oral	Inhibits DNA replication	Coliforms; not P. aeruginosa	Lower urinary infections	Side-effects include nausea; rarely visual disturbances
Nitrofurantoin*	Oral	Inhibits DNA replication	Enterococci but not proteus or P. aeruginosa	Lower urinary infections	Nausea; peripheral neuropathy sometimes seen
Spectinomycin	i.m.	Bactericidal	N. gonorrhoeae, other Gram-negative bacteria	Penicillin-resistant gonorrhoea	
Mupirocin (pseudomonic acid)	Topical	Bactericidal: arrests protein synthesis	Staphylococci and streptococci	Skin infections; elimination of nasal carriage of S. aureus (including MRSA)	High-level resistance in certain MRSA strains

i.m.: intramuscular; i.v.: intravenous.
* Serum levels inadequate for treatment of systemic infections, including pyelonephritis.

Antibacterial spectrum: mycobacteria. Also active in vitro against a wide range of Gram-positive and Gram-negative bacteria.

Clinical use: tuberculosis; prophylaxis of meningococcal meningitis; in combination with another drug, to treat severe staphylococcal infections (including MRSA strains).

Toxicity: low: liver function may be affected; often transient hypersensitivity; rarely, thrombocytopenia. Contraindicated in first trimester of pregnancy. Patients should be warned that urine, sputum and tears become coloured red with rifampicin therapy.

Pyrazinamide

Administration: oral.

Mode of action: bactericidal: acts on intracellular organisms; good meningeal penetration. Not active against *Mycobacterium bovis*.

Resistance: develops rapidly unless other drugs used in combination.

Clinical use: main effect in early phase of combination therapy: especially useful in tuberculous meningitis.

Toxicity: low: may be hepatotoxic.

Ethambutol

Administration: oral.

Resistance: uncommon.

Toxicity: optic neuritis may develop: reversible, and uncommon with low dosages.

Other (second-line) drugs

- Streptomycin
- Thiacetazone
- Capreomycin
- Cycloserine
- Ethionamide.

ANTIBIOTIC RESISTANCE IN BACTERIA

A major problem in antibiotic therapy is the emergence of drug-resistant bacteria. The frequency depends on the organism and the antibiotic concerned: some organisms rapidly acquire resistance, e.g. certain coliforms, *S. aureus*; others rarely do so, e.g.

S. pyogenes. Resistance to some antibiotics virtually never develops, e.g. metronidazole, whereas with others resistant strains readily emerge, e.g. penicillin, tetracycline, fusidic acid.

Drug resistance in clinical practice is associated with antibiotic use: when a small number of resistant bacteria have emerged, they will be at a selective advantage in the presence of the antibiotic and will multiply at the expense of sensitive bacteria. Widespread, often indiscriminate, prescribing of antibiotics in hospitals has therefore favoured the survival and increase of drug-resistant bacteria.

Drug resistance is of two types:

- **Primary**: an innate property of the bacterium unrelated to contact with the drug, e.g. resistance of *E. coli* to penicillin.
- **Acquired**: due to mutation or gene transfer.

Spontaneous mutation may be relatively infrequent or, as in the case of *M. tuberculosis* and streptomycin, common.

Gene transfer is a major cause of resistance in bacteria: it enables resistance to spread from bacterium to bacterium, within and between species (see Chapter 2).

Cross-resistance occurs when resistance to one antimicrobial drug confers resistance to other (usually chemically related) drugs, e.g. bacteria resistant to one tetracycline or one sulphonamide, are resistant to all tetracyclines or all sulphonamides respectively. Conversely, *dissociated resistance* occurs when resistance to one drug is not accompanied by resistance to closely related drugs, e.g. resistance to gentamicin is not always associated with resistance to tobramycin.

Mechanisms of antibiotic resistance

There are three main mechanisms: modification of the permeability of the cell wall or of the site of action of the drug, or inactivation of the drug.

Permeability

The cell wall may become altered – by modification of proteins in the outer membrane – so that antibiotics or other antimicrobial drugs cannot enter and be taken up by the bacterial cell. This is often associated with low-level resistance to several drugs, but occasionally with high-level resistance to a single drug (e.g. tetracycline): a common type of antibiotic resistance in *Pseudomonas aeruginosa.*

Modification of site of action

Modification of the enzyme, substrate as binding site with which the antibiotic reacts confirm resistance in a bacterium e.g. trimethoprim resistant bacteria acquire a plasmid or transposon coding for a resistant dihydrofolate reductase. An altered penicillin-binding protein, with a low affinity for methicillin is the mechanism of resistance in MRSA.

Inactivation of antibiotic

A common mechanism of resistance. The antibiotic is inactivated by enzymes produced by the bacterium, e.g. β-lactamase destruction of the β-lactam ring responsible for the antibacterial action of penicillins and cephalosporins. Some of these enzymes are plasmid coded, others chromosomal coded. Acetylating, adenylating and phosphorylating enzymes in the case of resistance to the aminoglycosides are plasmid coded.

PRINCIPLES OF ANTIMICROBIAL THERAPY

Administration

Antimicrobial therapy is indicated for an established infection that makes a patient sufficiently ill to require specific treatment: trivial, self-limiting infections in healthy individuals should not be treated with antibiotics.

Choice of drug

Successful chemotherapy depends on the infecting organism being sensitive to the drug chosen. Attempts to treat *viral* respiratory infections – a common practice – are doomed to failure unless there is secondary *bacterial* infection.

The choice of drug is based on:

Clinical diagnosis: implies prescribing on an informed 'best-guess' basis: most infections requiring antibiotics have to be treated before laboratory results are available; they vary in severity from exacerbations of chronic bronchitis to septicaemia.

Laboratory diagnosis: specimens adequate for diagnosis should, whenever possible, be taken before chemotherapy begins. Isolation of the pathogen and sensitivity tests take time – at least

24 h, and usually longer – and as soon as results are available treatment should be reviewed; laboratory monitoring can make the difference between success and failure of therapy.

Route of administration

Drugs must be given parenterally to seriously ill patients. Oral antibiotics for the treatment of systemic infections must be both acid stable (e.g. penicillin V is acid stable, but penicillin G is not) and absorbed from the gastrointestinal tract.

Dosage

Dosage must be adequate to produce a concentration of antibiotic at the site of infection greater than that required to inhibit the growth of the infecting organism. *In renal failure* the dosage of drugs eliminated by the renal route may require either major adjustment (e.g. aminoglycosides, vancomycin) or more minor modification (e.g. β-lactams), whereas those eliminated by the hepatic route (e.g. erythromycin) can usually be given in normal dosage.

Duration

Treatment of some severe infections, e.g. endocarditis, tuberculosis, needs to be prolonged and is aimed at eradication of the pathogen, but the majority of acute infections respond to a short course of antibiotics, leaving the body defence mechanisms to cope with any infection that remains.

Distribution

The drug must penetrate to the site of the infection, e.g. in meningitis the antibiotic must pass into the CSF. Deep-seated sepsis is a particular problem and an important cause of antibiotic failure: antibiotics cannot penetrate 'walled-off' abscesses or internal collections of pus, and treatment will probably fail unless the pus is drained. Surgical intervention is also necessary if there are established pathological changes, e.g. urinary obstruction due to stones, chronic tuberculous cavities.

Excretion

Agents used to treat urinary infections are excreted in the urine in high concentrations: some, e.g. nalidixic acid and nitrofurantoin, do not achieve useful serum levels: they are eliminated almost exclusively by the renal route, and are therefore indicated only for the management of lower urinary infections.

Urinary pH affects the activity of some drugs, e.g. the aminoglycosides are far more active in an alkaline medium. The reverse is true of nitrofurantoin, which therefore should not be used to treat infections caused by *Proteus* species, which raise the pH of the urine.

Erythromycin is excreted largely in the bile: only low concentrations can be detected in urine.

Toxicity

Although the antibiotics in general use are well tested and safe, patients should be warned of possible side-effects.

Serious toxicity can manifest itself in two ways:

• *Direct toxicity*, e.g. ototoxicity with the aminoglycosides; nephrotoxicity with vancomycin; (rare) bone marrow aplasia due to chloramphenicol.
• *Hypersensitivity*, most often due to the penicillins.

Other complications include *superinfection* with antibiotic-resistant microorganisms, e.g. coliforms and yeasts: a major problem in immunocompromised hosts. Antibiotic-associated pseudomembranous colitis is probably a special example: with the use of lincomycins restricted, broad-spectrum β-lactam antibiotics are often involved.

Use of drugs in combination

This may be necessary to treat a mixed infection if no single agent is active against all the causal organisms, e.g. in peritonitis due to coliforms and non-sporing anaerobes it is usual to give an aminoglycoside or cephalosporin along with metronidazole. In addition to this indication, there are two possible advantages:

1. *Emergence of drug-resistant bacteria will be prevented*: this applies in the treatment of tuberculosis, and may apply in infections due to *S. aureus*, an organism with a marked propensity to become resistant, especially during clinical therapy involving some antibiotics, e.g. fusidic acid.
2. *Enhanced antibacterial effect (synergism) will be achieved*: this is governed to some extent by the '*Jawetz Law*' (see below) on combined action, although there are exceptions. The combined

effect of two antibiotics depends on whether each is bacteriostatic or bactericidal in action, and the law predicts that the effect of a combination will be as follows:

Bactericidal + bactericidal: may be synergistic
Bactericidal + bacteriostatic: may be antagonistic
Bacteriostatic + bacteriostatic: will be additive.

This working rule has some value in clinical practice. For example, the combination of a penicillin and an aminoglycoside, both bactericidal, is often synergistic, with an increase in the efficacy of antibacterial action – and this may be essential, e.g. to treat septicaemia successfully in immunocompromised neutropenic patients, or to eradicate infection in endocarditis.

Antibiotic prophylaxis

Early but indiscriminate attempts to prevent infection by giving antibiotics for several days or more failed. This was because the infection to be avoided, e.g. pneumonia in unconscious patients, wound infection after surgery – was due to a number of different bacteria, not all of which were sensitive to the drugs chosen. Prolonged antibiotic administration therefore resulted in the selection of resistant organisms, which subsequently caused infection.

Prophylaxis should be considered when there is a high risk of infection, and the agent chosen must be active against the likely pathogens.

Short-term prophylaxis: one dose, or at most a few doses, of carefully chosen antibiotics given to cover the time when the risk of an infection being established is greatest – usually the perioperative period, e.g. use of cephalosporins during insertion of prosthetic joints.

Short-term (2–3 days) prophylaxis: e.g. use of rifampicin or ciprofloxacin in close contacts of a patient with *meningococcal meningitis*.

Long-term prophylaxis: may be continued for months or years.

Rheumatic fever: recurrence of rheumatic fever invariably follows throat infection with *S. pyogenes*. Incidence of further attacks is greatly reduced by giving penicillin.

Urinary tract infection: may be avoided in women who suffer repeated episodes, by administration of trimethoprim or nitrofurantoin.

Tuberculosis: close contacts of a case of open tuberculosis should be given rifampicin and isoniazid for 6 months.

Antibiotic policies

The large number of antimicrobial agents now available, many with similar properties and overlapping activity, may make the choice of drug difficult. Hospitals must have policies to improve the quality of antibiotic prescribing and enable clinicians to select the most effective therapy. These policies must be formulated in consultation with microbiologists, clinicians and pharmacists, and give guidance on suitable choices based on local resistance patterns, spectra of activity and efficacy, side-effects and cost. They should be regularly reviewed and audited. The aim is to prevent the indiscriminate use of antibiotics and inappropriate treatment. As a result, antibiotic costs, a major item in pharmacy expenditure, are decreased (sometimes substantially), and there is strong evidence that the emergence of resistant bacterial pathogens is reduced.

'Chemotherapy without bacteriology is guesswork'

Collaboration between clinician and bacteriologist is crucial, especially in combating the severe infections increasingly encountered in hospitals today. Frequent discussions are to be encouraged.

VIRUSES

20 Viruses: general properties, host response and replication

Viruses are the smallest known infective agents. Most forms of life – animals, plants and bacteria – are susceptible to infection with appropriate viruses.

Three main properties distinguish viruses from other microorganisms:

1. **Small size**: viruses are smaller than other organisms, although they vary considerably in size – from 10 nm to 300 nm. In contrast, bacteria are approximately 1000 nm and erythrocytes are 7500 nm in diameter.
2. **Genome**: the genome of viruses may be either DNA or RNA; viruses contain only one kind of nucleic acid.
3. **Metabolically inert**: viruses have no metabolic activity outside susceptible host cells. They do not possess active ribosomes or protein-synthesizing apparatus, although some contain enzymes within their particles.

Viruses, therefore, can *multiply only inside living cells*, not on inanimate media. Inside a susceptible cell, the virus redirects the cell's synthesizing machinery to the manufacture of new virus components. It does this by transcription of the virus genome or nucleic acid into virus-specific messenger or mRNA (sometimes the incoming genome can act as this), which then directs the cell to the replication of new virus particles.

VIRUS STRUCTURE

Viruses consist basically of a core of nucleic acid – the *genome* – surrounded by a protein coat. The protein coat protects the genome from inactivation by adverse environmental factors, e.g. nucleases in the bloodstream. It is antigenic and often responsible for stimulating the production of protective antibodies.

The *structures* that make up a virus particle are known as:

- *Virion*: the intact virus particle
- *Capsid*: the protein coat
- *Capsomeres*: the protein structural units of which the capsid is composed
- *Nucleic acid genome*: either DNA or RNA
- *Envelope*: the particles of many viruses are surrounded by a lipoprotein envelope containing viral antigens, but also partly derived from the outer membrane or, in some cases, the nuclear membrane of the host cell.

Virus particles show three types of *symmetry*:

1. *Cubic*: in which the particle is an icosahedral protein shell with the nucleic acid contained inside (Fig. 20.1).
2. *Helical*: in which the particle contains an elongated *nucleocapsid*; the capsomeres are arranged round the spiral of nucleic acid (Fig. 20.2). Most helical viruses possess an outer envelope, which invests the helical nucleoprotein.

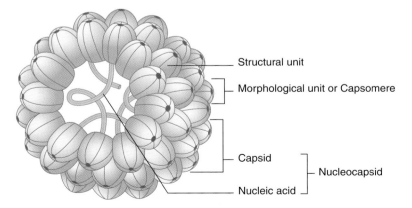

Fig. 20.1   Icosahedral virus particle with cubic symmetry. (Reproduced with permission from Madeley C R 1972 *Virus morphology*.)

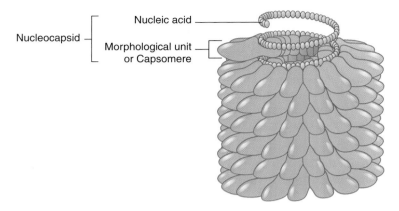

Fig. 20.2 Nucleocapsid of virus particle with helical symmetry. (Reproduced with permission from *Advances in Virus Research* 1960, p. 274.)

3. *Complex*: in which the particle does not conform to either cubic or helical symmetry.

CULTIVATION OF VIRUSES

Because viruses can only replicate within living cells, special methods have to be employed for culture in vitro. The three main systems used for their cultivation in the laboratory are described in Chapter 21.

EFFECTS OF VIRUSES ON CELLS

Viruses can affect cells in four ways:

1. *Death*: the infection is lethal: it causes a cytopathic effect (CPE) that kills the cell.
2. *Transformation*: the cell is not killed, but is changed from a normal cell to one with the properties of a malignant or cancerous cell.
3. *Latent infection*: the virus remains within the cell in a potentially active state, but produces no obvious effects on the cell's functions.
4. *Haemadsorption*: some viruses have protein (haemagglutinin) in their outer coats which adheres to erythrocytes, causing them

to agglutinate; in tissue culture these viruses produce haemagglutinin on the surface of infected cells, to which added erythrocytes adhere.

THE EFFECT OF PHYSICAL AND CHEMICAL AGENTS ON VIRUSES

- *Heat*: most are inactivated at 56°C for 30 min or at 100°C for a few seconds.
- *Cold*: stable at low temperatures; most can be stored satisfactorily at –70°C and most survive well at 4°C. Some viruses are partially inactivated by the process of freezing and thawing.
- *Drying*: variable: some survive well, others are rapidly inactivated.
- *Ultraviolet irradiation*: inactivates viruses.
- *Chloroform, ether and other organic solvents*: viruses with lipid-containing envelopes are inactivated; those without envelopes are resistant.
- *Oxidizing and reducing agents*: viruses are inactivated by formaldehyde, chlorine, iodine and hydrogen peroxide.
- *β-propiolactone and formaldehyde*: used to inactivate viruses for vaccine production.
- *Phenols*: most viruses are relatively resistant.

Table 20.1   Classification of DNA viruses and their diseases

Family	Viruses	Diseases
Poxviruses	Variola	Smallpox
	Molluscum	Molluscum contagiosum
Herpesviruses	Herpes simplex	Herpes simplex
	Varicella-zoster	Chickenpox, shingles
	Cytomegalovirus	Congenital infection in the immunocompromised
	EB (Epstein–Barr) virus	Infectious mononucleosis
	HHV-6 and -7	Exanthem subitum
Adenoviruses	Adenoviruses	Sore throat, conjunctivitis
Hepadnaviruses	Hepatitis B	Hepatitis
Papovaviruses	Papilloma	Warts
	JC virus	Progressive multifocal leukoencephalopathy
Parvoviruses	B19	Erythema infectiosum, aplastic crises

• *Virus disinfectants*: the best are hypochlorite solution (which is corrosive) and glutaraldehyde (which can cause sensitization and irritation to users); newer disinfectants include chlorine dioxide and peracetic acid.

CLASSIFICATION

Viruses are assigned to *groups*, on the basis mainly of the morphology of the virus particle, but also of their nucleic acid and method of RNA transcription. A simplified scheme of classification of the main groups of medically important viruses and the diseases they cause is shown in Tables 20.1 and 20.2.

Table 20.2 Classification of RNA viruses and their diseases

Family	Viruses	Diseases
Orthomyxoviruses	Influenza	Influenza
Paramyxoviruses	Parainfluenza	Respiratory infection
	Respiratory syncytial	
	Measles	Measles
	Mumps	Mumps
Coronaviruses	Coronavirus	Respiratory infection
Rhabdoviruses	Rabies	Rabies
Picornaviruses	Enteroviruses	Meningitis, paralysis
	Rhinoviruses	Colds
	Hepatitis A	Hepatitis
Caliciviruses	Norwalk-like viruses	Gastroenteritis
Togaviruses	Alphaviruses (Group A arboviruses)	Encephalitis, haemorrhagic fevers
	Rubivirus	Rubella
Flaviviruses	Flaviviruses (Group B arboviruses)	Encephalitis, haemorrhagic fevers
	Hepatitis C	Hepatitis
Bunyaviruses	Bunya arboviruses	Encephalitis, haemorrhagic fevers
	Hantavirus	Haemorrhagic fever, renal involvement
Reoviruses	Rotavirus	Gastroenteritis
Arenaviruses	Lymphocytic choriomeningitis	Meningitis
	Junin virus	Haemorrhagic fevers
	Lassa virus	
Retroviruses	HTLV-1	T-cell leukaemia/lymphoma, paresis
	HIV-1, 2	AIDS
Filoviruses	Ebola virus	Marburg and Ebola haemorrhagic fevers
	Marburg virus	

(*Note*: Virus families are now known by Latin names. The more widely used anglicized or vernacular names are used in this classification and throughout the text.)

Diagrams of some representative virus particles are shown in Figure 20.3.

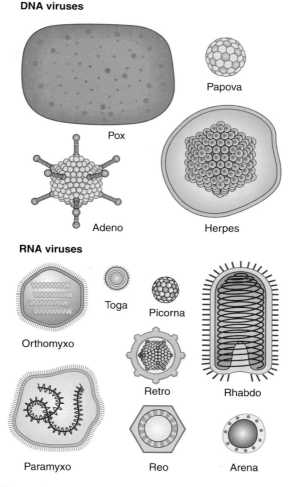

DNA viruses

Pox

Papova

Adeno

Herpes

RNA viruses

Orthomyxo

Toga

Picorna

Retro

Rhabdo

Paramyxo

Reo

Arena

Fig. 20.3 Diagram of the particles of different families of virus. *Note*: These drawings are schematic and are not drawn to scale, although differences in relative size are indicated.

VIRUS DISEASES

Viruses are important and common causes of human disease, especially in children. Most infections are mild and the patient makes a complete recovery; many are silent and the virus multiplies in the body without causing any symptoms at all. However, viral infections which are usually mild sometimes cause severe disease in an unusually susceptible patient. A few viral diseases are severe and always have a high case fatality rate.

Entry

Viruses enter the body in four main ways:

1. *Inhalation*: via the respiratory tract
2. *Ingestion*: via the gastrointestinal tract
3. *Inoculation*: through skin abrasions; mucous membranes (e.g. sexual transmission); transfusion; injections (e.g. medically administered or via shared syringes in drug abuse); organ transplants; via the bite of an arthropod or other animal
4. *Congenital*: or vertically, from mother to fetus.

Invasiveness

The main pathogenic mechanism of viruses is *invasion*. Disease is produced by the effect of viruses when they replicate in the cells of tissues and organs of the body: replication usually – but not always – kills the infected cells. This cytopathic effect in vivo causes lesions and hence dysfunction in the tissue or organ concerned, with associated symptoms and signs.

Note: In some virus infections the immune response contributes to the pathogenesis of virus lesions.

HOST RESPONSE TO VIRUS INFECTION

As with other infectious agents, the body defends itself against viruses by both non-specific and specific mechanisms.

The *non-specific mechanisms* are essentially those activated in response to other infections, such as the flushing effect of secretions in the respiratory tract, the conjunctivae and the urinary tract. Stomach acid, however, does not inactivate the acid-resistant enteroviruses but is active against their close relatives the rhinoviruses.

Non-specific defence mechanisms

The body has defences that are not specifically directed at particular infectious agents, but which act as non-immunological barriers to infection:

Phagocytosis: an important defence mechanism in virus infections: invading viruses are ingested by two types of scavenger cell:

1. *Neutrophil polymorphonuclear leukocytes* in the blood
2. *Macrophages* (or mononuclear cells of the reticuloendothelial system) – of two types:
   - free macrophages in lung alveoli and peritoneal cavity
   - fixed macrophages in lymph nodes, spleen, liver (Kupffer cells), connective tissue (histiocytes) and CNS (microglia).

Phagocytosis is enhanced by antibody (a specific immune mechanism) and complement, an effect known as *opsonization*. Macrophages 'activated' by the cytokines released by T lymphocytes (a specific immune mechanism) have increased phagocytic activity and are attracted by chemotaxis to the site of infection.

Specific (immunological) defence mechanisms

Immunological responses are of two types:

1. *Humoral* – in which antibody neutralizes viruses and renders them non-infectious: responsible for long-term protective immunity
2. *Cellular* – which eliminates virus-infected cells and localizes virus-induced lesions.

Antibody has a role in the cellular response (*antibody-dependent cell-mediated cytotoxicity* – see below) and also aids the elimination of virus directly, through its specific neutralizing activity.

Humoral (antibody) response

Like other infectious agents, viruses induce the production of antibodies in the blood.

Antibodies are *immunoglobulins* – *IgM*, *IgG* and *IgA*: IgG confers long-lasting protection; IgA is important in local immunity to respiratory viruses and, in the gut, to enteroviruses and other faecal viruses. IgM is the earliest antibody produced.

Cell-mediated immunity

Extremely important: clears virus from the body. Children with congenital deficiency of cellular immunity, for example, are abnormally susceptible to virus infection and often (although not always) develop unusually severe and often fatal disease; those with humoral immune deficiency, on the other hand, usually respond normally to virus infections (an exception is enteroviruses – agammaglobulinaemic children are at high risk of poliomyelitis).

Cell-mediated immunity eliminates virus-infected cells – and therefore virus – from the body. *T or thymus-dependent lymphocytes* are the principal cells involved in this. There are two main types:

1. **CD4 helper T cells**: carry CD4 receptors as markers on their surface. The most important cells in the cellular response, they liberate *cytokines* that activate and modulate cellular immune responses. Virus is recognized as antigen by helper T cells presented by a macrophage or dendritic cell (found in lymph nodes and skin) acting as an antigen-presenting cell: recognition is dependent on MHC class II antigens. They also interact with B lymphocytes for antibody production. They are target cells for HIV, the virus of AIDS, and become severely depleted in that disease.

2. **CD8 cytotoxic T cells**: carry the marker CD8 receptor on their surface. They lyse target cells such as virus-infected cells and tumour cells that express MHC class I antigen; the main mechanism for elimination of virus-infected cells from the body; also release cytokines.

Suppressor function: note that both CD4 and CD8 cells can suppress as well as activate the cellular response.

Lysis of virus-infected cells

This important defence mechanism is mediated via several different mechanisms:

1. **Non-antibody-dependent cytotoxicity**: carried out by two types of lymphocyte:
   - *Cytotoxic T cells* – mostly CD8 T cells
   - *Natural killer (NK) cells* – these are large granular lymphocytes present in the non-immune host.

2. **Antibody-dependent cellular cytotoxicity (ADCC)**. Virus-infected cells can also be lysed by T cells with Fc receptors for

IgG, which bind to target cells coated with viral IgG bound to virus on infected cell surfaces. These cells include:

- *Natural killer (NK) cells* – mainly responsible for this type of cell destruction: present in non-immune as well as immune hosts
- *Polymorphonuclear leukocytes*
- *Activated macrophages.*

CYTOKINES

Small protein molecules released by many cells, including lymphocytes and macrophages, which function as signals or mediators to activate, modulate and control the immune responses (and other activities) of cells. There are numerous cytokines, such as interferons (which are important in virus infections), interleukins and tumour necrosis factors: several act sequentially and interact with other cytokines. In addition to their role in the immune response, some cytokines have physiological functions such as tissue repair, differentiation and signalling activity in the CNS.

Interferons are cytokines which render cells refractory to virus infection. There are three main classes, which reflect the cells of origin:

1. α: originate in leukocytes
2. β: originate in fibroblasts
3. γ: originate in T lymphocytes.

Interferons have antiproliferative activity on cells and the immune system, as well as inhibiting virus replication.

Characteristics of interferons:

1. *Host specific*: so that only human interferon is fully active in human cells
2. *Wide antiviral spectrum*: most viruses are inhibited
3. *Induced* by viruses and nucleic acids
4. *Action*: both virus transcription and protein synthesis are prevented.

Interferons were long thought to be potentially ideal chemotherapeutic agents against viruses, but this potential has not been realized in practice. Side-effects (similar to those of pyrogens) have proved troublesome and, despite undoubted clinical response with some viruses, indications for their use remain fairly restricted. However, interferon therapy is proving useful in the treatment of some forms of chronic hepatitis due to viruses.

VIRUS REPLICATION

Viruses have no metabolic activity of their own: they replicate by taking over the biochemical machinery of the host cell and redirecting it to the manufacture of virus components. This takeover is achieved by *virus mRNA*, and once this is produced, successful virus replication is virtually assured.

VIRUS GROWTH CYCLE

Takes place in seven stages:

1. *Adsorption*: to specific receptors on the cell plasma membrane; best at 37°C but also at 4°C
2. *Entry*: by invagination of the cell membrane round the virus particle or, with syncytial viruses, by fusion between virus envelope and cell membrane
3. *Uncoating*: releases or renders accessible the incoming virus genome
4. *Transcription* is: subject to complex control mechanisms:
   • Patterns of transcription differ before (early) and after (late) virus nucleic acid replication
   • Many virus genomes contain promoters and enhancers that stimulate transcription
   • Primary transcripts are often spliced to remove intron sequences between expressed exons
   • Transcription sometimes overlaps, with different starting and/or termination points within one gene, to produce different proteins from the same nucleic acid sequence
Virus mRNA usually contains leader sequences, is capped at the 5′ end and is polyadenylated at the 3′ terminus
5. *Synthesis* of virus components:
Proteins: virus mRNA is translated on cell ribosomes into two types of virus protein:
   • structural – the proteins that make up the virus particle
   • non-structural – not found in the particle; mainly enzymes for virus genome replication
Nucleic acid: new virus genomes are synthesized:

- templates are either the parental genome or, in the case of single-stranded nucleic acid genomes, newly formed complementary strands
- synthesis is most often by a virus-coded polymerase or replicase: in the case of some DNA viruses a cell enzyme carries this out

6. *Assembly*: newly produced virus genomes and proteins are assembled to form new virus particles in the cell nucleus, cytoplasm, or (with most enveloped viruses) at the plasma membrane: this invests the new particles to form the virus envelope

7. *Release*: either by sudden cell rupture or by gradual extrusion (budding) of enveloped viruses through the cell membrane.

VIRUS GENOMES

Nucleic acid

- May be DNA or RNA
- Single- or double-stranded
- Intact or segmented
- Linear or circular.

Large viruses

- Have high molecular weight nucleic acid
- Code for many proteins
- Code for many of the enzymes involved in replication.

Small viruses

- Have low molecular weight nucleic acid
- Therefore limited coding capacity and must use some of the cell enzymes for replication.

Infectivity

In the case of many viruses, the purified nucleic acid is *infectious* when applied to cells – i.e. without the capsid, nucleic acid on its own can infect a cell and initiate a complete infectious cycle of virus replication. Where virions contain a transcriptase, the genomes are *non-infectious* because the process of nucleic acid extraction destroys the virion transcriptase and mRNA cannot then be produced to initiate a replicative cycle.

Table 20.3 Some properties of viruses and their genomes

Virus family	Example	Genome[a]	Transcriptase contained in virus particles
DNA			
Pox	Vaccinia	DS DNA	+
Herpes	Herpes simplex	DS DNA	0
Adeno	Adenovirus	DS DNA	0
Papova	Papilloma	DS DNA	0
Hepadna	Hepatitis B[e]	DS DNA[e]	+[b]
Parvo	B19	SS DNA	0
RNA			
Picorna	Poliovirus	SS RNA	0
Calici	Norwalk-like viruses	SS RNA	0
Toga	Rubella	SS RNA	0
Corona	Coronavirus	SS RNA	0
Orthomyxo	Influenza A	SS RNA[c]	+
Paramyxo	Measles	SS RNA	+
Arena	Lassa fever	SS RNA[c]	+
Bunya	Crimean–Congo haemorrhagic fever	SS RNA[c]	+
Flavi	Yellow fever	SS RNA	0
Filo	Marburg	SS RNA	0
Rhabdo	Rabies	SS RNA	+
Retro	HIV-1	SS RNA[d]	+[b]
Reovirus	Rotavirus[c]	DS RNA[c]	+

[a] DS = double-stranded; SS = single-stranded.
[b] Reverse transcriptase.
[c] Segmented genome (arena 2, Bunya 3, orthomyxo 8, rotavirus 11 unique subunits).
[d] Two identical subunits in the virion.
[e] Virion contains DNA polymerase with reverse transcriptase activity.

Properties

The properties of the main virus groups and their genomes are shown in Table 20.3.

Baltimore classification

This classifies viruses into six groups on the basis of their nucleic acid and mRNA production (Fig. 20.4).

BIOCHEMISTRY OF VIRUS REPLICATION

A complex subject: a few simplified examples are outlined below to highlight the main differences between the growth cycles of some representative groups of DNA and RNA viruses.

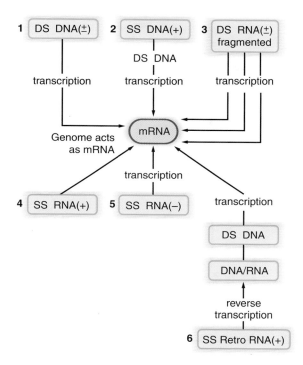

Fig. 20.4 Methods of transcription of the six different groups in the Baltimore classification of virus genomes. *Note*: (+) = positive-sense RNA, i.e. acts as a messenger; (−) = negative-sense RNA, i.e. transcribed to form complementary-sense strands, which then act as messengers.

Double-stranded DNA viruses

Examples: vaccinia, herpes simplex, adenovirus, papillomavirus. The principal steps in their growth cycle are detailed below and shown diagrammatically in Figure 20.5.

Transcription

Two main types of mRNA are produced:

1. *Early mRNA* – before virus DNA synthesis: codes mainly for enzymes required for DNA synthesis
2. *Late mRNA* – after virus DNA synthesis: codes mainly for structural proteins.

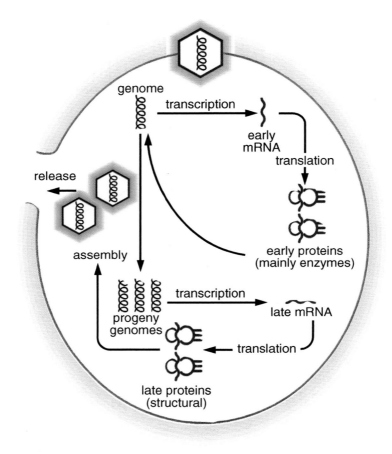

Fig. 20.5 Replicative cycle of double-stranded DNA virus.

Virus DNA synthesis

Enzymes: many are involved, but:

- The main DNA replicative enzyme is DNA-dependent DNA polymerase
- Larger viruses (e.g. vaccinia, herpes simplex) code for their own enzyme
- Smaller viruses (e.g. adenovirus, papillomavirus) use the host cell DNA polymerase.

Template: new progeny virus DNA is synthesized off the DNA genome of the input parental virus.

Site: nucleus (except poxviruses).
New progeny DNA: acts as templates for:

- transcription of late virus mRNA
- synthesis of more genomes for new virus particles.

Virus protein synthesis

A two-stage process:

1. *Production of early proteins* required for virus DNA synthesis (e.g. DNA-dependent DNA polymerase, thymidine kinase).
2. *Production of late proteins* produced after virus DNA synthesis: mostly the capsid proteins for new particles.

Site: virus proteins are synthesized on the ribosomes in the cell cytoplasm, and then transported to sites of assembly.

Assembly

Assembly of new DNA genomes and proteins into new infectious particles within the cell takes place in:

1. *Nucleus* (e.g. herpes simplex, adenovirus, papillomavirus) (*Note*: Herpes particles acquire an envelope by budding through the cell nuclear membrane modified by the incorporation within it of virus glycoproteins).
2. *Cytoplasm*: vaccinia replicates entirely in the cytoplasm in 'factories' which are based on clusters of ribosomes.

Other DNA viruses

Hepatitis B virus has an unusual and complex replication cycle. The genome is an incomplete double-stranded DNA molecule with a DNA polymerase, which can fill in the gap to produce a complete double-stranded molecule. The polymerase also has reverse transcriptase activity. Replication of the genome is unique in that it involves production of an RNA template which then, by reverse transcription, synthesizes an RNA/DNA intermediate which is subsequently converted to double-stranded DNA. The genes for the surface and core proteins are overlapped by the gene for the DNA polymerase.

Single-stranded DNA viruses: parvoviruses have a tiny single-stranded DNA genome. Some are autonomous in replication (e.g. human parvovirus B19); others are defective and require a helper virus for replication. B19 packages (in approximately equal proportions) both positive- and negative-strand DNA into virions, but separately, within different particles.

RNA VIRUSES

Because their genetic material is RNA, these viruses use biochemical mechanisms for their replication which are different from those of other forms of living organism. RNA virus genomes have different types of transcription:

- *Single-strand positive-sense (plus-sense) RNA*: the virus genome is the virus mRNA.
- *Single-strand negative-sense (minus-sense) RNA*: virus mRNA is transcribed from the parental genome.
- *Double-stranded segmented RNA*: individual virus mRNAs are transcribed separately off the parental RNA segments using a transcriptase associated with each segment.
- *Retrovirus*: an RNA virus whose genome alternates between RNA and DNA: virion single-stranded RNA is transcribed into double-stranded DNA, which is then integrated into the host chromosome as a 'provirus', from which virus RNA is later transcribed. But note, retrovirus genomes are inverted dimers of two complete genomes.

Below are examples of the replication cycle of some RNA viruses.

SINGLE-STRAND POSITIVE-SENSE RNA VIRUSES

Example: poliovirus.

With these viruses there is no transcription stage because the single-strand positive-sense genomic RNA itself acts as virus mRNA. The replication cycle is shown diagrammatically in Figure 20.6.

Translation

The virus genome is translated into one very large polypeptide, which is almost immediately cleaved into smaller proteins as follows:

1. *Structural viral capsid proteins*
2. *The RNA-dependent RNA polymerase* required for replication of virus RNA (no similar enzyme exists in cells)

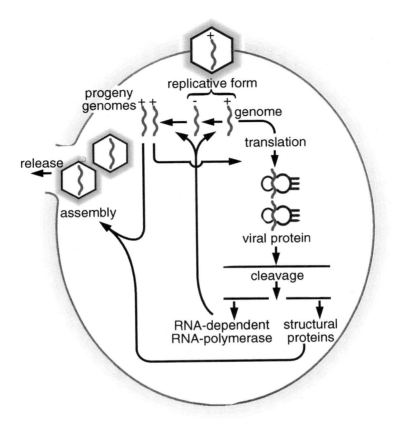

Fig. 20.6   Replicative cycle of single-strand positive-sense RNA virus.

3. *A protease* for cleaving the precursor polypeptide
4. *A genome-linked terminal protein.*

Virus RNA synthesis

New genome production takes place on a double-stranded *'replicative' form* of RNA made by the synthesis of a negative-sense RNA strand complementary to the input positive-sense parental RNA. New progeny positive-sense RNA strands are synthesized off the template of the negative RNA strand in the replicative form.

RNA-dependent RNA polymerase – synthesizes both the replicative form and also new positive-sense RNA strand genomes.

Progeny positive-sense RNA functions as:

- *templates* for the production of more replicative forms (and so for the synthesis of more genome RNA)
- *genomes* for new virus particles
- *virus mRNA.*

Assembly

New progeny virus particles are assembled on clusters of ribosomes from the cleavage products of the primary translation product and from progeny virus RNA in the cytoplasm: poliovirus replicates entirely in the cytoplasm.

SINGLE-STRAND NEGATIVE-SENSE RNA VIRUSES

Example: parainfluenza virus.
The replicative cycle is shown diagrammatically in Figure 20.7.

Transcription

Virus mRNA is synthesized off the parental (negative-sense strand) genome RNA using a transcriptase (RNA-dependent RNA polymerase) contained in the virus particle. Separate virus mRNAs are produced for each of the different virus proteins.

Virus RNA synthesis

Virus progeny genomes are produced – also by the transcriptase – using positive-sense RNA strands complementary to the parental genome as templates.

Virus protein synthesis

Virus proteins include:

- *Transcriptase*
- *Envelope proteins* (two are glycosylated and have haemagglutinin/neuraminidase and fusion/haemolysis activities, respectively)
- *Nucleocapsid.*

Assembly

New virus nucleocapsids are assembled at the cell membrane and become enveloped by budding through the plasma membrane.

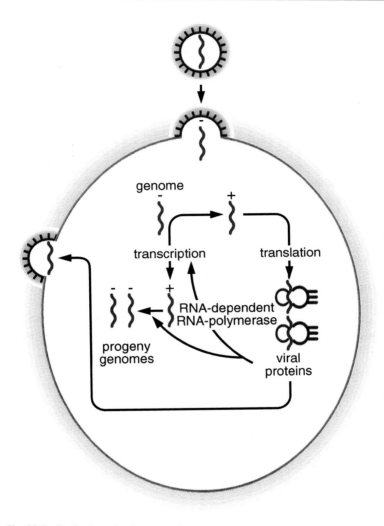

Fig. 20.7   Replicative cycle of single-strand negative-sense RNA virus.

Influenza virus

Influenza virus is unusual among single-stranded RNA viruses in that it has *a segmented genome*, each segment of which codes for a different virus protein.

Viral RNA is synthesized in the cell nucleus involving both host cell and viral transcriptase. Viral proteins are synthesized in the cytoplasm and migrate to the cell surface, where the envelope proteins become incorporated into the plasma membrane; new RNA genomes are also transported to the cell surface where, with the newly synthesized viral proteins, they become assembled into new virions. The virion envelope is acquired when the particles bud through the cell plasma membrane.

DOUBLE-STRANDED RNA VIRUSES

Example: reoviruses.

All double-stranded RNA viruses have segmented genomes. Each segment codes for a different protein and each is associated with a molecule of transcriptase (RNA-dependent RNA polymerase).

The replicative cycle starts with transcription of mRNA from each double-stranded RNA segment – the mRNAs produced are then translated into the different virus proteins.

These mRNA molecules later become enclosed within nucleocapsids, together with a transcriptase which directs the synthesis of a complementary RNA strand to produce the double-stranded segments that make up the genome.

Retroviruses

Example: HIV-1.

Most retroviruses are tumour viruses – HIV is an exception – which can replicate in cells without killing them and can also transform normal cells into malignant or cancer cells. Their replication involves the production of virus DNA, which integrates into the cell chromosome, an important mechanism for malignant transformation.

The retrovirus genome is *single-stranded dimeric RNA* with three principal genes and long terminal repeat regions that enable integration – in the DNA provirus form – into the host cell chromosome. The long terminal repeats contain promoter sequences.

The three principal genes are:

1. *Gag*: core proteins
2. *Pol*: polymerase, i.e. reverse transcriptase (an RNA-dependent DNA polymerase contained in the virion)
3. *Env*: envelope proteins.

Note: Retroviruses contain several other genes with regulatory functions in viral replication.

The replicative cycle is shown diagrammatically in Figure 20.8.

First stage

1. *Transcription* (by the reverse transcriptase contained in the virion) to produce a DNA/RNA genome heteroduplex
2. Conversion of the DNA/RNA heteroduplex into *double-stranded DNA*
3. *Integration* of the double-stranded virus DNA (known as *provirus*) into the cell chromosome.

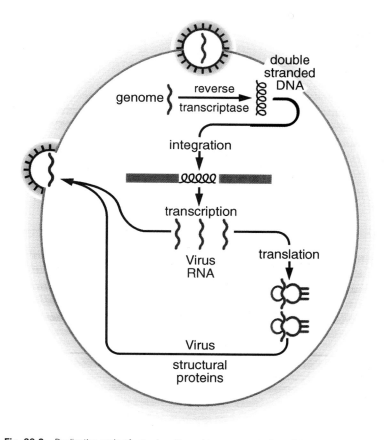

Fig. 20.8   Replicative cycle of retrovirus (the red bar represents the cellular chromosome).

Second stage

1. *Provirus DNA* is transcribed (by cell enzyme)
2. *The RNA transcripts* produced from this have two functions:
    (a) mRNA for translation into virus proteins
    (b) new virus genomes.

Virus protein synthesis

Virus proteins are produced on cell ribosomes by translation of mRNA transcribed off the provirus DNA: the *gag* gene product is synthesized as a large polyprotein and then cleaved by viral protease into the core and matrix proteins:

- Reverse transcriptase
- Core proteins
- Envelope proteins.

Assembly

Nucleocapsids are assembled from the progeny virus RNA genomes and proteins at the cell surface, and acquire their outer envelope by budding through the cell plasma membrane.

21 Laboratory diagnosis of virus diseases

Diagnostic techniques in virology have been revolutionized by the introduction of molecular technology. Because the nucleotide sequences of most viruses are known, it is possible by amplification methods to detect very specifically, minute quantities of virus nucleic acid sequences within patients' samples.

Nevertheless, older, more 'traditional' methods are widely used, and the majority of laboratory tests are still based on them.

The criteria of sensitivity and specificity for laboratory tests are:

Sensitivity: the extent to which a test detects the reaction under test – also reflects the false-negative rate.

Specificity: the quality of the test in detecting only the reaction being tested – also a measure of the false-positive rate.

The bedrock of virus diagnosis is immunological – that is, the demonstration of an antigen–antibody reaction as evidence of recent virus infection (the word 'recent' is important, as most virus infections are followed by long-lasting antibody in the blood).

Recent virus infection is shown by:

1. *Development of antibody* to the virus at the time of or just after the symptoms of disease (serology)
2. *Presence of virus or virus products* in the patient's blood or other tissues (isolation of virus or detection of virus or viral components directly in the specimen).

Serology

Showing that a patient has developed antibody at the same time (or shortly after) the symptoms of virus illness is the surest way to

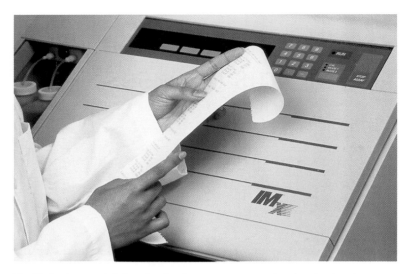

Fig. 21.1 Automated virology. Reading the computer-generated results printed out from an automated ELISA analyser and reader. (Reproduced with permission of Abbott Laboratories Ltd, Maidenhead, UK.)

confirm a diagnosis: this can be done by showing that early IgM antibody is present, or by looking for a fourfold rise in titre as the patient becomes convalescent. Virus serology is now almost entirely (but not quite always) automated.

Automated technology (Fig. 21.1):

- Usually based on enzyme-linked immunosorbent assay or ELISA (also known as EIA); sensitive, rapid, and economical of staff time.
- Carried out mainly using commercially available kits (nowadays generally of good quality).
- Enables large numbers of patients to be diagnosed accurately and rapidly.
- Detects IgM antibody, so that diagnosis can be made in the acute phase of illness.

ELISA

The principles of ELISA are shown in Figure 21.2: note that demonstration of the diagnostic antigen–antibody reaction depends on *labelling antibody with an enzyme* that reacts with an appropriate substrate to produce a measurable colour change.

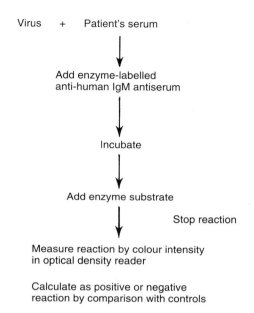

Virus   +   Patient's serum

↓

Add enzyme-labelled
anti-human IgM antiserum

↓

Incubate

↓

Add enzyme substrate

Stop reaction

↓

Measure reaction by colour intensity
in optical density reader

Calculate as positive or negative
reaction by comparison with controls

Fig. 21.2   ELISA test for virus IgM antibody (sandwich technique).

Most ELISAs are carrried out in the wells of microtitre plates, thereby facilitating handling and automation.

A *'sandwich' technique* is often used so that patient's antibody reacting with a known virus is identified by the addition of a second antibody, prepared in animals against the appropriate human immunoglobulin – such as IgM.

ELISAs can be varied by:

Competitive assay: in which patient's serum competes with known (i.e. labelled) virus antibody for combining sites on the virus antigen: inhibition of the activity of the known antibody shows the presence of antibody in the patient's serum.

Other serological techniques in virology

Western blot: in which virus proteins, separated on a cellulose membrane, are exposed to patient's serum: antibodies to individual proteins are detected by enzyme-linked antihuman antibody to analyse the immune response to different virus structural proteins and therefore identify the stage and progress of the viral illness.

Immunofluorescence

The label used is fluorescein dye: virus-infected cells are fixed on glass slides and the immune reaction is detected under UV light using a special microscope: liable to subjective interpretation and labour-intensive, but widely used.

Complement fixation test

When antigen reacts with antibody, complement (contained in guinea-pig serum) is used up or 'fixed'. After the addition of an indicator system such as red blood cells with anti-red-cell antibody, the red cells lyse if complement is present: that is, absence of haemolysis indicates a positive reaction (Fig. 21.3).

Haemagglutination inhibition

Antiviral antibody blocks the agglutination of red cells by haemagglutinating viruses: strain specific and mainly used in reference laboratories.

Single radial haemolysis

Related to haemagglutination inhibition but detects antibody by the appearance in agar gel of haemolysis round wells containing

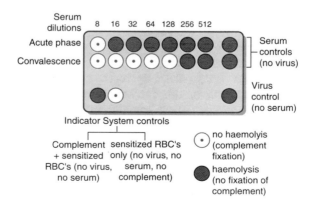

Fig. 21.3 Complement fixation test for viral antibody. Virus antigen is mixed overnight at 4°C with dilutions of the patient's serum and complement before the addition of sensitized sheep erythrocytes. Titre of complement-fixing antibody has risen from 8 in the acute phase to 128 in convalescence, a greater than fourfold rise, indicating recent infection.

patients' sera. The gel contains red cells, virus antigen and complement. Mainly used as a qualitative test.

Neutralization

Antibody blocks viral infectivity in the case of cell cultures (and laboratory animals): laborious and slow, but still sometimes necessary.

Interpreting the significance of virus antibody

Virus antibodies (particularly IgG) are common in healthy populations and usually remain at a high level for many years after infection. Diagnosis of recent infection depends on the following criteria:

1. ***Presence of IgM***: the earliest antibody to appear, and therefore proof of recent (or current) infection. Widely used as a rapid method of diagnosis: only one blood sample is required.

2. ***Rising titre***: increase in the level of IgG antibody (at least fourfold) over the course of infection from the acute phase into convalescence (10–14 days). *Titre* is the highest dilution of an antiserum at which activity is demonstrated: usually expressed as the reciprocal of the antiserum dilution, e.g. 64 rather than 1/64. Note that ELISA does not measure titre. Measurement of titre is best by complement fixation, haemagglutination inhibition, immunofluorescence or neutralization test.

3. ***High stationary titre of IgG***: unreliable, but if the titre of antibody is considerably higher than that found in the general population, and depending on the virus concerned, recent infection with the virus can often be assumed: detection of virus IgG even at low titre is often used to demonstrate pre-existing immunity or successful response to vaccination.

Direct demonstration of virus or virus components

Detection of virus, virus antigen or nucleic acid in specimens taken directly from the patient is used for rapid diagnosis and is particularly helpful if the virus is inactivated, latent, or does not grow in culture. Molecular techniques are increasingly used for this and for detection of the emergence of drug-resistant virus in patients on antiviral therapy.

Molecular methodology

The earliest tests detected virus nucleic acid (RNA or DNA) directly using a radioactive probe in fluids or tissue, i.e. Southern, Northern and dot blot, and in situ hybridization. These techniques were relatively insensitive and have largely been replaced by methods of nucleic acid amplification, such as the polymerase chain reaction (PCR) or signal amplification methods such as branched (b) DNA assay. This is a rapidly advancing field and many ingenious systems applicable to routine diagnostic laboratories have been, and are being, developed: most use non-radioactive detection.

PCR

This can detect either DNA or RNA – the latter by use of reverse transcriptase initially to convert the RNA into DNA (RT-PCR). The technique depends on the heat-stable *Taq* DNA polymerase, which can withstand the extremes of temperature required for the reaction:

1. DNA strands are first separated (i.e. denatured) at 95°C.
2. Then annealed at lower temperature, typically 40–65°C, with a pair of oligonucleotide primers which bind to sequences flanking the target area.
3. Primers are then extended by the *Taq* polymerase at 72°C so that the target sequence is replicated.
4. Cycle of replication is then repeated many times, yielding from 10^5 to 10^6 copies of the target DNA within 3–4 hours.

These heating and cooling step changes require an automated accurate thermal cycler – see Figure 21.4.

The reaction can be made more sensitive by *nesting* (Fig. 21.5): this adds, for a second round of PCR, two additional primers which bind internally within the target sequence, so giving more specific and sensitive amplification. PCR is exquisitely sensitive – one or only a very few copies of the target virus nucleic acid can be detected.

Multiplex PCR: uses multiple primers to detect a variety of viruses, e.g. in samples of CSF to screen for neurotropic viruses.

False positives: are the price paid for the extremely high sensitivity – even one molecule of extraneous DNA can lead to a false-positive reaction. Amplified product (the amplicon) carryover is therefore potentially a major problem.

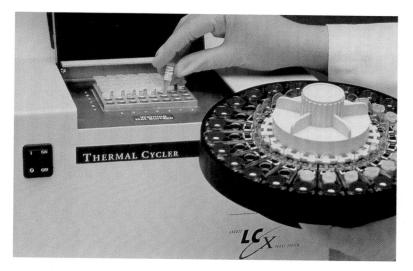

Fig. 21.4 Thermal cycler used for PCR: this allows the accurate temperature control needed for the synthesis of DNA by the thermostable enzyme *Taq* polymerase. DNA is denatured at high temperatures, alternating with cycles at lower temperatures for primer binding and the synthesis of specified regions of the DNA undergoing amplification. (Reproduced with the permission of Abbott Laboratories Ltd, Maidenhead, UK.)

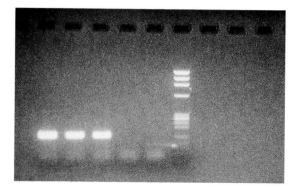

Fig. 21.5 Nested products analysed by agarose gel electrophoresis and viewed under ultraviolet light after staining with ethidium bromide. Counting from the left-hand side, the lanes contain PCR products derived fom 100, 10, 1, 0.1 and 0.01 copies of HTLV-1 DNA template. The lane furthest from the left contains a molecular weight marker. Note that the detection limit of this nested PCR is one copy. Photograph kindly provided by Dr J. Garson, Department of Virology, Royal Free and University College London Medical School.

False negatives: can be caused if the specimen contains inhibitors of *Taq* polymerase, e.g. heparin or haemoglobin.

These problems can for the most part be resolved by meticulous attention to detail, the inclusion of multiple controls and the use of separate rooms for different stages of the reaction.

PCR is the most generally useful test and is now available in many diagnostic laboratories, from where, if not available on site, specimens can be sent to more specialized centres for testing.

Other amplification methods are available, such as the ligase chain reaction (LCR) – especially for *C. trachomatis* detection in genital specimens and NASBA (nucleic acid sequence-based amplification), which is used to detect RNA and is an isothermal reaction and so does not require a thermal cycler.

AMPLICON ASSAY

The product (amplicon) of the viral nucleic acid amplification methods must be carefully identifed. This is usually done by capturing the product with complementary probes on to a solid phase (such as the wells of a microtitre plate). The amplicon has already been labelled with biotin at the 5′ end so that it can be detected (and specified) by reacting with streptavidin and horseradish peroxidase in a colorimetric assay. Amplicons can also be run in an agarose gel and their size compared to standards in a molecular weight ladder (Fig. 21.5).

QUANTITATIVE ASSAY

There is now considerable demand for quantification of the viral nucleic acids, not only to monitor progress of the infection but also to determine indications for therapy. The amplification techniques described above can be adapted for quantitative assay, but the *signal amplification assays* (such as branched (b) DNA or hybrid capture) are also commonly used.

bDNA

The reaction works through a series of probes, which first fix the viral target on to a solid phase (such as the wells of a microtitre plate). Then extender probes fix another set of branched and enzyme-labelled indicator probes, which react with a chemiluminescent substrate, dioxetane. Although the number of target viral sequences remains unaltered, each viral sequence is indirectly bound to many thousands of indicator probes and the signal (the light emitted) is directly proportional to the concentration of target nucleic acid. The bDNA assay is easier to perform than PCR and not so prone to false positives or inhibition.

Other direct tests for virus include:

1. Virus antigen tests
2. Electron microscopy
3. Inclusion bodies.

1. **Tests for virus antigen**
   - *ELISA*: basically the same method as that designed for antibody tests but adapted for antigen, for example by adsorbing antibody to the wells of the test plate to 'capture' the virus: monoclonal antibodies which have higher specificity are often used for this.
   - *Immunofluorescence*: fluorescein-labelled antibody detects virus antigen and enables the extent, localization within cells and distribution to be visualized. Still commonly used to detect respiratory viruses.

2. **Electron microscopy**

Laborious and insensitive (10^6 particles per mL are necessary for detection) but still used for the diagnosis of some faecal viruses and for detecting virus in vesicle fluid.

3. **Inclusion bodies**

Virus-induced masses seen in the nucleus or cytoplasm of infected cells in stained preparations: hardly ever used now as, with a few exceptions, e.g. rabies, they are too non-specific to be useful in diagnosis.

VIRUS ISOLATION

Virus isolation requires the use of living cells, as viruses cannot grow on inanimate media. Now used for diagnosis much less than formerly, with the advent of more rapid tests, but is still necessary to detect the unexpected virus. The rapidly expanding field of antiviral therapy also requires virus isolation and subsequent susceptibility testing to detect the emergence of resistant virus.

Three main systems of living cells are used for culturing viruses:

1. Tissue culture
2. Chick embryo ⎫
3. Laboratory animals ⎭ rarely used.

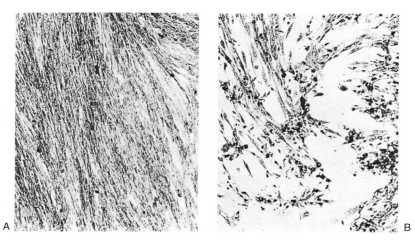

A   B

Fig. 21.6 CPE in a tissue culture of fibroblastic cells. (A) Uninoculated control; (B) culture showing viral cytopathic effect (CPE) with cell death.

Tissue culture

Tissue culture is really cell culture in vitro, and consists of a single layer (monolayer) or a suspension of actively metabolizing cells in a test tube, Petri plate or bottle.

Cultures may be: primary (e.g. monkey kidney); semicontinuous (e.g. human embryo lung) or continuous (e.g. HeLa cells) grown at 37°C in balanced and buffered salt solution with added amino acids, vitamins, serum and antibiotics; CO_2 is added if the containers are not stoppered.

Specimens: are collected on a wooden-shafted swab with the tip broken off into a bottle of transport medium and delivered rapidly to the laboratory; if this is impossible, keep at 4°C.

After inoculation: virus growth is recognized by cytopathic effect (CPE) or cell death; (Fig. 21.6), haemadsorption (adherence of erythrocytes to the cells), or by immunofluorescence with virus-specific antiserum.

Chick embryo: rarely used now for virus diagnosis. Useful for preparation of bulk virus, e.g. for antigen or vaccine production.

Laboratory animals: some viruses can only be isolated by inoculation of laboratory animals, usually mice. After inoculation the animals are observed for signs of disease or death.

VIRUS
DISEASES

22 Virus respiratory diseases

Virus infections of the respiratory tract are by far the commonest of human infections and, although usually not life-threatening, cause a large amount of morbidity and loss of time at work. Influenza is the most severe of these, but the numerous viruses that cause the common cold and related syndromes are important because they are so common. In addition to the viruses that primarily infect the respiratory tract, respiratory involvement is common with many other virus diseases, e.g. the childhood fevers, cytomegalovirus in the immunocompromised, and the non-viral agents chlamydiae and rickettsiae.

INFLUENZA

Influenza is the most important of the great epidemic diseases. From time to time, influenza becomes pandemic and sweeps throughout the world. The most severe pandemic recorded was in the winter of 1918–19, when more than 20 million people perished. Worldwide pandemics of influenza are due to the emergence of antigenically new strains of influenza virus.

Clinical features

Transmission: inhalation of respiratory secretions from an infected person.

Incubation period: 1–4 days.

Symptoms: fever, malaise, headaches, generalized aches, a characteristic non-productive hacking cough: sometimes with sore throat and hoarseness, nasal discharge and sneezing.

Duration: symptoms usually last for about 4 days, but tiredness and weakness often persist for longer.

Primary site of virus multiplication: superficial epithelium of the lower respiratory tract, with damage to the cilia and desquamation of the epithelium.

Complications

Two kinds of pneumonia may follow influenza:

1. *Primary influenzal pneumonia*: rare, almost always fatal: a patient with typical influenza suddenly deteriorates, with the onset of severe respiratory distress and symptoms of hypoxia, dyspnoea and cyanosis; circulatory collapse – and usually death – follows. The onset can be so sudden that typical symptoms of influenza have not developed. Post mortem there is congestion of the lungs, with desquamation of ciliated epithelium and hyperaemia of tracheal and bronchial mucosa; no significant bacteria are present.

2. *Secondary bacterial pneumonia*: more common, especially in the elderly or in patients with pre-existing cardiac or pulmonary disease; due to secondary invasion of the lungs by bacteria such as *Staphylococcus aureus*, *Haemophilus influenzae* or pneumococci. The signs and symptoms are those of severe bacterial pneumonia. Although there is a high case fatality rate, the disease is less lethal than primary influenzal pneumonia. Post mortem there is heavy invasion of the lungs by bacteria.

3. *Reye's syndrome*: a rare but serious complication (see also Chapter 28) seen in children after influenza (and other virus infections): neurological signs are prominent, with cerebral oedema and fatty degeneration of the viscera, especially the liver, causing raised transaminase levels in the blood. The mortality is 20–35%. Aspirin predisposes to the syndrome and children should not be treated with this drug.

Types of virus

There are three influenza viruses: A, B and C, differentiated by their nucleoprotein antigen:

- *A*: the principal cause of epidemic influenza
- *B*: usually a milder disease, but also causes winter outbreaks (especially in children)
- *C*: of doubtful pathogenicity for humans.

Influenza A viruses are also found in animals, notably birds, pigs and horses.

Epidemiology

Seasonal distribution: present every winter in varying prevalence in temperate and cold climates (but the pandemic of 'Asian' influenza started in Britain in the summer of 1957). Seasonal prevalence is much less marked in tropical countries.

Epidemic spread: more rapid than with any other infectious disease and associated with *antigenic shift* or *drift* in the haemagglutinin (and sometimes the neuraminidase also) on the virus surface (see below).

Virology

Orthomyxoviruses, pleomorphic enveloped particles (Fig. 22.1) with single-strand negative-sense RNA in eight separate segments,

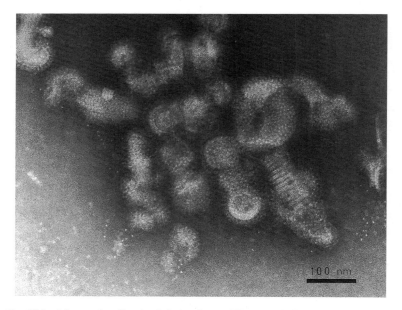

Fig. 22.1   Influenza virus. The virus helical nucleocapsid is surrounded by an envelope containing spikes of haemagglutinin and neuraminidase. This micrograph shows rarely observed morphology with the internal structure revealed by a particle with an extruded internal helix. ×66 000. (Reproduced by kind permission of Dr Anne Field, Central Public Health Laboratory, Colindale, London.)

each of which is a gene coding for a different protein, such as haemagglutinin, neuraminidase, or the internal protein of the nucleocapsid.

Antigenic structure

Influenza viruses have three main antigens:

1. **'S' or soluble antigen**: the internal protein of the nucleocapsid. All influenza A viruses share a common 'S' antigen which is different from that present in influenza B and C viruses; demonstrated by complement fixation test.

2. **Haemagglutinin**: a subtype-specific virus envelope protein; combines with specific receptors (sialic acid, also known as neuraminic acid) on respiratory epithelium: the main target of neutralizing antibodies and thus responsible for immunity to the virus. Haemagglutinin also combines with sialic acid on erythrocytes in vitro, which is inhibited by neutralizing antibody, giving a convenient test for diagnosis.

3. **Neuraminidase**: also a subtype-specific virus envelope protein which destroys neuraminic acid receptors on cells: it aids release of the virus from the cells during replication; also antigenic and plays a minor role in immunity to reinfection.

Virus subtypes: the subtypes of haemagglutinin and neuraminidase are used to characterize different subtypes (or strains) of influenza virus, e.g. H1N1, with further designations indicating the place, the culture number and year of isolation, e.g. A/Sydney/5/97.

Influenza A

Influenza A viruses are uniquely able to undergo *frequent antigenic change*. Epidemics are due to the emergence and spread of a new virus containing a haemagglutinin (and sometimes a neuraminidase also) different from those of previously circulating viruses: the population therefore lacks herd immunity (i.e. antibody) to the new haemagglutinin. Antigenic change may be:

- *major* – or shift
- *minor* – or drift.

Antigenic shift

This results from genetic reassortment of the RNA segments that code for haemagglutinin during replication, when two different influenza viruses infect the same cell and one virus acquires its haemagglutinin gene from the second virus. As a result, a new virus subtype emerges with a novel haemagglutinin to which human populations have no pre-existing antibody and which can cause a pandemic. Genetic reassortment can also result in the acquisition of a new neuraminidase.

Table 22.1 lists the main (shifted) influenza A viruses of the last 80 years.

Antigenic drift

Due to spontaneous point mutations in the haemagglutinin gene that cause minor substitutions in the amino acid sequence of the haemagglutinin protein, with consequent slight changes in antigenicity (although the haemagglutinin remains the same subtype). A drifted subtype of virus then becomes selected in a population of partially immune hosts. Antigenic drift increases progressively from season to season.

Epidemics

Pandemics of influenza A break out every few years when an epidemic new virus subtype spreads worldwide. The worst was in 1918–19, when it caused high mortality, especially in young adults. Nowadays, influenza is generally milder and is most severe in the elderly and in patients with chronic respiratory or cardiac disease.

Several pandemics of influenza have been recorded this century:

Table 22.1 Main influenza A viruses

Year of emergence	Haemagglutinin	Neuraminidase
1918	H1	N1
1957	H2	N2
1968	H3	N2
1977	H1	N1

- *1918–19*: due to an H1N1 swine influenza strain. This virus was never isolated, but its antigenic structure has been deduced from analysis of stored sera collected at the time and from genetic analysis of RNA recovered by PCR from stored lung tissue of fatal cases in the pandemic.
- *1933*: the first influenza virus (a drifted H1N1 strain) was isolated.
- *1957*: H2N2: the 'Asian flu' epidemic.
- *1968*: H3N2: the 'Hong Kong flu' epidemic.
- *1977*: H1N1 reappeared: 'Red flu', a mild form of influenza that infected young people, because older people had antibody from exposure to the virus before 1957.
- *1989*: H3N2 caused a widespread epidemic with many deaths in the UK in late 1989 after several years of low influenza activity.

Since 1977 both H3N2 and H1N1 strains (interspersed with B strains) have circulated together in countries throughout the world, but with considerable antigenic drift, particularly in the case of H3N2.

Influenza B

Influenza B also shows antigenic variation, but the changes are less dramatic than with influenza A. Although generally less severe than influenza A, B viruses can cause quite extensive epidemics.

Diagnosis

Detect virus by PCR or antigen by immunofluorescence in nasopharyngeal aspirate or respiratory secretions: *serologically* by complement fixation with the 's' antigen.

Isolation: necessary for tracking current circulating virus subtypes, now less used for diagnosis; virus is grown from respiratory secretions in monkey kidney tissue cultures.

Prophylaxis and treatment (see also Chapters 33 and 39)

Annual vaccination is recommended for high-risk patients, including the elderly: current vaccines contain recent subtypes of H3N2, H1N1 and one B virus.

Zanamivir (Relenza) can reduce the duration of symptoms and protect against influenza. Also Amantadine.

OTHER RESPIRATORY VIRUS INFECTIONS

Upper respiratory infections are the commonest illnesses seen in general practice, but predominantly upper respiratory syndromes usually show some involvement of the lower respiratory tract.

Incubation period: variable but generally short – from 12 hours to 8 days, depending on the virus.

Transmission: rapid, by inhalation of respiratory secretions and by surface contamination (including hands) with nasal secretions.

The principal viruses other than influenza that affect the respiratory tract are shown in Table 22.2.

PARAINFLUENZA VIRUSES

Clinical features

A wide spectrum of respiratory syndromes, from severe life-threatening lower respiratory tract disease to mild, self-limiting colds; generally more severe than rhinovirus infections but less severe than influenza.

Croup or acute laryngotracheobronchitis: mainly in infants and young children: preceded by symptoms of a common cold that worsen with increasing hoarseness, cough and the development of severe inspiratory stridor, which can lead to respiratory distress and cyanosis requiring tracheostomy.

Table 22.2 Viruses other than influenza that infect the respiratory tract

Virus	No. of serotypes	Disease
Parainfluenza viruses	4	Croup, colds, lower respiratory infections in children
Respiratory syncytial virus	1	Bronchiolitis and pneumonia in infants, colds
Rhinoviruses	100+	Colds
Adenoviruses	49	Pharyngitis and conjunctivitis
Coronaviruses	3	Colds

Common cold with coryza, sore throat, hoarseness, cough and, sometimes, fever.

Bronchiolitis and pneumonia in young children are also sometimes caused by parainfluenza viruses, particularly type 3.

Bone marrow transplant patients: parainfluenza type 3 has a predilection for these and other immunocompromised patients: nosocomial outbreaks have been reported in bone marrow transplant units, where there is a high death rate – often from giant-cell pneumonia: the patients cannot clear the virus and usually succumb to chronic, progressive infection.

Age: seen in both children and adults, but most common in children under 5 years old; the more severe infections are seen in preschool children.

Serotypes and disease: types 1, 2 and 3 (type 4 is rare and of low pathogenicity): there is considerable overlap, but type 3 virus is particularly associated with bronchiolitis and bronchopneumonia, and types 1 and 2 (especially type 1) with croup. Type 3 infects younger children than types 1 and 2.

Epidemiology: type 3 tends to be endemic in the community, with a peak incidence in the spring: types 1 and 2 used to be seen every second year – sometimes together – but this pattern has been less clear in recent years.

Immunity is not long-lasting and reinfection is common.

Virology

Paramyxoviruses, single-stranded negative-sense RNA, large enveloped particles: haemagglutinate and grow in monkey kidney tissue cultures.

Diagnosis

Detect virus in nasopharyngeal aspirates by immunofluorescence.

Serology: of little value because of frequent cross-reactions with pre-existing antibody.

RESPIRATORY SYNCYTIAL VIRUS (RSV)

Causes common colds, but its importance lies in its tendency to invade the lower respiratory tract in infants under 1 year old, causing bronchiolitis and pneumonia.

Clinical features

Colds: the most common manifestation of infection and especially frequent in children under 2 years of age: but also affects the elderly, sometimes with lower respiratory tract involvement.

Bronchiolitis: an important and life-threatening disease in infants, especially in the first 6 months of life: starts with nasal obstruction and discharge (i.e. the symptoms of a common cold) followed by fever, cough, rapid breathing, expiratory wheezes and signs of respiratory distress, with cyanosis and inspiratory indrawing of the intercostal spaces.

Pneumonia: also seen in small infants: the clinical picture is similar to that of bronchiolitis, with fever, cyanosis, prostration and rapid breathing, but without expiratory wheezing.

Bronchiolitis and pneumonia: have a case fatality rate of 2–5%.

Bone marrow transplant patients: like parainfluenza virus type 3, RSV causes severe illness in the immunocompromised, who are often unable to clear virus and succumb to chronic, progressive respiratory infection; sometimes seen in nosocomial outbreaks.

Virus shedding: infected children are infectious, i.e. they shed virus in respiratory secretions, for between 3 and 8 days: nosocomial outbreaks can be a problem in paediatric units.

Epidemiology: every year there are outbreaks of RSV, most often during the later winter months from December to March.

Immunopathology: vaccine containing RSV (there is one serological type, although two differing strains can be distinguished) enhanced the incidence of bronchiolitis and pneumonia in infant vaccinees compared to controls: this suggested that there may be an immunological component to the pathology of these diseases in infants – in whom maternal antibodies would still be present – possibly causing the formation of immune complexes; however, this remains controversial. Alternatively, the susceptibility of very young infants to serious disease may be mechanical owing to the narrowness of the bronchiolar lumen: when this is inflamed, serious obstruction may be produced more readily than in older infants with wider bronchioles.

Virology

A paramyxovirus with single-strand negative-sense RNA: pleomorphic enveloped particles (Fig. 22.2). Grows in cells with syncytial CPE: no haemagglutination. Two types distinguishable by serotyping.

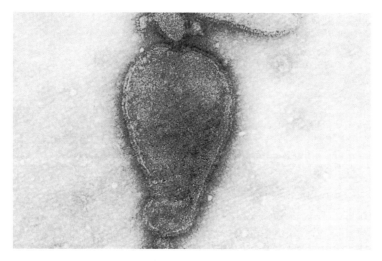

Fig. 22.2 Respiratory syncytial virus. The pleomorphic particle has a helical nucleocapsid. × 90 000. (Electronmicrograph courtesy of Dr E. A. C. Follett.)

Diagnosis

Detect virus in nasopharyngeal aspirates by immunofluorescence, or *isolate* virus from mouth washings or aspirates in tissue cultures.

Prevention and treatment: palivizumab, a monoclonal antibody, is used to protect especially vulnerable infants; ribavirin administered by inhalation is used to treat severe disease.

RHINOVIRUSES

The cause of roughly a third of common colds, with very numerous antigenically distinct types ensuring frequent infections.

Clinical features

Signs and symptoms: nasal discharge with nasal obstruction, sneezing, sore throat and cough; about half the patients are mildly febrile; hoarseness and headache are common, especially in adults.

Duration: on average symptoms subside in about a week, but are prolonged for up to 2 weeks in a proportion of cases; complications include sinusitis and otitis media.

Age: most frequent in preschool children; thereafter the attack rate falls, but infections are common even among adults.

Incidence: variable, but on average the attack rate is about one rhinovirus infection per person per year.

Seasonal prevalence: infections are found all year round, but the highest incidence is in the winter months.

Immunity: neutralizing antibody is formed after rhinovirus infection, both in blood and in respiratory secretions: respiratory IgA has the main protective effect against reinfection with the particular serotype responsible.

Epidemiology

This is complex, as would be expected from the numerous virus serotypes. In any community at any given time several serotypes can be found circulating, but over a period of time the serotypes present gradually change owing to increasing immunity within the population to earlier serotypes.

Virology

Picornaviruses, single-stranded, positive-sense RNA; more than 100 serotypes; grow in tissue culture, but at 33°C rather than the usual 37°C.

Diagnosis

Isolate virus from nasal secretions, mouth washings in human embryo cell cultures: rarely attempted although not difficult.

ADENOVIRUSES

Respiratory infection: clinical features

The main features of adenovirus respiratory infection are *pharyngitis* (often with tonsillitis) and *conjunctivitis*, but adenoviruses cause other syndromes as well. The main respiratory diseases and the types of virus that cause them are shown in Table 22.3.

Epidemic infection: with high attack rates seen where susceptible young people are crowded together, e.g. in army recruit camps (where attack rates of 70% have been recorded) and in children's institutions.

Table 22.3 Respiratory syndromes associated with adenoviruses

Syndrome	Adenovirus types
1. *Epidemic infection* Pharyngoconjunctival fever, acute respiratory disease	3, 4, 7, 14, 21
2. *Endemic infection* Pharyngitis, follicular conjunctivitis	1, 2, 5, 6
3. *Epidemic keratoconjunctivitis or 'shipyard eye'*	8, 19, 37

Endemic infection: adenovirus infections are endemic at a low level in the general population: they cause around 3% of the respiratory infections in the community at large; typically associated with types 1, 2 and 5, but infections due to types 3 and 7 are also common in the community and tend to be found in clusters.

Pneumonia: adenoviruses – particularly types 3 and 7 – are a significant cause of pneumonia in preschool children: the illness starts with fever, dyspnoea, cough and wheezing, and is sometimes followed by residual lung damage.

Epidemic keratoconjunctivitis: a more severe infection than the more common adenovirus conjunctivitis; due to infection of the cornea and conjunctiva spread by contaminated instruments at eye clinics and surgeries; epidemics are seen in patients attending these clinics, and also in shipyard and metal workers who are prone to minor eye injuries; the disease is mainly associated with adenovirus type 8, although other types, especially types 19 and 37, have been reported.

Intestine: adenoviruses are often found in the faeces during respiratory infection, but not often with intestinal symptoms.

Other syndromes

Intestinal: types 40 and 41 cause viral gastroenteritis and are 'fastidious' in that they do not grow in routine cell cultures (see also Chapter 23); adenoviruses probably play a part in mesenteric adenitis and intussusception in children.

Bone marrow transplantation: adenovirus infection, sometimes disseminated, has been reported in transplant patients; AIDS patients are also vulnerable to severe adenovirus infection.

Acute haemorrhagic cystitis: has also been described associated with adenovirus types 11 and 21: this can be a problem in renal transplant patients, but is also seen in the immunocompetent.

Persistent infection: adenoviruses tend to persist for long periods in tissues such as the tonsils, adenoids and, less often, kidneys: this may not be true latency but rather a low grade chronic infection.

Oncogenic properties: several adenoviruses cause cancer on injection into hamsters; the most highly oncogenic are types 12, 18 and 31. However, adenoviruses do not cause tumours in humans.

Virology

Double-stranded DNA viruses with classic icosahedral particles, with fibres topped by knobs projecting from the vertices (Fig. 22.3). There are 49 types.

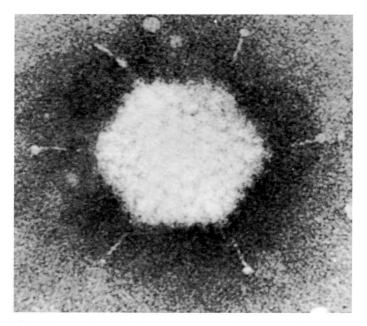

Fig. 22.3 Adenovirus. Icosahedral-shaped particle with cubic symmetry and fibres that project from the vertices. × 200 000. (Reproduced with permission from Valentine R C, Pereira H G 1965 *Journal of Molecular Biology* **13**: 13.)

Diagnosis

Isolate: from mouth washings, throat swabs, in cell culture; also s*erology* by complement fixation test, which is not type-specific.

Other viruses causing common colds

CORONAVIRUSES

Quite a common cause of colds in the community but not often diagnosed because they require specialized techniques for isolation. Single-stranded, positive-sense RNA viruses with characteristic enveloped particles surrounded by a fringe of club-shaped projections (toroviruses, similar to coronaviruses and not a cause of respiratory disease, are found in the stools of children and adults with diarrhoea).

ENTEROVIRUSES

Also cause respiratory infection; a variety of echo and coxsackie viruses have been reported.

23 Viral gastroenteritis

Viruses are an important cause of acute diarrhoea – most often (but not exclusively) in young children. In developing countries viral gastroenteritis is a major cause of the high infant mortality; in Britain the disease is now generally mild. Four main viruses are responsible; growth in cell culture is difficult and, with some, impossible: most were discovered and are still diagnosed by electron microscopy.

Clinical features

Viral gastroenteritis presents a broadly similar clinical picture no matter what virus is the cause.

Incubation period: short: 1–2 days.

Symptoms: acute onset of watery diarrhoea, often with vomiting – which may be projectile – and sometimes with fever: abdominal cramps are common; dehydration – with hyponatraemia – can be life-threatening in small children (see Fig. 7.1 of a child with infantile gastroenteritis), but the disease is usually self-limiting, with a relatively short duration of from 3 to 5 days.

Symptomless infection: is a frequent feature with most of these viruses.

Age: seen in all age groups (including the elderly), but much more common in children.

Pathology: diarrhoea is due to the destructive effect of virus on the epithelium of the small intestine.

The main viruses causing acute diarrhoea are listed in Table 23.1, which also indicates some features of the disease they cause.

Table 23.1 Viruses causing gastroenteritis

Virus	Family	Epidemiological features
Rotavirus	Reovirus	Major cause of childhood diarrhoea
Norwalk-like viruses	Calicivirus	Causes outbreaks in adults
Adenovirus types 40 and 41	Adenovirus	Second most common cause of childhood diarrhoea
Astrovirus	Astrovirus	Less common cause of childhood diarrhoea; sometimes outbreaks

Epidemiology

Two patterns of disease are seen:

Endemic infection: common in young children, especially with group A rotaviruses and adenoviruses 40 and 41.

Epidemic: outbreaks of infection are seen, often in adults and most often due to Norwalk-like viruses.

Season: generally most common in the winter months.

Geographical distribution: worldwide distribution, but highest incidence in conditions of poor sanitation, overcrowding and poverty.

Transmission: often difficult to determine – probably mainly faecal–oral, via contaminated fomites or food and water.

Immunity

Second attacks of viral gastroenteritis are common, even with the same virus: this may be due to the plethora of different serotypes, or perhaps because immunity to these viruses is short-lived.

Diagnosis

Electron microscopy: still widely used but depends on large numbers of virus particles in a stool sample – more than 10^6/mL are necessary, preferably obtained early in infection. Now being replaced or supplemented by ELISA for virus antigen detection or RT-PCR for RNA detection.

Isolation: not an option: Norwalk-like viruses do not grow in cell culture and the other viruses with difficulty, or only with the use of specialized cell culture techniques.

Treatment

Symptomatic: rehydration, with care to correct sodium loss (hyponatraemia).

ROTAVIRUS

The first virus found to cause infantile gastroenteritis: mainly affects small children, but occasional outbreaks have been reported in adults – most often among the elderly in hospitals or in residential homes. The commonest strains are of group A, but group Bs have caused large outbreaks in children and adults in China. Note that in infants less than 3 months of age rotavirus infection is often symptomless.

Pathogenicity: there is no doubt that rotavirus causes diarrhoea, but infection is often symptomless – with virus being found in the stools of healthy controls.

Epidemiology

Infection is mainly endemic, but is both widespread and world-wide.

Transmission: faecal–oral from case to case, but respiratory symptoms have been described in rotavirus infection, raising the possibility that respiratory secretions may also be a source of spread.

Virology

Electron microscopy: characteristic double-shelled particles (Fig. 23.1) with double-stranded RNA in 11 segments (Fig. 23.2).

Classified into five groups (A–E) based on the antigenicity of the inner capsid protein: group A is further subdivided into a variety of different serotypes based on the G (glycoprotein) and P (protease) proteins.

Vaccine: an oral, live tetravalent vaccine containing reassortant virus based on rotavirus from Rhesus monkeys has been developed, but early reports indicate that its use may be associated with intussusception.

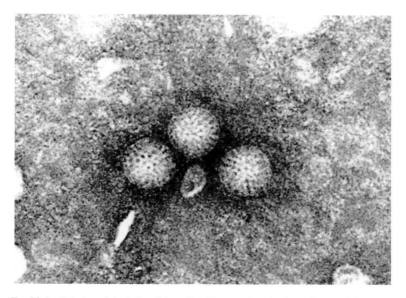

Fig. 23.1   Rotavirus. Spherical particles with cubic symmetry, showing a characteristic outer layer like the spokes of a wheel, which distinguishes the virus from other reoviruses. × 200 000. Electronmicrograph courtesy of Professor C. R. Madeley.)

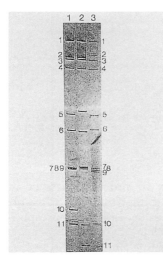

Fig. 23.2   The 11 RNA segments of the rotavirus genome can be separated by gel electrophoresis. The three rotavirus strains shown here are distinguishable by differences in the size – and hence the migration into the gel – of their RNA segments. (Photograph courtesy of Dr U. Desselberger.)

NORWALK-LIKE VIRUSES

Formerly known as SRSVs, these human caliciviruses are an important cause of diarrhoea, both in childhood as well as in outbreaks in adults. Many are still known by the place where they were first isolated.

Norwalk *gastroenteritis* is often accompanied by abdominal cramps and vomiting is prominent, often projectile – sometimes without diarrhoea, when the disease has been called 'winter vomiting disease'.

Epidemiology

Transmission: faecal–oral, i.e. case-to-case, and also via polluted water and food contaminated by a food handler: but contamination of the environment with virus-containing vomit is also probably a route of infection; virus is excreted in the faeces for only up to 72 h.

Outbreaks are common and have been reported associated with shellfish (especially oysters) and faeces-contaminated water; SRSVs are a common problem in hospitals and in residential homes for the elderly, in whom the infection can occasionally prove fatal, doubtless owing to the frailty of the inhabitants. Also the cause of not infrequent outbreaks in cruise ships, and of vomiting among the American military during the Gulf War.

Virology

Electron microscopy: small particles having a six-pointed star surface structure with a central hole (Fig. 23.3); single-strand positive-sense RNA: five serotypes have been identified and, with the advent of sequencing, three genotypes.

Culture: Norwalk-like viruses do not grow in any cell cultures.

ADENOVIRUSES

Diarrhoea-causing adenoviruses, types 40 and 41 (classified as group F adenoviruses) are 'fastidious' in that they are cultivable only by specialized techniques; serologically distinct from respiratory strains.

Endemic: adenovirus diarrhoea is endemic and adenoviruses are second only to rotaviruses as a cause of diarrhoea: the infection

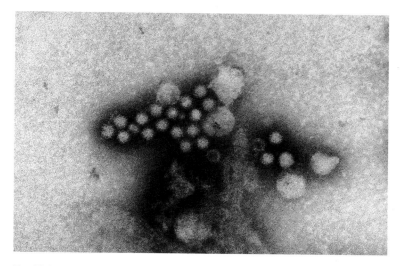

Fig. 23.3 Norwalk-like virus. × 200 000. (Electronmicrograph courtesy of Dr Hazel Appleton.)

tends to be milder, but the diarrhoea also tends to last longer than that due to rotavirus.

Virology

Electron microscopy: characteristic adenovirus particles (see Fig. 22.3): double-stranded DNA.

Culture: although these viruses grow with specialized technique in cell cultures, isolation is not usually attempted in routine laboratories.

ASTROVIRUSES

Many animal species have their own astroviruses, which are strongly host species specific. Human astroviruses cause diarrhoea – usually somewhat milder than that due to rotavirus – mainly in children, and have been reported in several outbreaks in hospitals and within families. They are responsible for between 5 and 10% of cases of infantile gastroenteritis, and improved techniques for diagnosis show the incidence to be greater than previously thought.

Virology

Electron microscopy: small virus particles with a six-pointed star surface structure and distinguishable (but with difficulty) from those of Norwalk-like viruses which they resemble: single-stranded positive-strand RNA: seven serotypes have been identified.

Culture: astroviruses can be grown in some cell cultures, but isolation is not usually attempted in routine laboratories.

OTHER VIRUSES

Several other viruses, some of which cause gastroenteritis in animals, have been found in human stools in patients with diarrhoea, but their role in the human disease is not proven.

These include:

• Toroviruses
• Coronaviruses
• Enteroviruses
• Adenovirus serotypes (other than types 40 and 41).

24 Enteroviruses

Enteroviruses primarily infect the gut but, unlike their fellow picornaviruses, the rhinoviruses, enteroviruses are resistant to acid and so can infect the gastrointestinal tract. Surprisingly, they rarely cause intestinal symptoms: enterovirus diseases are the result of viral spread to other sites of the body, particularly the CNS.

Table 24.1 lists the various viruses included in the enterovirus family.

Pathogenesis

Enteroviruses invade and spread in the following ways:

Enter the body via ingestion by mouth.

Table 24.1	Enteroviruses				
	Polioviruses	**Coxsackie⁺ A**	**Coxsackie B**	**Echo#**	**Enteroviruses (unclassified)**
Types*	1–3	1–22, A24	1–6	1–9,11–27 29–33	68–71
Total number of types	3	23	6	31	4

* *Note*: The types are not entirely sequential, as with further knowledge some have had to be reassigned to other groups.
⁺ Coxsackie is the village in New York where these viruses were first isolated.
Enteric, cytopathic, human, orphan (orphan because originally (and wrongly) thought not to be associated with any human disease).

Table 24.2 Enterovirus diseases

Syndrome	Main viruses responsible
Neurological	
(1) Paralysis (poliomyelitis)	Polioviruses, coxsackie A7, enteroviruses 70 and 71
(2) Aseptic meningitis	Most enteroviruses
Febrile illness, sometimes with rash	Most enteroviruses
Herpangina, hand, foot and mouth disease	Coxsackie A, especially A16
Myocarditis, pericarditis	Coxsackie B
Bornholm disease	Coxsackie B
Acute haemorrhagic conjunctivitis	Enterovirus 70, coxsackie A24
Neonatal infection	Coxsackie B2 and 4, echo 11

Primary site of multiplication is the lymphoid tissue of the alimentary tract, including the tonsils and, more importantly, the Peyer's patches of the small intestine.

Spread from the gut is in two directions:

- *Outwards* into the blood (viraemia), and so to other tissues and organs
- *Inwards* into the lumen of the gut, and so to shedding into the faeces.

Clinical features

The main enterovirus diseases are shown in Table 24.2.

General features of enterovirus infections

Most infections are confined to the alimentary tract and are symptomless: enteroviruses do not cause diarrhoea.

A small proportion of infections give rise to febrile illness due to viraemia, often with a rubella-like rash.

Fewer cases still progress to aseptic meningitis (and more rarely still to paralysis) and other non-neurological syndromes: spread of virus to the CNS or other organs and tissues is a relatively rare complication of enterovirus infection.

INFECTIONS OF THE CNS

The most important and potentially the most serious enteroviral infection; most enterovirus types can cause CNS disease, although some are more neurotropic than others.

The illness is typically *biphasic*: initially a febrile illness (due to viraemia) followed by an intervening period of wellbeing for a day or two before the onset of neurological symptoms, when the virus spreads through the blood–brain barrier to invade the CNS.

The two main neurological syndromes due to enteroviruses are:

1. **Paralysis** (or *poliomyelitis,* because most often due to the polioviruses): an acute illness with pain and flaccid paralysis, generally affecting the lower legs. Sometimes bulbar paralysis, when the muscles of breathing and swallowing are involved. Paralysis is always accompanied by the signs and symptoms of aseptic meningitis.

2. **Aseptic meningitis**: is much more common; CNS damage is minor, with fever, headache and nuchal rigidity (stiffness of the neck muscles owing to meningeal irritation). Lymphocytes and protein in the cerebrospinal fluid (CSF) are increased. In contrast, the CSF in bacterial meningitis has a higher cell count and neutrophils predominate. Most patients with viral meningitis (sometimes called lymphocytic meningitis) recover completely (see also Chapter 38).

Pathology: the paralysis is due to the destruction of the cells of the anterior horn of the spinal cord by the virus, causing lower motor neuron dysfunction and so a flaccid paralysis. If damage to the nerve cells is severe, the paralysis becomes irreversible (Fig. 24.1).

Post-polio syndrome: many years after acute poliomyelitis a proportion of patients develop a recurrence of progressive muscle weakness: probably not due to virus persistence.

Eradication. *Polioviruses*: are the most paralytogenic enteroviruses, especially poliovirus type 1. Poliomyelitis was formerly common as infantile paralysis (and still is in a few remaining areas of the world). WHO is at present mounting a campaign to eradicate polioviruses worldwide by means of large-scale vaccination programmes; there are no animal hosts of the virus.

NON-NEUROLOGICAL DISEASES

Febrile illness: common with any enterovirus infection, and due to viraemia.

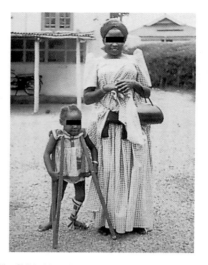

Fig. 24.1 Poliomyelitis. Child with residual paralysis and wasting in affected leg. (Photograph courtesy of Dr Eric Walker.)

Rash: many enteroviruses cause a rubelliform maculopapular rash, but this is particularly common with coxsackieviruses A9 and A16 (see below) and echovirus 9.

Herpangina: typically a painful eruption of vesicles in the mouth and throat, but seen as part of the syndrome of hand, foot and mouth disease, in which there are vesicles also on the hands and feet (Fig. 24.2); caused by group A coxsackieviruses (especially A16); enterovirus 71 also causes hand, foot and mouth disease sometimes with encephalitis.

Bornholm disease: also known as pleurodynia or epidemic myalgia: a painful inflammation of the intercostal muscles. The disease is named after the Danish island where there was an extensive outbreak in 1930; caused by group B coxsackieviruses.

Myocarditis and pericarditis: caused by group B coxsackieviruses; myocarditis is characterized by rapid pulse, enlargement of the heart and ECG abnormalities, and pericarditis by pericardial friction or effusion; seen mainly in adult males and may be mistaken for myocardial infarction; although most patients recover completely, cardiomyopathy may supervene and is a serious complication sometimes requiring cardiac transplantation.

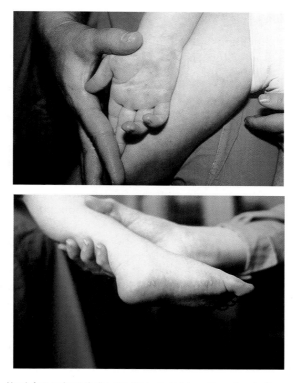

Fig. 24.2 Hand, foot and mouth disease: the typical blisters. Reproduced with permission from Bannister B A, Begg N T, Gillespie S H *Infectious disease*, 2nd edn. Blackwell Science, Oxford, 2000.

Neonatal infection: acquired from mothers or via cross-infection from other babies in the ward; varies from a mild but generalized infection to a severe, life-threatening illness, with myocarditis, pneumonia and meningoencephalitis. Most often associated with coxsackie B viruses or echoviruses, especially echo 11.

Acute haemorrhagic conjunctivitis: due to enterovirus 70 and a variant of coxsackievirus A24; appeared in widespread epidemics in the Far East, Africa and the Americas in the past 30 years. The incubation period is short – 24 h–3 days and the disease lasts about 10 days; subconjunctival haemorrhage is particularly associated with coxsackie A24. Most patients recover completely: the disease spreads rapidly via eye discharges and contaminated towels etc. A few patients in the large outbreaks have developed a polio-like paralysis.

Epidemiology

Enterovirus infections are common, especially in children and in conditions of poor hygiene. In children in tropical or developing countries, multiple infection of the gut with several different enteroviruses simultaneously is common, so that most people have acquired immunity by adulthood.

Spread: mainly by the faecal–oral route from virus shedders to contacts; virus in pharyngeal secretions may also be a source of infection. High standards of living, in countries such as the USA, diminish the chance of childhood infection and therefore of immunity being acquired early.

Gut immunity: after infection the gut becomes resistant to reinfection with the same virus type, owing to production in the gut of virus-specific neutralizing IgA antibody.

Seasonal distribution: infection is more common in the summer months.

Epidemics of aseptic meningitis are seen, with one, or sometimes two, viruses predominating – traditionally 4 years apart, when enough children have been born into the community to act as susceptible hosts. Nowadays the epidemiology is more of sporadic infections, which increase in incidence during the summer months, and with several different viruses responsible. Echovirus 9 is often seen in outbreaks and, before the widespread use of poliovaccine, polioviruses were a major cause of epidemic aseptic meningitis and paralysis. Echoviruses 4, 6, 11, 14, 16 and 30, and coxsackieviruses A9 and B5, also cause epidemics of aseptic meningitis, sometimes with other non-neurological syndromes also.

Epidemic poliomyelitis: before the advent of polio vaccines, countries with a high standard of living had a relatively high proportion of non-immune adults and suffered from repeated and widespread epidemics of paralytic disease, involving adults as well as children. Adults are more liable to develop severe paralysis in poliovirus infection than are children, and the risk of this is increased by pregnancy, tonsillectomy, fatigue, trauma, or inoculation with bacterial vaccines.

Virology

Picornaviruses with single-strand positive-sense RNA and small featureless particles (Fig. 24.3): grow in tissue cultures with rapid CPE (except coxsackie A viruses, many of which can only be isolated in suckling mice). Pathogenic for primates.

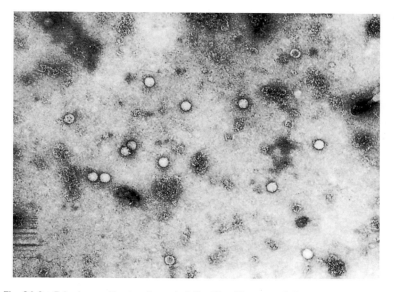

Fig. 24.3 Echoviruses. All enteroviruses look like this, with very small virus particles and cubic symmetry. × 90 000. (Electronmicrograph courtesy of Dr E. A. C. Follett.)

Diagnosis

Isolate virus in monkey kidney cultures from faeces, throat swabs: sometimes CSF – useful for some viruses (e.g. echovirus 9) but not for polioviruses.

Serology: not generally useful, except for neutralization tests used for the diagnosis of poliomyelitis (and especially the rare cases of paralysis following vaccination) and with ELISA to detect IgM to group B coxsackieviruses.

PCR to detect enterovirus RNA in tissues and CSF.

Vaccines

Two vaccines are available against the three polioviruses – *Sabin* live attenuated virus vaccine (the most widely used) and *Salk* inactivated virus vaccine (see Chapter 39).

25 Viral hepatitis

Hepatitis is a feature of many viral diseases, usually as part of a generalized infection which involves the liver, e.g. yellow fever, cytomegalovirus and Epstein–Barr infection, and congenital rubella. However, some viruses primarily target the liver to cause *viral hepatitis*. The five main hepatitis viruses are listed in Table 25.1.

Viral hepatitis presents a similar clinical picture even when caused by different viruses. Laboratory tests, however, can now differentiate between them, and this is important for prognosis.

Clinical features of viral hepatitis

Long incubation period: although variable, this tends to be several weeks.

Symptoms: jaundice (Fig. 25.1), with low-grade fever, anorexia, nausea and malaise – the latter symptoms may precede the jaundice. Jaundice is obstructive in type, with raised bilirubin, dark bile-containing urine and pale stools.

Transaminases: liver function tests are abnormal, with raised transaminase levels, e.g. ALT (alanine aminotransferase) in the serum.

Duration: variable, but usually 2–3 weeks.

Anicteric hepatitis: seen in all forms of viral hepatitis: with disturbance of liver function tests, fever, and other constitutional signs and symptoms, but no frank jaundice.

Symptomless infection in the acute stage and *persistent infection* (equivalent to a carrier state) are also common, making control difficult because the sources of infection are not recognized.

Table 25.1   Hepatitis viruses

Virus	A	B	C	D	E
Family	Picornavirus	Hepadnavirus	Flavivirus	Deltavirus	Calicivirus
Genome	SS positive-sense RNA	DS DNA	SS positive-sense RNA	RNA (defective-hepatitis B acts as helper)	SS positive-sense RNA
Transmission	Faecal–oral	Sexual, parenteral, blood, perinatal, intrapartum	Parenteral, blood, vertical	As for hepatitis B	Faecal–oral, water, food
Chronic hepatitis	No	Yes	Yes	Yes (increases risk of chronicity with hepatitis B)	No

SS: single-stranded; DS: double-stranded.

Complications

Fulminant hepatitis with massive liver necrosis ('acute yellow atrophy'), leading to liver failure, coma and, very often, death. A rare complication of hepatitis A, more common with hepatitis B, and a particular problem in pregnancy with hepatitis E.

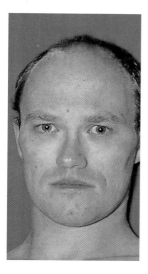

Fig. 25.1   Jaundice due to acute viral hepatitis: the sclera show typical yellow discoloration. (Photograph courtesy of Dr A. K. Chaudhuri.)

Sequelae

1. *Chronic hepatitis*: associated with persistent infection with either hepatitis B or hepatitis C (see below); associated with increased risk of cirrhosis and liver failure.

2. *Primary hepatocellular carcinoma*: chronic hepatitis B and C lead to a relatively high risk of liver cancer.

HEPATITIS A

A form of hepatitis endemic in many communities, with enteric spread mainly in children: sometimes epidemic, especially if foodborne.

Clinical features

Incubation period: about 2–6 weeks.

Onset: usually quite abrupt.

Clinically: milder than hepatitis B; fulminant hepatitis is a rare complication: overall case fatality rate in hepatitis A is 0.1%.

Alimentary infection: site of entry and primary multiplication is the gut; virus then spreads to infect the liver, where it multiplies in hepatocytes.

Shedding: virus is shed in the faeces for about 2 weeks before the onset of jaundice, but for only up to 8 days after the onset of symptoms.

Viraemia: blood is briefly infectious, but is an uncommon source of infection. Antibody appears around the time of onset of jaundice.

Age incidence: mainly seen in children 5–15 years old, but foodborne outbreaks often predominantly affect adults.

Hepatitis A does not become a chronic infection.

Epidemiology

Geography: worldwide: endemic in most countries and especially common in the tropics. Outbreaks appear from time to time, some of which are associated with faecal contamination of food or water.

Transmission: the routes of infection are:

1. *Case-to-case spread* via the faecal–oral route: the most common route of the spread of the disease; symptomless or anicteric

patients can be important – because undetected – sources of infection.

2. *Via contaminated food and water*: numerous outbreaks have been described due to contamination of foodstuffs by food-handlers shedding virus in their stools, or due to pollution of water by infected sewage. Raw shellfish (especially oysters), contaminated by growing in sewage-polluted water, have been responsible for several outbreaks.

3. *Blood*: outbreaks in haemophiliacs have been traced to contamination of batches of the blood product factor VIII – a reminder that hepatitis A involves a period of viraemia.

Seasonal prevalence: more common in autumn and winter.

Decline: the incidence of hepatitis A increased during the late 1980s in the UK, to reach a peak in 1990, but has since declined sharply; the reasons for this are unclear. This decline has not been observed in tropical countries, where the prevalence is always higher than in developed countries.

Virology

A picornavirus, single-strand positive-sense RNA, one serological type: can be grown – with difficulty – in tissue cultures; infects chimpanzees and other primates.

Diagnosis

Serology: *ELISA* to detect virus-specific IgM.

Prophylaxis

Hepatitis A vaccine for travellers and those at high risk; passive immunization with normal immunoglobulin for family contacts of cases and others at special risk (see Chapter 39).

HEPATITIS B

A more severe form of hepatitis, most often transmitted vertically, sexually or via blood. Blood for transfusion is now screened in many countries, but there remain many millions of carriers worldwide.

Clinical features

Incubation period: long – from 2 to 3 months, sometimes much longer – up to 6 months.

Onset: typically rather insidious.

Clinical course: generally more severe than hepatitis A: although most patients recover, fulminating hepatitis and liver failure are seen more often than with hepatitis A or the other forms of viral hepatitis.

Viraemia: virus and virus surface antigen (Figs 25.2 and 25.3) are present in the blood during the acute phase but often persist for much longer; virus is also present in body fluids, secretions and discharges.

Carriers: persistent infection is a feature of hepatitis B. The prevalence of chronic infection in the general population is 0.2–0.5% in western countries, but in Africa and Asia it is higher, ranging up to 20% in some areas.

Epidemiology

Worldwide, hepatitis B is transmitted mainly vertically from mother to child; in the UK it used to be the major cause of post-transfusion hepatitis, but this is now rare owing to the screening of blood donations.

Blood: is highly infectious and minute traces can infect, e.g. by the use of communal or inadequately sterilized syringes and needles. Although rare, infection has been transmitted to patients from infected surgeons during invasive surgery, and those infected may be barred from operating if highly infectious.

Drug abusers: at high risk, especially if sharing syringes for intravenous administration: infection is endemic in the drug-abusing community, with a high prevalence of either virus surface antigen in their blood or antibody – indicating past infection.

Haemophiliacs: used to be at high risk because of contaminated factor VIII: no longer a problem because of screening of blood donations.

Renal dialysis units: in the past, hepatitis B was a particular problem in renal units: vaccination and screening of blood donations have controlled this.

Tattooing and acupuncture: have also been the source of outbreaks.

Sexual transmission: an important route of infection, especially among male homosexuals.

Non-parenteral spread: some cases of hepatitis B, especially in young children, are clearly due to non-parenteral transmission – almost certainly through close personal contact.

Pregnancy: infection is passed from mother to infant, but intrapartum (rather than transplacentally in utero). Perinatal infection probably also plays a part: the risk is increased if the mother has had acute hepatitis B during pregnancy and, if a carrier, is HBe antigen-positive (see below).

Antigenic structure

Hepatitis B virus has the following antigens:

1. *HBsAg*: the 's' or surface antigen – the coat protein of the virus particle
2. *HBcAg*: the 'c' or core antigen – the nucleoprotein core of the virus
3. *HBeAg*: the 'e' antigen and part of the core protein: associated with infectivity.

HBsAg and HBeAg are present in the acute stage of hepatitis B, as is ***anti-HBc IgM***, a useful marker of active infection as it becomes negative on convalescence.

Anti-HBc IgG is also useful to distinguish between previous infection from vaccine-induced antibody, as the vaccine does not induce core antibody.

The antigens and the antibodies that are markers for the disease and its progression are summarized in Table 25.2 and illustrated diagrammatically in Figure 25.2.

Table 25.2 Markers of hepatitis B

	Acute infection	Convalescence	Carriers	Chronic hepatitis
HBsAg	+	−	+	+
HBeAg	+	−	+/−	+/−
Anti-HBc IgM	+	−	−	−
Anti-HBc IgG	+	+	+	+
Anti-HBs	−	+	−	−
Anti-HBe	−	+	+/−	+/−

a) **Serological profile of acute, resolving hepatitis B**

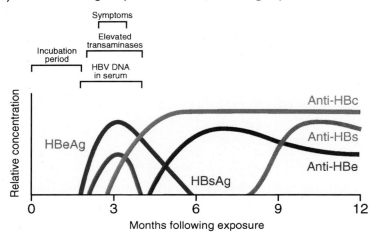

b) **Serological profile of chronic hepatitis B with seroconversion**

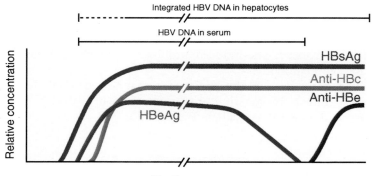

Fig. 25.2 Serological profiles of (a) acute, resolving hepatitis B and (b) chronic hepatitis B accompanied by seroconversion with the appearance of anti-HBe antibody. (Reproduced with permission from Zuckerman A J, Banatvala, J E, Pattison J R, eds *Principles and Practice of Clinical Virology*, 4th edn Chichester, John Wiley, 2000.)

Sequelae

CHRONIC HEPATITIS B

Persistent infection is common, and around 1–5% of adults fail to clear the virus in the months after acute hepatitis B (a much higher percentage – around 90% – of neonatally infected babies fail to do so): these patients remain HBsAg positive, often throughout life. However, some HBsAg carriers eventually clear the virus and become HBsAg negative.

HBsAg-positive carriers may be:

- **HBeAg negative with seroconversion to HBeAb positive**: indicates low infectivity but, note, they are still capable, albeit at a lower level, of transmitting infection; although often symptomless they usually have minor disturbance of liver function, such as slightly raised ALT levels.
- **HBeAg positive and HBeAb negative**: this indicates a high level of infectivity and that the patient is replicating virus, with circulating hepatitis B DNA in the blood. These patients are at risk of developing *chronic active hepatitis*, leading to *cirrhosis, liver failure* and, possibly, *primary hepatocellular cancer*.

LIVER CANCER

Primary hepatocellular carcinoma is much more common – as high as 200 times – in carriers of hepatitis B virus than in antigen-negative people, but after a period of possibly 20 years. Liver cancer is more common in men than in women. The virus DNA integrates into liver cell chromosomes (a prerequisite for onco-genicity). Hepatocellular cancer is rare in Europe but common in Africa and Asia, and hepatitis B virus is now recognized as a major cause of cancer worldwide.

Virology

1. *Hepadnavirus*, double-stranded DNA but with single-stranded regions: four subtypes, based on the HBsAg: *adw, adr, ayw* and *ayr*: all share the group-specific determinant *a* in addition to allelic *d* and *y*, and *w* and *r* (which are mutually exclusive).
2. *Electron microscopy* of infected blood shows the larger hepatitis B virus particles (also known as Dane particles) with numerous smaller particles that are aggregates of the virus coat protein (HBsAg): see Figure 25.3.
3. *Animals*: diseases similar to human hepatitis B exist in the animal world, where species of ducks, squirrels and woodchucks are natural hosts to viruses resembling hepatitis B in their properties. Liver cancer is associated with infection in woodchucks and ducks.

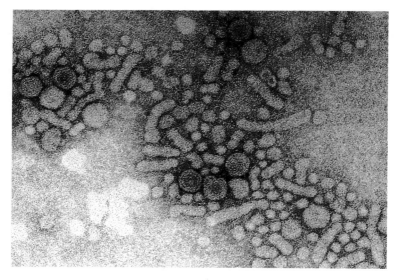

Fig. 25.3 Electron micrograph of hepatitis B virus, showing large 42 nm Dane particles, with smaller 22 nm spherical and tubular particles. (Photograph courtesy of Dr Anne Field, Central Public Health Laboratory, Colindale, London.)

Diagnosis

Serology:

1. *ELISA* test for HBsAg: if positive, test for anti-HBc IgM and for HBeAg: anti-HBc IgG without IgM is evidence of past infection; conversely, anti-HBc IgM indicates acute infection; anti-HBeAb correlates with low infectivity. Anti-HBs IgG is evidence of immunity after vaccination and is also present after natural infection (Table 25.2 and Fig. 25.2).
2. *PCR* for virus DNA detection and also for quantitative estimate of viral load.

Prophylaxis and vaccination (see also Chapter 39)

Hepatitis B vaccine with hepatitis B-specific immunoglobulin – give at birth to babies born to HBeAg-positive mothers, or after an accident involving a high risk of infection, e.g. needle-stick injury with known or suspected hepatitis B-positive blood (with active immunization started as soon as possible). Vaccinate at birth babies born to HBsAg-positive but anti-HBeAg-negative mothers.

All healthcare workers and others in high-risk occupations should be vaccinated.

Treatment

Chronic hepatitis B: interferon-α, lamivudine.

HEPATITIS C

With effective control of transfusion-transmitted hepatitis B, it became clear that there was another form of transfusion hepatitis. This was transmissible to chimpanzees, and with some brilliant molecular technology using animal serum the causal virus was discovered and characterized. It is now known as *hepatitis C*. Most countries now screen blood for transfusion for this virus.

Clinical features

A milder acute disease than hepatitis B – only about 10% of patients have jaundice – but much more likely to cause chronic infection; a shorter incubation period (usually 6–12 weeks).

Chronic hepatitis C: follows acute infection in around 50–90% of patients, most of whom have virus RNA in their blood and are infectious: possibly as many as half of those chronically infected will go on to develop cirrhosis (with risk of liver failure) or hepatocellular carcinoma.

Hepatocellular carcinoma: chronic hepatitis C is now recognized – like hepatitis B – as an important cause of primary liver cancer, although generally a long time after the acute disease – around 20 years.

Epidemiology

Transmission: mainly parenterally by blood.

Haemophiliacs: many have evidence of past infection (i.e. the presence of antihepatitis C antibody), indicating contamination of human factor VIII concentrate – now prevented by screening and treatment in the preparation of concentrates.

Drug abusers: now the most common victims of and sources of hepatitis C: show a high prevalence of antibody owing to frequent exposure to infection through sharing of syringes and needles.

Pregnancy: from 5 to 10% of infected mothers transmit the virus to their babies.

Sexual transmission: has been reported, but the virus appears much less infectious sexually than hepatitis B.

Normal populations: there is a low prevalence (around 0.2–0.5%) of antibody to hepatitis C in Western Europe but higher – up to more than 10% – in parts of Africa and Asia.

Virology

Flavivirus: RNA genome: single-strand positive-sense RNA; six genotypes (with subtypes) and with different geographical distribution and less clear correlation with severity of infection. Infects chimpanzees; does not grow in cell culture.

Diagnosis

Serology:
ELISA for antibody detection: confirm by RIBA (recombinant immunoblot assay).
PCR to detect viral RNA in blood and for quantitative estimate of viral load.

Treatment

Acute hepatitis C: interferon can be effective in resolving infection and preventing carriage.
Chronic hepatitis C: interferon-α and ribavirin: response is related to genotype, with cases of genotype 1 (common in western Europe and the USA) being the poorest responders; relapse is frequent and further long-term evaluation is required (see Chapter 33).

HEPATITIS D (δ AGENT)

This interesting virus is defective and can only replicate in the presence of hepatitis B acting as *helper virus* to supply the virus coat – the defective gene product. Therefore, hepatitis D is found only in patients also infected with hepatitis B.

Pathogenicity: exists as a superinfection (i.e. infects patients chronically infected with hepatitis B) or as a coinfection (acquired at the same time as hepatitis B); probably increases the severity of hepatitis B, especially when superinfecting rather than coinfecting.

Epidemiology

Found mainly among drug abusers infected with hepatitis B – less often among other groups infected with hepatitis B. The ecology of the virus is unknown – for example, it is unclear how it maintains itself in populations, where it originated, and so on. Some populations in areas in South America, Russia, Italy, Romania, the Middle East and Africa have a high prevalence of hepatitis D (and, of course, also hepatitis B).

Virology

RNA genome: single-stranded RNA; small particles coated with HBsAg surrounding the internal or δ antigen; three genotypes: transmissible to hepatitis B-infected chimpanzees – and woodchucks (if also infected with woodchuck virus).

Diagnosis

Serology: *ELISA* tests for antigen and antibody – available in specialist laboratories.

HEPATITIS E

An enteric virus causing community outbreaks which are sometimes very large and usually due to waterborne spread – but hepatitis E also causes sporadic infections.

Clinical features

Transmission: faecal–oral, by contaminated water – occasionally food.

Incubation period: around 6 weeks.

A generally milder form: of hepatitis (except in pregnancy) clinically resembling hepatitis A and often anicteric.

Pregnancy: particularly severe in women in the third trimester, causing fulminant hepatitis, and in whom case fatality rates as high as 20% have been recorded; the reasons for this are not understood.

Age: predominantly a disease of young to middle-aged adults.

Geographical distribution: mainly seen in India, southeast Asia, Africa and the Middle East, especially where the water supply is liable to sewage contamination. In 1993 a large epidemic was recorded in the Indian state of Uttar Pradesh, involving more than 3000 cases.

Animal hosts: there is some evidence that pigs may act as a reservoir for the virus, but this is not yet proven.

Virology

RNA genome: single-stranded positive-sense RNA: provisionally designated as a calicivirus, with morphologically similar particles seen in patients' stools on electron microscopy. Transmissible to primates.

Diagnosis

Serology: refer to reference laboratories for: *ELISA* for total HEV antibody (i.e. IgG and IgM) and HEV IgM.

HEPATITIS G

There are certainly other transfusion-associated viruses. One, known as hepatitis G virus or HGV (and identical to another which was independently isolated and named GB-C virus), causes viraemia in high-risk groups such as drug abusers and recipients of blood products, but its role in causing hepatitis is uncertain, with conflicting reports in the literature. Two similar viruses, GB-A and GB-B, may not be human but be derived from primates during the laboratory procedures used to identify them. All three viruses are similar to flaviviruses and resemble, but are distinct from, hepatitis C virus.

Role in disease: uncertain: may cause a few cases of post-transfusion hepatitis.

TTV

TT virus is named after the patient from whom it was isolated in Japan; although it has been reported in association with post-transfusion hepatitis, its role in that disease remains unproven.

26 Childhood fevers

Measles, mumps and rubella, together with parvovirus B19 and varicella (the latter described with the other herpesviruses in Chapter 27), are known as the childhood fevers. The introduction of a combined measles, mumps and rubella (MMR) vaccine has resulted in a sharp decline in these three diseases. Nevertheless, it must be remembered that many individuals, for one reason or another (e.g. immigrants from overseas), may not be immunized, and small outbreaks of childhood fevers are still seen in some communities in the UK.

MEASLES

Clinical features

Now generally a mild disease in the UK, although complications used to be relatively frequent; measles is still a severe disease in developing countries (especially in Africa), where it is an important cause of childhood mortality and morbidity.

Incubation period: 10–14 days.

Prodromal symptoms: respiratory, e.g. nasal discharge and suffusion of the eyes.

The main illness is fever, with a maculopapular rash lasting 2–5 days (Fig. 26.1): the rash is an enanthem (as well as an exanthem), and characteristic spots (Koplik's spots) in the buccal mucosa inside the cheek and mouth are a diagnostic feature.

Immunity following natural infection is lifelong: measles itself has a suppressive effect on the immune system, especially on cell-mediated immunity.

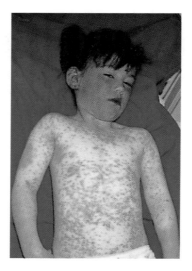

Fig. 26.1 Child with measles, showing the characteristic rash: note the intensity of the dusky red maculopapular rash on the face. (Photograph courtesy of Dr A. K. Chaudhuri.)

Complications

Respiratory: the most common: bronchitis, bronchiolitis, croup and bronchopneumonia, otitis media; before the advent of antibiotics, these were largely responsible for the mortality associated with measles.

Giant cell pneumonia: a rare complication, seen in immunodeficient patients – children and adults; direct invasion of the lungs by measles virus and usually fatal: there are numerous multinucleated giant cells in the lungs at post mortem.

Neurological: two types of encephalitis are seen (see also Chapter 28):

1. *Subacute sclerosing panencephalitis*: a rare, fatal neurological disorder seen after – sometimes long after – uncomplicated measles; progressive personality and behavioural changes, with myoclonus, convulsions and increasing neurological deterioration, leading to death. Due to cerebral infection with defective measles virus.

2. *Postinfectious encephalitis*: follows measles in about one in every 1000 cases; the mortality rate can be as high as 50% and many survivors have residual neurological symptoms; commonly presents with drowsiness, vomiting, headache and convulsions. Virus is not demonstrable in the CNS.

Epidemiology

Infectiousness is high; before vaccination virtually everybody in Britain under 15 years old had had the disease. When introduced into isolated communities, where the disease has not been endemic and the entire population was susceptible, attack rates of more than 99% have been recorded.

Transmission: by inhalation of respiratory secretions from patients.

Epidemics: in Britain and other countries with universal vaccination measles is now rare, but clusters of cases, usually in unvaccinated immigrants, are still seen. Measles remains a major cause of childhood morbidity and death in developing countries.

Virology

Paramyxovirus, enveloped particle with helical symmetry (Fig. 26.2); single-strand negative-sense RNA, one serological type.

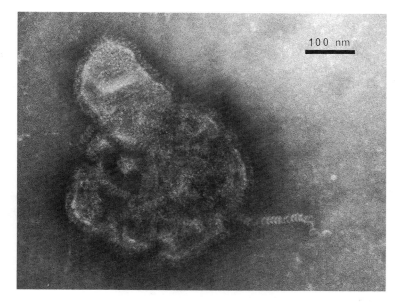

Fig. 26.2 Measles virus. Pleomorphic enveloped particle showing extrusion of the internal helical nucleocapsid. × 66 000. (Electronmicrograph courtesy of Dr Anne Field, Central Public Health Laboratory, Colindale, London.)

Diagnosis

Detection of measles IgM in serum by ELISA. In subacute sclerosing panencephalitis, by demonstration of measles antibody in the CSF.

MUMPS

Mumps is a generalized infection by a virus with a predilection for the CNS (*neurotropism*) and for glandular tissue.

Clinical features

Incubation period: relatively long: 14–21 days.

Classic mumps is a febrile illness, with parotitis causing characteristic swelling of the parotid and submaxillary glands (Fig. 26.3).

Aseptic meningitis: mumps is an important cause of viral meningitis, with signs of meningeal irritation, fever, headache and vomiting: rarely, the CNS involvement becomes more severe with the onset of meningoencephalitis and convulsions and altered consciousness. In around 50% of cases mumps meningitis is not accompanied by parotitis (see also Chapter 28).

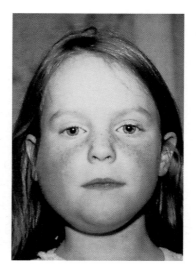

Fig. 26.3 Child with mumps, showing swelling of the parotid and submandibular glands on the right-hand side of the face. (Photograph courtesy of Dr A. K. Chaudhuri.)

Immunity: an attack is followed by solid and long-lasting immunity; second attacks are very rare.

Complications

Orchitis, pancreatitis and – rarely – oöphoritis and thyroiditis are seen with mumps: about 20% of adult males who contract mumps develop orchitis (but not usually causing sterility). Deafness was not uncommon in prevaccination mumps; although it usually resolved spontaneously, permanent hearing defects occasionally resulted.

Adults: tend to have more severe disease: orchitis and oöphoritis are more common after puberty.

Epidemiology

Transmission: by inhalation of infectious respiratory secretions.

Seasonal prevalence: most common in winter and spring.

Age distribution: mainly in children from 5 to 15 years old, but not uncommon in young adults.

Infectiousness: less infectious than measles; as a result, infection in childhood is less frequent, and before vaccination a significant proportion of adults were non-immune.

Epidemics of mumps used to be seen every 3 years, followed by years when the prevalence of infection was low. MMR vaccine has had an impact, and the incidence of mumps is now very low.

Virology

Paramyxovirus: single-strand negative-sense RNA, one serological type; grows in tissue culture with haemadsorption.

Diagnosis

Serology: by complement fixation test: two antigens are used: 'V' or viral surface protein: associated with long-lasting immunity; and 'S' or 'soluble' nucleoprotein: 'S' antibody appears early but fades early: can be useful for diagnosing acute infection. ELISA for IgM (but cross-reactions with other paramyxoviruses may be a problem).

Isolation: mainly for diagnosis of mumps meningitis: culture CSF or throat washings in monkey kidney tissue culture.

RUBELLA

Rubella is a mild disease, but if contracted in early pregnancy the virus can cause severe congenital abnormalities and disease in the fetus.

Clinical features

Incubation period: 14–23 days (average 18 days).

A mild febrile illness with a macular rash which spreads down from the face and behind the ears; there is usually pharyngitis and enlargement of the cervical – especially the posterior cervical – lymph glands: arthralgia (painful joints) are a common symptom. Infection is symptomless in some cases.

Complications: rare, postinfectious encephalitis, thrombocytopenic purpura.

Immunity after rubella: good, after both natural and vaccine-acquired immunity, but it is not solid and reinfections are well documented. Rarely, congenital infection has been reported as a result of maternal reinfection.

Virus is present in both blood and pharyngeal secretions, and is shed during the incubation period for up to 7 days before the appearance of the rash, and for 2 weeks after the rash appears.

Congenital infection (see also Chapter 38)

The teratogenic properties of the virus were first discovered in Australia in 1941, when Gregg (an ophthalmologist) noticed an increased number of cases of congenital cataract following an epidemic of rubella: affected infants had been born to mothers with a history of rubella in early pregnancy.

Congenital defects: result when rubella virus crosses the placenta to infect the developing fetal tissues during the first 16 weeks of pregnancy; after this, damage is unlikely.

The main defects are a **triad** of:

• Cataract
• Nerve deafness
• Cardiac abnormalities (such as patent ductus arteriosus, ventricular septal defect, pulmonary artery stenosis, Fallot's tetralogy).

However, affected infants also have generalized infection which, together with the defects, constitutes the *rubella syndrome*

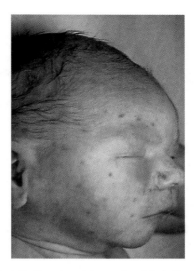

Fig. 26.4 Congenital rubella. Purpuric rash in a newborn infant with congenitally acquired rubella, who was subsequently found to have congenital heart disease and cataract as well. (Reproduced with permission from Topley and Wilson's *Principles of Bacteriology, Virology and Immunity*, 7th edn 1984. Edward Arnold, London, vol 4.)

(Fig. 26.4). The signs of this are: hepatosplenomegaly, thrombocytopenic purpura, low birth weight, mental retardation, jaundice, anaemia, lesions in the metaphyses of the long bones and retinopathy.

Incidence of defects after maternal rubella in the first 3 months of pregnancy has varied in different studies, but it now appears that it is around 80–85%. The severity and multiplicity of defect increase the earlier the maternal rubella.

Deafness and defective vision increase as congenitally infected children grow up, doubtless owing to easier recognition of these defects in older children: deafness is a particular problem after congenital rubella.

Insulin-dependent diabetes mellitus (juvenile onset; type 1): a late complication of congenital rubella and has been reported in around 12–20% of patients.

Immunity: infants with the rubella syndrome have IgM antibody to rubella virus (the maternal antibody that crosses the placenta is IgG antibody).

Subacute sclerosing panencephalitis: has been reported as a rare, late complication of congenital rubella.

Epidemiology

Age: mainly seen in children under 15 years old. Before the introduction of vaccination programmes a proportion of people reached adult life without being infected, and about 15% of women of childbearing age were non-immune.

In the UK: following the introduction of the MMR vaccination programme, rubella has declined sharply in prevalence.

Virology

A non-arthropod borne togavirus, single-strand negative-sense RNA, one serological type.

Diagnosis

Used mainly to confirm suspected rubella in a pregnant woman, congenital rubella, and to detect non-immune pregnant women (tested when attending antenatal clinics).

Serology: recent infection, including congenital rubella in the newborn, is best diagnosed by detection of IgM by ELISA.

Single radial haemolysis: widely used for detecting immunity (the test detects only IgG antibody) in pregnant women or in women at special risk.

PCR: for detection of viral RNA for the diagnosis of congenital rubella in the fetus or newborn infant.

MMR vaccine (see also Chapter 39)

Live, attenuated virus vaccine given in UK to all babies in the second year of life, with a booster at school entry.

B19 INFECTION (ERYTHEMA INFECTIOSUM)

This disease (also called *slapped cheek* or *fifth disease*) is caused by the human parvovirus B19.

Clinical features

Fever and an erythematous rash, most intense on the cheeks, where there is marked redness, hence the name 'slapped cheek disease', with circumoral pallor. The rash on the body and limbs becomes maculopapular and lesions fade from the centre, leaving the periphery red, so developing a characteristic reticular or lace-like pattern. There is mild generalized lymphadenopathy and, especially in women, arthralgia, with swelling and pain in the joints. Clinically, the disease resembles rubella.

Aplastic crises: the parvovirus B19 has a predilection for the haemopoietic cells of the bone marrow, causing aplastic crises; mainly seen in children with chronic haemolytic anaemias, such as sickle cell anaemia, hereditary spherocytosis, thalassaemia. There is evidence that previously healthy people also show transient bone marrow 'arrest' during the course of infection.

Symptomless infection: appears to be common – probably around 20% of those infected have no symptoms.

Congenital infection (see also Chapter 38)

Non-immune hydrops fetalis: B19 virus can infect the fetus during the course of maternal infection. Many congenital infections are symptomless and the fetus develops normally; however, up to the 20th week of pregnancy, when the fetus is most vulnerable, the virus can cause severe fetal infection and death, with a catastrophic fall in the haemoglobin level. The severely anaemic fetus – with gross oedema and congestive cardiac failure – resembles the hydrops fetalis associated with rhesus blood group incompatibility – hence the name non-immune hydrops fetalis.

Immunodeficiency: persistent B19 infection can cause persistent infection with chronic anaemia in children with leukaemia and other forms of immunodeficiency; also reported in patients with organ transplants.

Epidemiology

Epidemics: outbreaks of infection are seen in the community approximately every 4 years. Between outbreaks, B19 virus is endemic, causing sporadic infection.

Transmission: by inhalation of infected respiratory secretions.

Seasonal prevalence: most common in late winter and early spring.

Age: the peak incidence of infection is in childhood, during the early school years – from 5 to 10 years old.

Virology

Human parvovirus B19 is an autonomously replicating parvovirus (other parvoviruses are defective and require helper viruses for replication). Single-stranded DNA. The virus genetic organization is interesting, because populations of virus show, in roughly equal measure, particles that contain either positive- or negative-sense DNA molecules.

Diagnosis

Serology: ELISA (or radioimmunoassay) for virus-specific IgM.

Detection of viral DNA in tissues and blood by molecular techniques.

POXVIRUS DISEASES

By far the most dangerous childhood fever was smallpox, one of the most fatal of all virus infections, yet it was defeated, for three reasons:

1. Humans were the only hosts.
2. There was an effective vaccine against it, originally discovered by Jenner (Fig. 26.5) in 1796.
3. By the mid-20th century there were only a limited number of areas of endemic infection.

SMALLPOX

Clinical features

A severe febrile illness characterized by a profuse vesicular rash, progressing from macules, papules, and vesicles to pustules, with scabbing and eventual scarring; marked malaise and a high mortality of around 30%; survivors were left with disfiguring facial scars.

Eradication: in 1967 the World Health Organization (WHO) embarked on a smallpox eradication campaign based on a policy of 'search and containment', i.e. the isolation of cases and the tracing and vaccination of contacts. There was continuing and

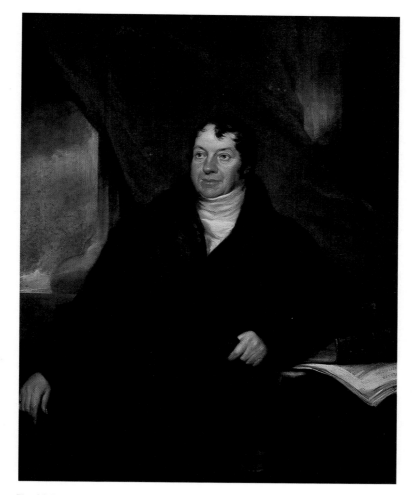

Fig. 26.5   Portrait of Edward Jenner, who discovered that vaccination with cowpox protected against smallpox. (Reproduced with permission of the Royal Society of Medicine Press Ltd, London.)

long-term surveillance of previously endemic areas (India, Pakistan and Bangladesh and, in Africa, Ethiopia and Somalia) before these were declared smallpox free. The campaign was outstandingly successful and in May 1980 WHO declared the world free of smallpox. Fear of bioterrorism has prevented the planned destruction of the last stocks of virus (held in only two laboratories).

OTHER POXVIRUS DISEASES

Molluscum contagiosum

A low-grade infection in humans, with reddish, waxy papules on the skin – usually in the axilla or on the trunk; a fairly common infection in children, spread by close contact, e.g. at swimming pools. Lesions contain numerous poxvirus particles, visible on electron microscopy; the lesions resolve spontaneously in 4–6 weeks; sometimes disseminates in immunocompromised patients (e.g. with AIDS).

Orf (contagious pustular dermatitis): an infection of sheep and goats: occasionally transmitted to the hands of animal workers, causing chronic granulomatous lesions; diagnosed by characteristic oval particles with criss-cross surface banding, seen on electron microscopy.

Paravaccinia (pseudocowpox): the virus is similar to orf virus, but causes lesions on the udders of cows and is occasionally transmitted to the hands of animal workers.

Monkeypox: a disease resembling mild smallpox caused by a natural poxvirus of monkeys. Seen in West Africa among people with frequent contact with monkeys; however, the main animal reservoir seems to be squirrels.

Tanapox: probably also acquired from contact with monkeys and, in humans, produces scanty vesicular lesions on the skin which do not progress to pustules. Outbreaks have been reported in East Africa.

Cowpox: this disease seems nowadays to be surprisingly rare in both cows and humans. There has been a suggestion that it may be a natural infection of horses.

Virology

Human poxviruses include smallpox (variola), alastrim (a milder form of smallpox, due to a related but distinguishable virus known as variola minor) and molluscum contagiosum (vaccinia virus, used for vaccination against smallpox, is of uncertain origin). Large DNA viruses with double-stranded DNA.

27 Herpesvirus diseases

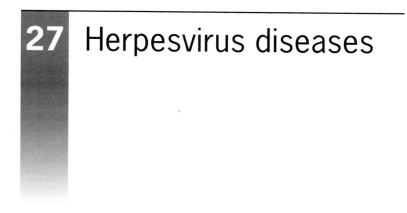

Most animal species, including humans, are hosts for their own herpesvirus – and sometimes for two or more. All herpesvirus particles are morphologically identical (Fig. 27.1) and contain double-stranded DNA; they vary in their ability to grow in cell culture.

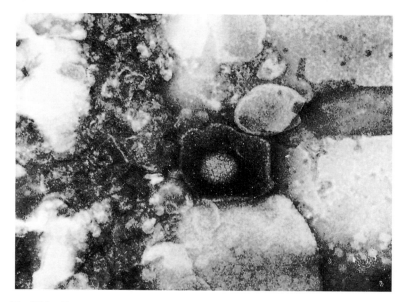

Fig. 27.1 Herpes simplex virus. The particle has cubic symmetry and the capsid is composed of hollow-cored capsomeres. There is a loose, baggy envelope. × 108 000. (Electronmicrograph courtesy of Dr E. A. C. Follett.)

Herpesviruses have the important property of remaining *latent* within the cells of the host, but with the potential to reactivate at some later time after the primary infection.

Reactivation with recurrent infection is therefore a feature of herpes infections.

THE HUMAN HERPESVIRUSES

- Herpes simplex virus types 1 and 2
- Varicella-zoster virus
- Cytomegalovirus
- Epstein–Barr (EB) virus
- Human herpesvirus 6
- Human herpesvirus 7
- Human herpesvirus 8.

HERPES SIMPLEX VIRUS

Unusual among viruses in causing a wide variety of clinical syndromes: the basic lesions are vesicles, but these can take different forms.

There are two types of herpes simplex virus:

- Type 1: the commonest; causes mainly oro-facial lesions
- Type 2: the main cause of genital herpes.

Diseases fall into two categories:

- *Primary*: when the virus is first encountered
- *Reactivation*: recurrent infections, due to reactivation of latent virus.

Primary infections

Most are symptomless. Below are the main diseases where primary infection is symptomatic.

Gingivostomatitis: vesicles inside the mouth on the buccal mucosa and on the gums: these ulcerate and become coated with a greyish slough (Fig. 27.2): the commonest primary disease, but vesicles may be produced at other sites, most often on the head or neck. *Herpes gladiatorum*, or scrum pox, with a herpes eruption on the back and shoulders, has been described in rugby players who exchange shirts after the game.

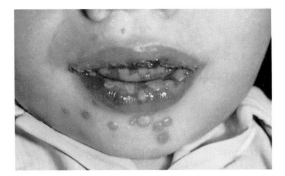

Fig. 27.2 Primary herpes simplex infection. Stomatitis with satellite vesicles over the chin. (Reproduced with permission from Grist N R, Ho-Yen D O, Walker E, Williams G R 1988 *Diseases of infection*. Oxford, Oxford University Press.)

Herpetic whitlow: due to implantation of the virus into the fingers: the lesion produced looks similar to a staphylococcal whitlow, but the exudate is serous rather than purulent; an occupational hazard of doctors and nurses, especially of anaesthetists or neurosurgical nurses, who deal with unconscious patients who are intubated; infection is acquired through contamination of the hands by virus in saliva or respiratory secretions.

Conjunctivitis and keratitis: primary herpes can involve the eye, both conjunctiva and cornea: the eyelids are generally swollen and there are often vesicles and ulcers on them.

Kaposi's varicelliform eruption: a superinfection of eczematous skin: mainly seen in young children; sometimes a serious disease with a significant fatality rate.

Acute necrotizing encephalitis: a rare but severe disease: presents with the sudden onset of fever, mental confusion and headache; the main site of infection is the temporal lobe, where the disease causes necrosis. Recently a milder form of herpes encephalitis, with a better prognosis, has been described – usually in children. It seems that herpes encephalitis can be either a primary infection or a reactivation (see also Chapter 28).

Genital herpes: typically a vesicular eruption of the genital area but which may also involve the cervix in women: sexually transmitted and most often due to herpes simplex virus type 2, but type 1 virus causes between a quarter and a third of cases.

Neonatal infection: in neonates herpes infection takes the form of severe generalized infection and is usually acquired during birth from primary genital infection in the mother (i.e. when no maternal antibody is present to protect the child). Affected infants have jaundice, hepatosplenomegaly, thrombocytopenia and large vesicular lesions on the skin: there is a high case fatality rate; usually due to herpes simplex virus type 2, but in around a third of cases to type 1, which may also be acquired from the mother's genital tract (or from the hands or face of a nurse or other patient suffering from a type 1 lesion).

Generalized infection in adults: a rare manifestation of primary infection with type 1 virus, with disseminated vesicular skin lesions and virus throughout viscera and other body organs and tissues; *herpes hepatitis* has also been described.

Erythema multiforme: a rash with 'target' lesions surrounded by a red erythematous halo: most commonly seen on the extremities; often precipitated by streptococcal or *Mycoplasma pneumoniae* infection or by drugs, but sometimes due to herpes simplex and then responds to antiherpes drugs.

Latency

During primary infection the virus travels via sensory nerves from the site of infection in the mouth to the trigeminal ganglion – and to other cranial and cervical ganglia as well. Virus remains in ganglia in a potentially viable state, and in a proportion of people reactivates to cause recurrent infection. Virus can be isolated from the trigeminal ganglia of people who suffer reactivation – and from some who do not. In genital herpes, type 2 becomes latent in the sacral ganglia.

Stimuli: such as common colds, sunlight (possibly a result of exposure to ultraviolet light), pneumonia, stress and menstruation can provoke reactivation. This recurs sporadically, sometimes often, throughout life.

Neutralizing antibody: is produced after primary infection, but does not prevent reactivation: virus is protected from serum antibody within the axons of sensory nerves as it travels to the site of recurrent infection. Reactivation does not stimulate a rise in titre of herpes antibody.

Clinical reactivation

Cold sores: vesicles at mucocutaneous junctions of the nose and mouth are the commonest forms of reactivation (Fig. 27.3), with progression to pustules and crust formation; reactivated latent

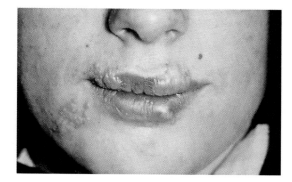

Fig. 27.3 Vesicular cold sores – the commonest disease due to herpes simplex virus. The virus has reactivated from the latent state in the trigeminal ganglion. (Reproduced with permission from Topley and Wilson's *Principles of Bacteriology, Virology and Immunity* 8th edn 1990. Edward Arnold, London, vol 4.)

virus travels from the trigeminal ganglion down the maxillary or mandibular branches of the trigeminal nerve to reach areas of the skin supplied by these nerves. Herpetic vesicles can recur – but more rarely – at other sites on the skin; genital lesions also recur, most often with type 2 virus: less often when the primary genital infection is due to type 1 virus.

Dendritic ulcer of the cornea: reactivation less often affects the eye: recurrent lesions are – at least at first – restricted to the cornea: virus reaches the cornea via the ophthalmic branch of the trigeminal nerve. Lesions take the form of a branching or dendritic ulcer, a form of keratitis (Fig. 27.4); if recurrence is frequent, scarring develops and the disease may progress to a severe, destructive uveitis.

Immunosuppressive therapy: patients with organ transplants are liable to develop severe, extensive cold sores, usually in the mouth; these can become necrotic and spread on to the face and into the oesophagus; due to deficient cell-mediated immunity, but note that the majority of transplant patients have the usual self-limiting herpes reactivations.

Epidemiology

Prevalence: infection is virtually universal in human populations, and in elderly people the prevalence of antibody (indicating previous infection) is almost 100%.

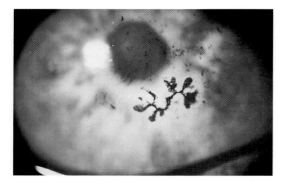

Fig. 27.4 Dendritic (branching) ulcer of the cornea, stained with rose Bengal – another disease due to recurrent herpes simplex. (Photograph courtesy of Professor) W. R. Lee, University of Glasgow.)

Transmission: by close personal contact, e.g. kissing (type 1 virus), sexual intercourse (type 2 virus).

Sources: generally people with herpetic lesions; however, carriers of latent virus from time to time shed virus in their saliva without any symptoms, and this may act as a source of (undetected) infection.

Age: infection is most common in childhood and is usually symptomless: there is another peak in incidence during adolescence, due to kissing as contact with the opposite gender increases.

Virology

Types 1 and 2 share group-specific antigens, but can be differentiated by tests for type-specific antigens and by DNA restriction enzyme analysis; both types grow well in a variety of cell cultures.

Diagnosis

Isolate virus from swab or fluid from vesicles, skin, saliva, conjunctiva; corneal scrapings, brain biopsy in cell cultures.

PCR to detect virus DNA in CSF or other tissue; or detect virus particles in skin lesions by electron microscopy.

Treatment

Aciclovir, famciclovir (see also Chapter 33).

VARICELLA-ZOSTER VIRUS

Varicella (chickenpox) and zoster (shingles – but also sometimes called 'herpes zoster') are different diseases caused by the same virus:

Varicella is the primary illness and one of the common childhood fevers.

Zoster is a reactivation.

VARICELLA

Clinical features

Incubation period: 10–21 days.

A mild febrile illness with a characteristic vesicular rash: vesicles appear in successive waves, so that lesions of different ages are present together: the vesicles (in which there are giant cells) develop into pustules; virus is shed in respiratory secretions from 48 h before the rash appears, and is also present in the vesicular lesions. May be severe and life threatening in the immunocompromised e.g. leukaemic children.

Complications: pneumonia, which in adults is a relatively common and serious complication and may be followed by pulmonary calcification: pulmonary involvement is dangerous in pregnancy. Rarely, postinfectious encephalitis and severe haemorrhagic (fulminating) varicella.

Immunity: attack is followed by solid and long-lasting immunity to varicella, but *not to zoster*.

Varicella and pregnancy (see also Chapter 38)

Congenital varicella: very rare: maternal varicella in early pregnancy is occasionally followed, in the infant, by a syndrome of limb hypoplasia, muscular atrophy and cerebral and psychomotor retardation.

Perinatal or neonatal varicella: maternal varicella near the time of delivery may also affect the child. If the mother contracts varicella more than 7 days before delivery, the disease in the child is usually mild: this is because the child's disease is modified by placentally transmitted early maternal antibody; within 7 days of delivery there is no maternal antibody and the child is liable to develop severe disease.

Pregnancy: varicella can be unusually severe in pregnant women.

Epidemiology

Transmission: via inhalation of respiratory secretions, or via virus present in skin lesions.

Seasonal distribution: highest incidence is in late winter and early spring.

Varicella (unlike zoster) is an epidemic disease acquired by contact with cases of varicella or (less commonly) of zoster.

ZOSTER

A reactivation of virus latent in dorsal root or cranial nerve ganglia following – and usually many years after – childhood varicella. Virus travels down sensory nerves to produce painful vesicles in the area of skin (dermatome) innervated from the affected ganglion. A particular problem in the immunocompromised.

Clinical features

Vesicles: in a band – almost always unilateral – corresponding to a dermatome, with pain, reddening of the skin, and progressing to pustules and crusting.

Ganglia: dorsal root ganglia – and therefore the thoracic nerves supplying dermatomes of the chest wall – are most often affected: there is a segmental rash which extends from the middle of the back in a horizontal strip round the side of the chest – 'a belt of roses from hell' (Fig. 27.5).

Cranial zoster: reactivation in the trigeminal ganglion involving the ophthalmic nerve causes a sharply demarcated area of lesions down one side of the forehead and scalp: in about half the patients there are lesions in the eye.

Ramsay Hunt syndrome is a rare form of zoster: the eruption is on the tympanic membrane and the external auditory canal, and there is often a facial nerve palsy and sometimes loss of taste on the anterior two-thirds of the tongue; zoster has also been implicated in Bell's palsy.

Neurological signs are sometimes seen, e.g. paralysis and rarely encephalitis.

Residual neuralgia – which may be severe – often follows zoster in the elderly.

Age: incidence rises with age: zoster is much more common in the elderly, as are second attacks.

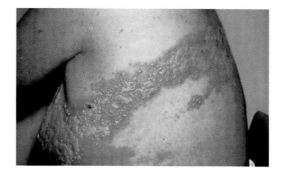

Fig. 27.5 Zoster. Thoracic rash with characteristic distribution of lesions: 'a belt of roses from hell'. (Photograph courtesy of Dr Alan Lyell.)

Virus: is present in the skin vesicles and in the ganglia involved (where there are cytopathic changes of cell destruction and marked inflammatory infiltration).

Epidemiology

Cases are sporadic: there is no seasonal incidence.

Zoster – unlike varicella – is *not acquired by contact* with cases of either varicella or zoster, although it may give rise to varicella in susceptible contacts.

Diagnosis

Serology: *ELISA* for IgM is useful for both varicella and zoster: unlike reactivations of herpes simplex, zoster usually causes a rise in antibody titre detectable by complement fixation test.

Rapid latex test: for detection of antibody indicating pre-existing immunity – useful to detect non-immune women in contact with a case of varicella or zoster in pregnancy.

Detection of herpesvirus particles in vesicle fluid by electron microscopy is a quick method of confirming a clinical diagnosis (but note, this does not distinguish varicella-zoster from herpes simplex virus).

Treatment and prophylaxis

Aciclovir, famciclovir, valaciclovir, zoster immune globulin (see also Chapters 33 and 39).

CYTOMEGALOVIRUS

An almost universal virus infection which in the previously healthy is generally (but not always) symptomless. Cytomegalovirus can infect the fetus during maternal infection in pregnancy: cytomegalovirus infection is a major problem in transplant patients.

Latency: the virus can reactivate from the latent state in cells of the monocyte lineage (and perhaps in other organs and cell types also).

Cytomegalovirus disease is either:

• Congenital
• Postnatal.

Congenital disease (see also Chapter 38)

A more difficult problem than congenital rubella because:

• maternal infection is almost always symptomless
• the fetus can be damaged by infection in any of the three trimesters of pregnancy
• fetal infection can follow reactivation as well as primary maternal infection
• approximately 0.4% of British children are congenitally infected, but most do not suffer sequelae (termination therefore presents ethical problems).

Clinical features

The majority of congenitally infected neonates show no signs or symptoms, and diagnosis is made by virological tests. Many of the children develop normally, although some show neurological sequelae later in life, principally deafness and/or mental retardation.

About 7% of infected infants develop severe generalized (or cytomegalic inclusion) disease:

Signs and symptoms: jaundice, hepatosplenomegaly, blood dyscrasias such as thrombocytopenia and haemolytic anaemia; the brain is almost always involved and some infants have microcephaly: motor disorders are common; surviving infants are usually deaf and mentally retarded. Cytomegalovirus probably causes about 10% of cases of microcephaly.

Affected organs: show characteristically enlarged cells (hence the prefix 'cytomegalo') with large intranuclear 'owl's eye' inclusions.

Postnatal disease

Hepatitis

In young children, primary infection with cytomegalovirus can – although rarely – cause hepatitis, with enlargement of the liver and disturbance of liver function tests; jaundice may or may not be present.

Infectious mononucleosis syndrome

In adults and in older children, infection can give rise to infectious mononucleosis (see below), but with a negative Paul–Bunnell reaction and no lymphadenopathy or pharyngitis. There is fever, hepatitis and lymphocytosis, with atypical lymphocytes in the peripheral blood; sometimes seen after transfusion with fresh unfrozen blood or platelets – screening of donors for cytomegalovirus is now carried out to prevent this, and also to prevent infection being transmitted to recipients of transplants.

Infection in the immunocompromised

Disseminated infection is sometimes seen in immunocompromised patients, with widespread lesions in lungs as well as other organs and tissues, e.g. adrenals, liver and alimentary tract; a major complication of transplantation surgery.

Transplant patients are subject to frequent infections with cytomegalovirus – sometimes reactivations, sometimes due to primary infection acquired from the donor organ: not infrequently symptomless with renal transplants, but a major problem with bone marrow and heart transplant patients.

Pneumonia is the main disease associated with cytomegalovirus in transplant patients. Cytomegalovirus retinitis is a particular problem in AIDS patients (Fig. 27.6).

Diagnosis

Isolate: virus from urine, throat gargle, in human embryo lung cell cultures: detect early virus by the direct early antigen fluorescent foci test (DEAFF) test.

Serology: ELISA tests for IgM (or IgG to test for pre-existing immunity).

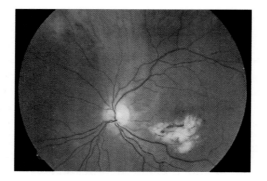

Fig. 27.6 Cytomegalovirus retinitis in an AIDS patient, showing a triangular focus of retinal necrosis above the macula in the right fundus. (Photograph courtesy of Professor W. R. Lee, University of Glasgow.)

Treatment

Ganciclovir; foscarnet and cidofovir for retinitis (see also Chapter 33).

EPSTEIN–BARR (EB) VIRUS

EB virus is named after the virologists who first observed it when examining cultures of lymphoblasts from Burkitt's lymphoma in the electron microscope. Infection is widespread in human populations, and most people have antibody to the virus by the time they reach adulthood.

Most infections are symptomless, especially if acquired during childhood: if infection is delayed until adult life there is greater likelihood of disease: this takes the form of *infectious mononucleosis* (glandular fever).

Persistence of virus: EB virus persists in latent form within lymphocytes following primary infection: the virus is present in cell cytoplasm in the form of unintegrated viral DNA. EB virus has oncogenic properties, and transforms cells in vitro.

Human cancer: EB virus has a causal association with Burkitt's lymphoma and nasopharyngeal carcinoma (see below).

INFECTIOUS MONONUCLEOSIS

Clinical features

Incubation period: long, from 4 to 7 weeks.

Signs and symptoms: low-grade fever with generalized lymphadenopathy and sore throat due to exudative tonsillitis; malaise, anorexia and tiredness to a severe degree are characteristic; splenomegaly is common and most cases have abnormal liver function tests; a proportion have palpable enlargement of the liver, and frank jaundice is not uncommon.

Mononucleosis: (or, more correctly, a relative and absolute lymphocytosis) is a diagnostic feature; at least 10% (and usually more) of the lymphocytes are atypical, with enlarged misshapen nuclei and excess cytoplasm; the atypical lymphocytes are both B and T cells, but mainly T cells stimulated in a cytotoxic response against EB virus-infected B cells.

Duration: in most cases of infectious mononucleosis symptoms last 2–3 weeks, but in a proportion tiredness and malaise persist for weeks or even months.

EB virus infection in the immunocompromised: can cause severe lymphoproliferative disease, which may be frankly malignant or fatal and is characterized by infiltration of organs and tissues by immature B lymphocytes.

Duncan's syndrome: fatal infectious mononucleosis, with malignant lymphoma due to EB virus, has been described in boys who suffer from this rare, congenital X-linked lymphoproliferative syndrome associated with immunodeficiency.

Transmission: close contact, mainly kissing: the virus is present in cells in salivary secretions. The disease is most prevalent among young adults, especially student populations (of whom a sizeable minority have no antibody).

Diagnosis

Paul–Bunnell test: heterophil antibodies to sheep erythrocytes are a good diagnostic test for infectious mononucleosis. Development of other non-specific antibodies (e.g. rheumatoid factor and anti-i cold agglutinin) are also features of the disease.

Anti-EB virus antibody: is produced during infection, but antibody is usually present before symptoms develop; the detection of IgM to virus capsid antigen and of antibody to early antigen is a useful diagnostic test.

HUMAN CANCER

Burkitt's lymphoma

A highly malignant tumour common in African children (Fig. 27.7). Primarily a tumour of lymphoid tissue, the earliest

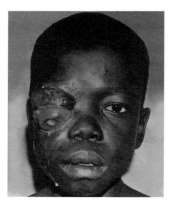

Fig. 27.7 A 9-year-old girl with a typical Burkitt lymphoma of the right upper maxilla presenting through the orbit. The Epstein–Barr virus was first identified in cultures of malignant lymphoblasts from this tumour. (Epstein M A, Barr Y M Characteristics and mode of growth of a tissue culture strain (EB1) of human lymphoblasts from Burkitt's lymphoma. Reproduced with permission from the Journal of the National Cancer Institute, 1965, *34*, 231–240.)

manifestations are often large tumours of the jaw and, in girls, sometimes of the ovaries; it spreads rapidly, with widespread metastases.

Geography: the tumour shows a striking geographical distribution: Burkitt's lymphoma is virtually confined to areas in Africa with holoendemic malaria and in which disease-carrying mosquito vectors are found. Outside Africa, e.g. in western Europe and the USA, reported cases are sporadic and rare. The geographical distribution may be because malaria can act as a cofactor with EB virus to produce malignant transformation in lymphoid tissue.

Nasopharyngeal carcinoma

This also shows a striking geographical and probably racial distribution, and is particularly common among the southern Chinese. Nasopharyngeal carcinoma is also associated with EB virus, and virus DNA is regularly present in the malignant epithelial cells of the tumour.

HUMAN HERPESVIRUS 6 (HHV 6)

Discovered in recent years, HHV 6 is a latent infection of monocytes. Infection is widespread, as there is a high incidence of antibody in normal populations acquired in early life, and is mostly symptomless. However it does cause some diseases.

Clinical features

Exanthem subitum (also known as *roseola infantum*): a mild rash in small babies is associated with primary HHV 6 infection. The virus probably also causes febrile convulsions, and occasionally encephalitis in babies.

Mononucleosis with cervical lymphadenopathy: has been described in a few adults undergoing primary infection.

Immunocompromised: HHV 6 can cause encephalitis in transplant patients, in whom viral reactivation has been reported, sometimes with fever and signs of generalized infection.

HUMAN HERPESVIRUS 7 (HHV 7)

Recently described and can also cause exanthema subitum and febrile convulsions: infection is widespread (as judged by the prevalence of antibody) and is acquired in childhood, although not as early in life as HHV 6.

HUMAN HERPESVIRUS 8 (HHV 8)

This virus is associated with Kaposi's sarcoma in AIDS and other patients. Infection with the virus is fairly common in some areas of the Mediterranean and Africa – usually asymptomatically. It is also associated with lymphoproliferative disorders such as primary effusion lymphoma (characterized by malignant effusions of lymphoma in pleural or abdominal cavities) and multicentric Castleman's disease (or angiofollicular lymph node hyperplasia), both of which are found as rare complications of HIV infection.

28 | Virus neurological disease

Viruses are important causes of neurological disease, often as a complication of infection elsewhere in the body.

Spread: viruses generally invade the CNS via the bloodstream, but some (e.g. rabies) reach the CNS by the neural route, i.e. by spread along peripheral nerves.

There are three main types of virus neurological disease:

1. Acute virus infections of the CNS
2. Chronic virus neurological disease
3. Neurological syndromes precipitated by virus infection.

ACUTE VIRUS INFECTIONS OF THE CNS

The two principal acute infections are:

1. **Aseptic meningitis**
2. **Encephalitis.**

Table 28.1 summarizes some features of acute viral neurological disease.

ASEPTIC MENINGITIS

Relatively common and can be due to many different viruses (and also to *Mycobacterium tuberculosis*, *Listeria monocytogenes*, *Leptospira* and *Cryptococcus neoformans*).

Viral meningitis is rarely severe and patients usually make a complete recovery: but paralysis is often seen with polioviruses (see Chapter 24).

Table 28.1 Acute virus neurological disease

| Disease | Aseptic meningitis | Encephalitis | |
		Primary	Postinfectious
Lesions	Meningeal inflammation, occasionally progresses to destruction of anterior horn cells with paralysis	Varied: perivascular cuffing, may be necrotizing (herpes simplex) or minimal (rabies); inclusions often present	Multifocal perivenous demyelination
Pathogenesis	Direct invasion of brain by virus	Direct invasion of brain by virus	Probably immunological, follows 2–14 days after disease or vaccination
CSF	Virus often present Lymphocytes ++	Virus DNA or RNA detectable Lymphocytes +	No virus Lymphocytes +
Viruses	Enteroviruses, mumps	Herpes simplex, mumps, arthropod-borne viruses, rabies	Measles, rubella, varicella, influenza

Clinical features

Sudden onset: with fever, headache and malaise.

Signs of meningeal irritation: stiffness of neck (nuchal rigidity), Kernig's sign (the leg cannot be straightened at the knee because of hamstring spasm), photophobia and nausea and vomiting.

Convulsions: relatively common in children.

CSF: shows a lymphocytosis, although polymorphs often predominate in the early stages.

Pathogenesis

Most often bloodborne from virus disease elsewhere: thus enteroviruses – the commonest cause of virus aseptic meningitis – invade the CNS as a result of secondary viraemia from infection of the gut. Mumps virus spreads from the parotid and other glands, but also from the respiratory tract (in approximately half the cases there is no accompanying parotitis).

Pathology: little is known of the pathology, which may be merely invasion of the subarachnoid space by lymphocytes and virus.

Epidemiology

Epidemics of aseptic meningitis are common, especially in the summer when enteroviruses are prevalent: echoviruses are the most common cause. The incidence of mumps has declined steadily since the introduction of MMR vaccine.

Virology

Apart from enteroviruses and now, less commonly, mumps, aseptic meningitis can, although rarely, be due to a variety of other viruses, such as herpes simplex types 1 and 2, EB virus, adenoviruses and lymphocytic choriomeningitis virus.

Diagnosis

CSF examination for cells, glucose (usually normal) and PCR for detection of viral nucleic acid: also virus culture.
    Serology: less useful.

ACUTE VIRUS ENCEPHALITIS

A severe disease caused by direct invasion of the brain by virus; with a variable but sometimes high case fatality rate and often neurological sequelae in the survivors. Many different viruses cause encephalitis, but in the UK the main cause is herpes simplex type 1, although this is nevertheless a rare disease. In most British cases the cause is unknown. Sometimes accompanied by meningitis, when the syndrome is known as meningoencephalitis.

Clinical features

Early symptoms: fever, irritability, headache.
    Neurological: photophobia, vomiting, behavioural changes, confusion and disorientation; focal neurological signs with paralysis of cranial and other nerves; drowsiness, with lowered level of consciousness leading to convulsions and coma.

Pathology

Herpes encephalitis: necrosis mainly in the temporal lobe, and often presents as a space-occupying lesion. The brain tissue shows cuffing with lymphocytes round blood vessels and microglial clusters; there is infarction (and so necrosis) of the grey and white matter, and infected cells show characteristic intranuclear inclusions.

Virology

Numerous viruses cause encephalitis. Worldwide, arboviruses are the most important cause and the disease is seen in many – in fact most – countries. Other causes include enteroviruses, EB virus, mumps (usually a meningoencephalitis), rabies and cytomegalovirus in the immunocompromised.

Diagnosis

CSF examination appropriate to the geographical and clinical probability, e.g. in UK, test by PCR for herpes DNA; in an immunocompromised patient consider PCR for cytomegalovirus or EB virus.

CHRONIC VIRUS NEUROLOGICAL DISEASES

Viruses also cause chronic neurological diseases (Table 28.2). Although rare, these are severe, often fatal diseases, and in two instances are associated with immune deficiency.

1. *Subacute sclerosing panencephalitis*
2. *Progressive multifocal leukoencephalopathy*

Table 28.2 Chronic virus neurological diseases

Disease	Subacute sclerosing panencephalitis	Progressive multifocal leukoencephalo- pathy	Tropical spastic paraparesis	HIV/ dementia encephalo- pathy
Site	Brain	Brain	Spinal cord	Brain
Lesions	Neuronal degeneration, intranuclear inclusions	Multiple foci of demyelination	Demyelination, perivascular cuffing	Cerebral atrophy, degenerative change
Infectious agents	Measles, congenital rubella	JC virus	HTLV-1, 2	HIV-1, -2

3. *Tropical spastic paraparesis*
4. *HIV dementia and encephalopathy*.

SUBACUTE SCLEROSING PANENCEPHALITIS (SSPE)

A rare, severe, chronic neurological disease seen in children and young adults as a late sequela of measles: very rarely, a late complication of congenital rubella.

Clinically: presents with personality and behavioural changes and intellectual impairment; progresses to convulsions, myoclonic movements and increasing neurological deterioration, leading to coma and death.

Cause: persistent infection with defective measles virus following primary (and usually uncomplicated) measles several years previously; affected children have high titres of measles antibody in their serum and both IgM and IgG measles-specific antibody in the CSF.

At post mortem: there are numerous intranuclear inclusions throughout the brain: measles virus can be grown from brain tissue.

PROGRESSIVE MULTIFOCAL LEUKOENCEPHALOPATHY

A rare disease due to the papovavirus *JC*, one of two human poly-omaviruses (the other is *BK virus* and is not neurotropic). JC virus is 'opportunistic' in that it does not cause disease in normal people, but only in the immunocompromised. BK virus is also an opportunistic pathogen and has been isolated from immunodeficient patients, mainly from urine – sometimes in association with ureteric stenosis.

Clinically: a variety of neurological signs: such as hemiparesis, dementia, dysphasia, incoordination, impaired vision and hemi-anaesthesia; usually fatal in 3–4 months.

Pathology: multiple foci of demyelination in cerebral hemi-spheres and cerebellum: brain stem and basal ganglia are also sometimes affected: oligodendrocytes with swollen nuclei and intranuclear inclusions are characteristic.

Cause: reactivation of latent virus. Infection is common in the community as around 50–60% of adults in Britain have antibody to it.

Symptomless viruria: with either JC or BK virus is not uncom-mon in pregnancy – around 3–7% of pregnant women shed human polyomaviruses in urine; transplant patients also shed these viruses, which apparently usually cause no urinary symptoms.

Diagnosis: electron microscopy or viral DNA detection by molecular technology.

TROPICAL SPASTIC PARAPARESIS (HTLV-1 ASSOCIATED MYELOPATHY; HAM)

Due to HTLV-1.

Clinically: chronic, progressive spastic paraparesis of the legs; initially stiff gait with back pain, urinary incontinence and, in men, impotence; increasing spasticity, leading to lower limb weakness and ataxia.

Age and sex ratio: twice as common in women as in men, and usually appears in the third to fourth decades of life.

Pathology: demyelination of the neurons of the motor tracts of the spinal cord.

HIV DEMENTIA/ENCEPHALOPATHY

HIV is known to infect neural tissue and CNS macrophages. Progressive infection with HIV is sometimes associated with a subacute encephalopathy, and dementia is a well-recognized feature of full-blown AIDS.

NEUROLOGICAL SYNDROMES PRECIPITATED BY VIRUS INFECTION

Three potentially serious neurological diseases are associated with common virus diseases, although the mechanism of the development of neurological complications is unclear:

1. *Postinfectious encephalitis*
2. *Reye's syndrome*
3. *Guillain–Barré syndrome.*

POSTINFECTIOUS ENCEPHALITIS

A rare complication of the childhood fevers but does not seem to be due to direct viral invasion of the CNS.

Clinical features

Onset: usually 1–2 weeks after the acute disease.

Symptoms: are of drowsiness, vomiting, headache, convulsions, and sometimes focal neurological signs.

Prognosis: about 10–20% of patients die after measles postinfectious encephalitis, and the majority of survivors have residual neurological sequelae.

Pathogenesis: virus cannot be isolated from the brain and the disease is thought to be the result of some abnormal immune response to the virus: pathology shows demyelination and perivascular cuffing.

Cause: follows – although rarely – infection with measles, rubella, varicella, influenza.

Measles: before vaccination the incidence of this complication was 1 in 1000 cases: it was less common after the other childhood fevers. Note that measles can also cause subacute encephalitis in the immunocompromised by direct invasion of the brain.

REYE'S SYNDROME

A disease characterized by fatty degeneration of the CNS and liver: seen only in children; aspirin increases the risk of developing the disease.

Clinical features

Onset: usually follows 4–6 weeks after a virus infection.

Symptoms: nausea and vomiting, with CNS symptoms progressing from lethargy, mental change, convulsions, to coma, hepatomegaly.

Mortality is high – case fatality rate around 10–40%.

Cause: associated with various virus infections – influenza B, varicella, less often influenza A, and rarely, a variety of other viruses.

GUILLAIN–BARRÉ SYNDROME

An acute demyelinating polyneuropathy involving the peripheral nerves; probably immunologically mediated; seen at all ages.

Clinical features

Onset: approximately two-thirds of patients have had a viral infection some 4–6 weeks before onset.

Symptoms: flaccid, symmetric paralysis of the legs, sometimes ascending to involve muscles of respiration.

Prognosis: spontaneous recovery is usual, but some patients require assisted ventilation before symptoms subside.

Cause: various viruses have been incriminated, including cytomegalovirus and EB virus – and influenza vaccination (although the virus in this vaccine is inactivated); can also follow surgery and campylobacter enteritis, and sometimes associated with lymphoma.

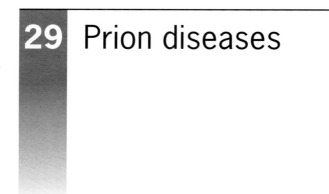

29 Prion diseases

Prions are not viruses: they contain no detectable nucleic acid and are exceptionally resistant to heat and other inactivating agents. They are proteins but are conformationally altered forms of a normal protein – PrP. Surprisingly, this form of the protein is infectious, and can cross species barriers.

Prions cause disease in humans and other animal species, such as sheep and cows. Most, but not all, of the diseases they cause are neurological, and have the following features:

- Rare
- Long incubation period
- Protracted, severe progressive course: always fatal
- Pathology: degeneration of the CNS with *status spongiosus*
- No antibody or other immune response
- Transmissible to experimental animals such as chimpanzees and, after passage, to mice and hamsters.

The four human prion diseases are:

1. Creutzfeldt–Jakob disease and its variant form
2. Kuru
3. Gerstmann–Sträussler–Scheinker disease
4. Fatal familial insomnia.

Pathology: The spongiform encephalopathies are associated with the presence in the brain (and sometimes other tissues) of characteristic fibrils composed of a cell protein coded by a gene, the PrP gene, on human chromosome 20. This protein is present in normal brain and tissues but exists in an abnormal form in the spongiform encephalopathies. The abnormal prions seem to combine with the normal cellular protein to induce replication of the abnormal form. The abnormal form is infectious.

Susceptibility: susceptibility to infection is associated with mutations in the PrP gene.

CREUTZFELDT–JAKOB DISEASE (CJD)

A rare progressive neurological disease characterized by a combination of presenile dementia and symptoms caused by lesions in the spinal cord.

Clinical features

Prodromal stage: the disease starts with tiredness, apathy and vague neurological symptoms.

Second stage: dementia is prominent and the patient develops ataxia, dysarthria and progressive spasticity of the limbs, with involuntary movements such as myoclonic jerks or choreoathetoid movements.

Steady progression until death: usually from about 6 months to 2 years after the onset of symptoms.

Pathology: diffuse atrophy with *status spongiosus* in the cerebral cortex and marked astrocytic gliosis; atrophy also in basal ganglia, cerebellum, substantia nigra and anterior horn cells. Amyloid plaques are scanty.

Epidemiology

Sporadic: seen mainly as a sporadic disease affecting mostly the middle-aged to elderly; a few cases are familial; in both types of case there are mutations in the PrP gene.

Iatrogenic: CJD has been transmitted to patients via the insertion into the brain of electrodes contaminated from use in a previous patient; dura mater grafts and corneal transplants have also been responsible for transmission.

Human growth hormone: use of this product prepared from often thousands of pooled human pituitary glands removed at post mortem has also transmitted CJD: the patients involved are, of course, younger.

VARIANT CJD

During 1996, a new type of CJD, 'v' or variant CJD, was reported: this affected a younger age group with early psychiatric and behavioural disorders, a prolonged course, and was characterized by large, florid, amyloid or kuru-like plaques in the brain: this form of the disease appears to be due to the prion of bovine spongiform encephalopathy (BSE), ingested in beef and having crossed the species barrier from cows to humans. The variant appeared in 1994, and since then the number of cases has increased steadily although, fortunately, not yet to epidemic level.

KURU

Kuru is a fatal human disease found only among the Foré-speaking people in New Guinea. It seems to have appeared about 60 years ago. The incidence increased up to the late 1950s, when kuru was responsible for about half the deaths of the Foré-speaking people. The incidence declined rapidly from the early 1960s, and it is now rare.

Clinical features

Kuru is a native word meaning 'trembling with cold and fever'.
Incubation period: around 4–20 years.
The disease has three stages:

- *First or ambulant stage* of the disease starts with unsteadiness in walking, postural instability, cerebellar ataxia and tremor; facial expressions are poorly controlled and speech becomes slurred and tremulous.
- *Second or sedentary stage* is reached when the patient cannot walk without support, but can still sit upright unaided.
- *Tertiary stage*: the patient cannot sit upright without clutching a stick for support: even a gentle push makes the patient lurch violently; the patient becomes progressively more paralysed and emaciated until death, which is due to bulbar depression or intercurrent infection.

Duration averages 1 year, but ranges from 3 months to 2 years.
Pathology: neuronal degeneration in cerebellum, with astrocytic hyperplasia, gliosis and *status spongiosus*; demyelination is minimal or absent; florid amyloid plaques and fibrils are characteristic features.

Epidemiology

Incidence: kuru was uncommon in adult males; most patients were women or children of either sex.

Transmission: cannibalism of dead relatives is thought to have been responsible for the spread of kuru among the Foré people. The women and children (but not men) eat the viscera and brains of relatives, including those who have died of kuru. Even if cooked, the causal agent would not be inactivated. Cannibalism stopped around 1957, and kuru has now declined sharply in incidence.

GERSTMANN–STRÄUSSLER–SCHEINKER DISEASE

An atypical form of CJD, most often seen as an inherited disorder, in which cerebellar ataxia is a feature: occasionally sporadic; also transmissible to primates.

FATAL FAMILIAL INSOMNIA

Another familial human spongiform encephalopathy in which encephalitis is associated with progressive sleep disorder and loss of autonomic functions.

Prion disease in animals

Scrapie is the best- and most-studied naturally occurring prion disease in animals. Indeed, it may be the source of bovine spongiform encephalopathy (BSE), although this is far from certain.

SCRAPIE

A neurological disease of British sheep, known to exist for more than 200 years. Natural scrapie affects both sheep and goats. Long recognized as infectious, it can be transmitted experimentally not only to sheep but to laboratory mice and hamsters. However, scrapie is *non-infectious to humans*.

Clinical features

Long incubation period: 2–5 years.

Signs and symptoms: excitability, incoordination, ataxia, tremor and continuous scratching or rubbing owing to sensory

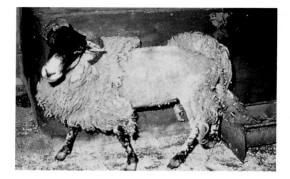

Fig. 29.1 Scrapie-infected sheep: the loss of fleece is due to rubbing ('scrapie') – a neurological rather than a dermatological disorder. (Photograph courtesy of M. Stack, Pathology Research Discipline, Central Veterinary Laboratory, Weybridge.)

neurological disturbance (Fig. 29.1); the symptoms progress to paralysis and death.

Pathology: cerebellar neuronal degeneration, with astrocytic proliferation and *status spongiosus*.

Heredity: a major gene controls whether or not sheep develop disease after experimental inoculation. The operation of the gene is complex; however, different strains of scrapie have distinctive incubation periods, indicating genetically determined control over some features of the disease.

Route of infection: the disease seems to be maintained in flocks by vertical transmission from ewes to lambs, possibly mainly perinatally through contact with infected placentas.

Transmissible mink encephalopathy

A disease also spread from sheep products and due to scrapie agent: mink bred in mink farms became infected when fed on the heads of scrapie-infected sheep.

BOVINE SPONGIFORM ENCEPHALOPATHY (BSE)

First recognized in 1986, and a major epidemic disease in British cattle through the 1980s and much of the 1990s: possibly due to scrapie transmitted from inadequately treated sheep carcasses, rendered down and used to supplement cattle feed as a source of protein; or, alternatively, to recycled infected cattle tissues contaminating cattle feed. However, the agent has altered properties from sheep scrapie (which might be due to selection as a result of passage in another species).There is also the possibility that BSE is due to a naturally occurring prion disease of cattle which can, unlike scrapie, infect humans by ingestion of infected tissues.

Clinical features

Incubation period: 2.5–8 years.

Signs and symptoms: abnormal gait, ataxia, apprehension and anxiety, slipping and falling, licking nose; progresses to frenzy and aggression.

Duration: between 2 weeks and 6 months.

Pathology: degeneration with spongiform vacuolation, especially in medulla oblongata; neuronal loss and gliosis.

Epidemiology

Transmission to other animal species: spongiform encephalopathies have been reported in some zoo animals, presumably transmitted by eating beef or bovine offal; BSE has also appeared in domestic cats.

Epidemic: the disease in cattle is now declining sharply, but has not disappeared: although probably rare, transmission from infected cows to calves has been reported.

30 Viral zoonoses

There are numerous virus diseases that are acquired from animals – sometimes via an insect or arthropod vector, sometimes not. The huge problem they pose in terms of human disease is described in this chapter.

ARTHROPOD-BORNE VIRUSES

Many hundreds of viruses (called *arboviruses*) infect arthropods. Many are not pathogenic for humans, but the diseases caused by the pathogenic members are found worldwide and are of major importance in terms of human illness, causing large-scale epidemics with thousands of cases of illness, death and residual morbidity.

Some of the most important arboviruses are listed in Table 30.1, together with their vectors and the diseases they produce.

Most arboviruses belong to three virus families:

- *Alphavirus* (formerly group A arboviruses)
- *Flavivirus* (formerly group B arboviruses)
- *Bunyavirus*.

ARTHROPOD VECTORS

Vectors: mosquitoes, ticks and sandflies are the principal arthropod vectors that transmit arboviruses.

Reservoirs: the primary or natural hosts are usually wild birds and small mammals, although other animal species may act as intermediate hosts: horses, for example, are intermediate hosts for the three equine encephalitis viruses, and human epidemics are

Table 30.1 Some important arboviruses

Virus	Disease	Vector
Alphaviruses		
Eastern equine encephalitis	Encephalitis	Mosquito
Western equine encephalitis	Encephalitis	Mosquito
Venezuelan equine encephalitis	Fever	Mosquito
Chikungunya	Fever with polyarthritis	Mosquito
Ross River	Fever with polyarthritis	Mosquito
Barmah	Fever with polyarthritis	Mosquito
Sindbis	Fever with polyarthritis	Mosquito
Flaviviruses		
St Louis encephalitis	Encephalitis	Mosquito
Japanese encephalitis	Encephalitis	Mosquito
Murray Valley encephalitis	Encephalitis	Mosquito
Tick-borne encephalitis	Encephalitis	Tick
Yellow fever	Haemorrhagic fever	Mosquito
Omsk haemorrhagic fever	Haemorrhagic fever	Tick
Kyasanur Forest disease	Haemorrhagic fever	Tick
Dengue	Haemorrhagic fever, shock	Mosquito
West Nile fever	Fever	Mosquito
Bunyaviruses		
La Crosse	Encephalitis	Mosquito
Crimean–Congo haemorrhagic fever	Haemorrhagic fever	Tick
Rift Valley fever	Fever	Mosquito
Oropouche	Fever	Mosquito
Sandfly (Phlebotomus) fever	Fever	Sandfly
Reovirus		
Colorado tick fever	Fever	Tick

often preceded by an epidemic of disease in horses. The reservoirs of many arboviruses are unknown.

Transmission: via the bite of an insect vector.

Geographical distribution: is of great importance – because of their mode of transmisssion, the distribution of the different arboviruses corresponds both to that of their arthropod vectors and to the prevalence of virus in animal hosts and reservoirs. Britain is one of the few countries in the world where arboviruses are not a problem (although there is one indigenous and pathogenic arbovirus responsible for the tickborne disease *louping ill* in sheep).

EPIDEMIOLOGY

Epidemics: in the countries affected are recurring (although not necessarily annual) and seasonal – being more frequent in summer and in autumn, to coincide with the active biting seasons of their vectors.

Season: before and during a human epidemic there is usually a seasonal increase in the arthropod vector population – in most cases mosquitoes – with concomitant infection spreading in the animals that are the natural and intermediate hosts of the virus.

ARBOVIRUS DISEASES

Arboviruses cause acute febrile disease but with features that define four main syndromes. The syndromes often overlap – for example, all are associated with fever, and several viruses in all categories can cause a rash or haemorrhagic complications or arthralgia leading to frank arthritis. This simplified classification into disease categories is based on the main or most serious clinical or presenting feature:

• Encephalitis
• Fever
• Haemorrhagic fever
• Fever with arthritis and rash.

ARBOVIRUS ENCEPHALITIS

Arbovirus encephalitis is a worldwide and serious public health problem. Table 30.2 lists the most important of the viruses responsible, together with their geographical distribution.

Clinical features

Fever: with progressively severe headache, nausea, vomiting, stiffness of neck, back and legs: progressing to convulsions, drowsi-

Table 30.2 Arboviruses causing encephalitis and their geographical distribution	
Arbovirus encephalitis	**Geography**
Eastern and western equine, La Crosse, St Louis	North and South America
Japanese	Far East
Central European tickborne	Europe
Far Eastern tickborne	Eastern part of former Soviet Union
Murray Valley	Australia

ness, deepening coma and varied neurological signs, such as paralysis and tremor.

Mortality: can be high: the case fatality rate varies but is highest with Japanese, eastern equine and Murray Valley encephalitis. In Europe, Central European tickborne encephalitis has a low case fatality rate (1–2%), whereas the similar virus of Far Eastern encephalitis (formerly known as Russian Spring–Summer fever) has a case fatality rate of around 20%.

Neurological sequelae: often follow arbovirus encephalitis – again variably, depending on the virus involved: a particular problem in young children and infants infected with Japanese and western and eastern equine encephalitis. Far Eastern tickborne encephalitis is often associated with residual focal epilepsy and flaccid paralysis of the arm and shoulder muscles.

Symptomless infection with these viruses is common: after (and often before) an epidemic, arbovirus antibodies are present in a considerable proportion of the population concerned, even though the incidence of encephalitis has been low. Some viruses, e.g. eastern equine encephalitis virus, cause CNS symptoms in a higher proportion of people infected than other arboviruses.

Age: affects people of all ages, although variation is seen with different viruses. For example, St Louis and eastern equine viruses are more likely to cause encephalitis when they infect the elderly. Western equine encephalitis, on the other hand, is more likely to cause symptomatic infection in infants. La Crosse virus encephalitis particularly affects children less than 15 years old.

ARBOVIRUS FEVERS

These are found worldwide and are caused by viruses in different families (see Table 30.1): their severity varies from mild to life-threatening. The syndromes overlap in their clinical features with arbovirus haemorrhagic fevers and some of the diseases listed here often show some haemorrhagic signs. Some of the most important viruses causing these are listed in Table 30.3, together with the countries or continents in which they are found.

Clinical features

Febrile disease: which may be severe, with high fever, chills, often headache, myalgia, nausea and vomiting, sometimes rash (West Nile fever): meningoencephalitis is sometimes seen with West Nile fever and Oropouche; Rift Valley fever can be complicated by

Table 30.3 Main arbovirus fevers and their geography

Arbovirus fever	Geography
Venezuelan equine encephalitis	Central and South America
Rift Valley fever	Africa
West Nile fever	Africa, India, Middle East, southern Europe, recently USA
Oropouche	South America, Caribbean
Colorado tick fever	Western USA, Canada
Sandfly (phlebotomus) fever	Southern Italy, Mediterranean, Far East

retinitis, hepatitis or encephalitis with haemorrhage; retro-orbital pain is a characteristic feature of Venezuelan equine encephalitis (in which, despite its name, encephalitis is comparatively uncommon); Colorado tick fever is moderately severe, typically diphasic, with leukopenia and thrombocytopenia.

Fatality rate: generally low – in most cases the patient recovers without sequelae.

Rift Valley fever: infects domestic animals such as sheep, goats and cattle, and these can be a source of human infection acquired during butchery.

Symptomless infection: is common with all these infections – detected by a relatively high prevalence of antibodies in the general population concerned.

ARBOVIRUS HAEMORRHAGIC FEVERS

These are listed in Table 30.4, which includes yellow fever and dengue, two diseases with important, because severe and life-threatening, clinical features.

YELLOW FEVER

The most important arbovirus haemorrhagic fever, because the most severe, in which liver involvement and jaundice are prominent. Historically the cause of many deaths ('yellow jack') among early European colonialists settling in Central and South America. Still a problem despite an effective vaccine and the susceptibility (at present theoretical) to mosquito control measures.

Table 30.4   Arbovirus haemorrhagic fevers and their geography

Arbovirus	Geography
Yellow fever	Central and South America, Africa
Dengue	Southeast Asia, India, South America, Pacific Islands, Australia, Caribbean
Crimean–Congo haemorrhagic fever	Southern part of former Soviet Union, Balkans, Middle East, Far East, Africa
Omsk haemorrhagic fever	Western Siberia
Kyasanur Forest disease	India

Clinical features

Fever with chills of sudden onset and severe prostration and malaise, myalgia, and nausea and vomiting; a relatively slow pulse and leukopenia are characteristic.

Jaundice: a defining feature, appears after a day or two, intensifying to liver failure.

Renal involvement with albuminuria, sometimes leading to anuria.

Haemorrhages associated with thrombocytopenia and prolonged clotting time, resulting in epistaxis, melaena, haematemesis, petechiae and bleeding from gums etc.

Death follows intensification of signs and symptoms leading to stupor and coma.

Case fatality rate: variable, around 20%, but rates as high as 50% have been recorded.

Epidemiology

There are two epidemiologically different forms of yellow fever:

1. *Urban*: the reservoir of the virus is humans and the vector the mosquito *Aedes aegypti*.
2. *Sylvan or jungle*: the reservoir is tree-dwelling monkeys and the vector various species of forest mosquito.

Vaccine: an extremely effective, live attenuated vaccine (17D virus) is available: previously always regarded as safe, although there have been recent reports of rare but fatal yellow fever due to vaccine virus in vaccinees.

DENGUE

A major and growing health problem in many areas of the world because the disease is spreading beyond its traditional boundaries. There are four antigenic types of virus (types 1–4).

Clinical features

Febrile disease: with headache, retro-orbital pain, prostration, nausea, myalgia, pain in the limbs (which is often severe) and a generalized maculopapular rash; minor bleeding signs such as petechiae and epistaxis are seen in some patients. The case fatality rate of this type of dengue is low.

Dengue haemorrhagic fever and dengue shock syndrome: are serious complications seen mainly in young children. A typical attack of dengue deteriorates to severe disease characterized by haemorrhages, thrombocytopenia, increased vascular permeability with haemoconcentration; even more serious is the development of *dengue shock syndrome*, with the onset of hypotension, profound weakness and shock, with pale, clammy extremities, weak rapid pulse and restlessness.

    Case fatality rate: of dengue shock syndrome untreated can be around 40–50%.

    Pathogenesis: dengue haemorhagic fever/shock syndrome seems to be immunologically mediated in children who have had a previous attack and later become infected with a different subtype of virus: antibody-mediated enhancement of infection is probably responsible for this, but the precise immunological mechanism involved is unclear.

Epidemiology

Reservoirs: often humans, in a man–mosquito–man cycle in which the vector is *Aedes aegypti*; in southeast Asia and west Africa monkeys are the reservoir.

OTHER HAEMORRHAGIC FEVERS

Crimean–Congo haemorrhagic fever: a tickborne bunyavirus disease which can also spread case-to-case to medical and nursing staff via contact with infected blood. Clinically, the disease has a variable but sometimes high mortality: the most serious cases are

Table 30.5 Arbovirus fevers with arthritis and rash

Arbovirus	Geography
Ross River fever	Australia
Chikungunya	Africa
Barmah fever	Australia
Sindbis	Africa, India, Southeast Asia, Australia, Russia

marked by haemorrhages, sometimes with extensive skin ecchymoses and circulatory collapse.

Omsk and *Kyasanur Forest fevers*: both are tickborne fevers – often severe, with rash and haemorrhages: the reservoirs of Omsk fever are muskrats (most cases of the disease are in muskrat hunters) and other rodents; the reservoirs of Kyasanur Forest fever are monkeys, rats and other animals, and the disease mainly affects forest workers.

ARBOVIRUS FEVERS WITH ARTHRITIS AND RASH

Several arboviruses cause fever with marked arthralgia, often progressing to polyarthritis and typically accompanied by a rash; often seen in large-scale epidemics and listed in Table 30.5.

Clinical features

Febrile but self-limiting diseases in which pain in the joints (which can be excruciating) due to a polyarthritis is prominent, with a maculopapular rash and often cervical lymphadenopathy. Minor haemorrhages are common in Chikungunya. Sindbis is one of the mildest of arbovirus infections.

ARBOVIRUS VIROLOGY

The following are some properties of the main arbovirus families:

Alphaviruses (Fig. 30.1) and *flaviviruses*: single-strand positive-sense RNA. *Bunyaviruses*: single-strand negative-sense RNA in three segments. *Reovirus*, Orbivirus (Colorado tick fever) double-stranded RNA in 12 segments.

Most viruses grow in certain cell cultures, sometimes in mosquito larvae, and are pathogenic for suckling mice.

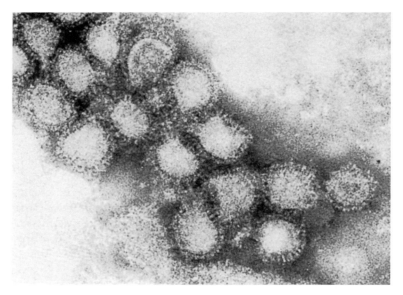

Fig. 30.1 An alphavirus. This electronmicrograph of sindbis virus shows roughly spherical particles with cubic symmetry and a surface fringe. × 200 000. (Photograph courtesy of Professor C. R. Madeley.)

Diagnosis

Generally requires facilities of a specialist reference laboratory for *serology* or attempted *isolation* – usually from blood.

Vaccines

The most widely used vaccine available for arboviruses is against yellow fever, but effective vaccines are also available for Japanese and tickborne encephalitis and, on a limited basis for those at special risk, for eastern and western equine encephalitis. Research into a vaccine for dengue is ongoing.

Treatment

Only supportive – there is no specific antiviral therapy.

NON-ARTHROPOD BORNE VIRAL ZOONOSES

Many other viral *zoonoses* are acquired from animals but not by the bite of an insect vector. The viruses responsible are shown in Table 30.6.

Table 30.6   The main virus causes of non-arthropod borne zoonoses

Virus family	Virus	Disease	Animal host	Geography
Lyssa	Rabies	Rabies	Foxes, dogs, wolves, bats	Worldwide except for a few island countries
Filo	Ebola, Marburg	Ebola, Marburg fevers	Possibly rodents	Africa
Arena	Lassa	Haemorrhagic fever	Multimammate rats	West Africa
	Tacaribe complex	S. American haemorrhagic fevers	Mice, rats	South America
	Lymphocytic choriomeningitis	Aseptic meningitis	Mice	Worldwide
Bunya	Hantaviruses	Haemorrhagic fevers, with renal, pulmonary syndromes	Rodents	Worldwide
Paramyxo	Hendra	Encephalitis, pneumonia	Horses, fruit bats	Australia
	Nipah	Encephalitis	Pigs, fruit bats	Malaysia

RABIES

Rabies is a lethal encephalitis caused by a virus that affects a wide variety of warm-blooded animals: rabies is transmitted to humans via the bite of an infected animal, which is usually (but not always) a dog.

Clinical features

Incubation period: long: usually 4–12 weeks, sometimes much longer; if the bite is on the head or neck the incubation period is shorter than for bites on the limbs. Virus spread from the wound to the CNS is via the nerves.

Symptoms: initially non-specific, often early psychological symptoms, such as personality changes, apprehension; paraesthesia around the wound is a common early symptom. Thereafter there are two forms of rabies:

1. *Furious*: the more common; symptoms are excitement, with tremor, muscular contractions and convulsions; typically, spasm

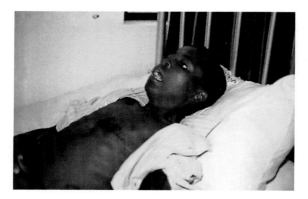

Fig. 30.2 Rabies. Patient in hydrophobic spasm. (Photograph courtesy of Dr D. A. Warrell.)

of the muscles of swallowing (hence the older name for the disease of 'hydrophobia', or fear of water) and increased sensitivity of the sensory nervous system (Fig. 30.2).

2. *Dumb* or *paralytic*: symptoms of ascending paralysis, eventually involving the muscles of swallowing, speech and respiration.

Virus is present in saliva, skin and eyes, as well as the brain.

Prognosis: the disease is virtually always fatal; death often follows a convulsion.

Pathology: despite the severity of the clinical disease, lesions in the CNS are minimal, with little evidence of destructive effects on cells, but with intracytoplasmic inclusions known as *Negri bodies* within neurons – diagnostic of rabies.

Epidemiology

Enzootic and often epizootic in many species of carnivorous wild animals (e.g. foxes in Europe, wolves in the former Soviet Union, and skunks and racoons in the USA), but also found in bats, rodents and cattle (especially in South America, where the virus is spread by the bite of infected vampire bats). Spreads from wild animals to infect domestic animals.

Dogs are the main danger to humans because of their close contact with humans: virus is present in the saliva of infected dogs for up to 7 days (but rarely for more than 4 days) before the onset of symptoms; dogs and cats remaining healthy for 10 days after biting can be regarded as being free of virus at the time of biting.

Incidence of rabies after biting: most dog bites are, of course, from non-rabid animals; only about 15% of people bitten by a rabid animal develop the disease; bites on the head or neck carry a greater risk of rabies than those on the limbs. Postexposure vaccination now offers effective prophylaxis.

Britain and some other countries in western Europe, Australia, New Zealand and Japan are free from indigenous animal rabies. Quarantine is no longer compulsory in Britain for pets travelling from western Europe and some other rabies-free countries if vaccinated and with certification from veterinary surgeons. The main danger is the establishment of a reservoir of infection in wild animals – and Britain has a large fox population.

European rabies: the virus has been spreading in Europe as an epizootic in foxes since 1945, slowly moving westward from eastern Europe to France over the past 50 years or so; however, this epizootic is being controlled by effective wildlife vaccination programmes.

Bats: are reservoirs of classic serotype 1 rabies virus in the USA and South America: some species of lyssavirus, related to but antigenically distinct from classic rabies virus, are presently epizootic in bats in Europe and have been found in other countries – notably in Africa, and recently in Australia. Although less likely to be transmitted to humans than carnivorous animal rabies, occasional cases of human infection have been attributed to them.

Aerosol infection: has been recorded as a result of a laboratory accident and also by exposure in bat-infested caves: a rare event.

Case-to-case spread: human patients do not seem to be infectious to others, including medical attendants, despite the presence of virus in saliva; nevertheless, vaccination is advisable.

Corneal transplant: cases of rabies in recipients of corneas from donors with undiagnosed rabies have been reported.

Virology

Classic rabies virus is a lyssavirus (serotype 1) within the rhabdovirus family: enveloped bullet-shaped particles (Fig. 30.3): single-strand negative-sense RNA; haemagglutinates, grows in certain cell cultures and is pathogenic for mice and other laboratory animals. The bat lyssaviruses comprise another six serotypes of lyssavirus.

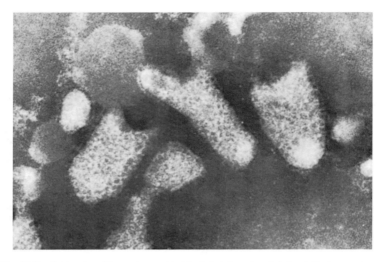

Fig. 30.3 Rabies virus. The nucleocapsid of the bullet-shaped particle has helical symmetry and is surrounded by an envelope. × 108 000. (Electronmicrograph courtesy of Professor C. R. Madeley.)

Diagnosis (refer to specialized reference laboratories)

Detect rabies virus antigen by immunofluorescence in hair-bearing skin (e.g. back of neck), corneal impression smears, brain tissue.

Isolation: inoculate: mice with brain tissue, saliva, CSF, urine; examine brain post mortem for virus antigen by immunofluorescence and for Negri bodies.

PCR: the most sensitive method of diagnosis.

Dogs

If rabies is suspected, the dog should be kept under observation to see if the disease develops. If killed before dying from the disease Negri bodies may not have developed in sufficient numbers to be detected. After death, send the dog's head to a specialist laboratory.

Vaccination (see also Chapter 39)

Human: diploid cell vaccine containing inactivated virus is used for both pre- and post-exposure immunization. Human antirabies immunoglobulin is also available and should always be given with post-exposure vaccination.

Animal vaccines

Inactivated: used for dogs and also available for cats and cattle in endemic areas, and occasionally other animals: for example, those in zoos, or particularly valuable stock, should be vaccinated.

Live attenuated: used for wild animals; trials in Europe of attenuated virus vaccine in bait have proved successful in eradicating rabies in wildlife.

EBOLA AND MARBURG VIRUS DISEASES

Both are severe diseases caused by similar but antigenically different viruses. Marburg disease first appeared in 1967 in an outbreak initially involving laboratory workers in Marburg, Frankfurt and Belgrade who had handled the tissues from a batch of African green monkeys. Ebola – an equally or even more severe disease – has appeared in outbreaks in different areas in Africa.

Clinical features

Very severe haemorrhagic febrile illness: with headache, myalgia and maculopapular rash; other features are vomiting, diarrhoea, hepatitis, pharyngitis, and signs of renal and CNS involvement. Haemorrhage from various sites in the body – gastrointestinal tract, lungs, vagina, gums and needle puncture sites – is a major feature. There is leukopenia, with atypical lymphocytes and plasma cells in the blood and signs of vascular damage.

Case fatality rate is high – considerably more than 50% in the Ebola outbreaks.

Infectiousness: to contacts, including medical and nursing personnel, is a feature: sexual transmission has been recorded, with long-term persistence of virus in body fluids.

Animal reservoirs

Although several outbreaks have involved monkeys they are thought to be intermediate hosts rather than the main reservoir of the viruses: no other animal hosts have been found despite extensive search.

Epidemiology

There have been several outbreaks of Ebola haemorrhagic fever in Africa in recent years: all have been associated with a high mortality. Marburg disease outbreaks appears less common and to involve fewer patients. Ebola virus was identified in monkeys imported from the Philippines to the USA in 1989–90, indicating that the virus was present outside Africa, although this strain appeared to be less pathogenic than the viruses isolated in earlier human outbreaks.

Virology

Filoviruses: negative-sense single-strand RNA; unusual elongated virus particles: grow in various tissue cultures without CPE but with intracytoplasmic inclusions; pathogenic for guinea-pigs.

Diagnosis (refer to specialized reference laboratories)

Isolate from blood in guinea-pigs or cell cultures.

Serology: ELISA and PCR for detection of virus in blood or tissues; ELISA for IgG or IgM detection.

ARENAVIRUSES

There are three main human pathogenic arenaviruses or arenavirus groups:

1. *Lassa fever* virus
2. *The Tacaribe complex* of viruses associated with South American haemorrhagic fevers
3. *Lymphocytic choriomeningitis.*

The natural hosts of all the viruses are mice or rats.

Transmission: infection is acquired by inhalation or ingestion of materials contaminated with rodent excreta, or direct contamination of cuts. Lassa fever can also be acquired by direct contact with a case of the disease.

LASSA FEVER

A febrile disease endemic in west Africa which was first reported from Lassa, Nigeria. The virus is highly infectious and spreads readily to contacts, including medical and nursing personnel.

Clinical features

Illness starts with fever and sore throat, then vomiting, cough, weakness and malaise, ulcers in the mouth and pharynx, and cervical lymphadenopathy; facial oedema is a prominent sign; abdominal pain, myalgia with diarrhoea; headache and encephalopathy; late features are haemorrhage and shock; deafness is a late complication.

Case fatality overall is 1%, although it is higher (15%) in hospitalized patients and in women in the third trimester of pregnancy. Not all cases are severe – many infections are mild.

Symptomless infection: common in rural populations.

Epidemiology

The virus seems to be fairly widespread in west Africa, where the animal host is the multimammate rat. Cases have also been reported in central Africa.

Diagnosis (refer to specialized laboratory)

Isolation: in cell culture from blood, urine, throat washings.

Serology: by ELISA and PCR for detection of virus; ELISA for IgM detection.

Note: In the UK the diagnosis may be missed unless a history of recent travel to west Africa is sought. Patients in hospital wards need to be nursed in a high security infectious diseases unit, as they represent an infectious hazard to staff.

Treatment

Ribavirin: effective if given early.

SOUTH AMERICAN HAEMORRHAGIC FEVERS

Below are the four related arenaviruses, which together form the Tacaribe complex, together with the countries in which they are found:

- *Junin*:   Argentina
- *Machupo*:   Bolivia
- *Guanarito*: Venezuela
- *Sabia*:   Brazil.

Clinical features

Severe diseases with haemorrhagic, renal, cardiovascular and some-times neurological symptoms. The reservoirs of the viruses are rats or mouse-like rodents.

The Argentinian disease is rural and spreads mainly during the maize harvest from mice which inhabit the maize fields: there have been large and severe annual outbreaks of the disease among the corn harvesters there, although vaccination is helping to control these.

The Bolivian disease was mostly acquired in houses and is now rare.

Guanarito and Sabia viruses have caused outbreaks of severe disease in Venezuela and Brazil, respectively.

Vaccine

An attenuated Junin virus vaccine has been developed for use in at-risk populations in Argentina.

LYMPHOCYTIC CHORIOMENINGITIS

A common natural infection in mice but also present in some hamsters: the virus is shed in the urine and faeces of infected animals; transmission to humans is a rare event. The disease has been acquired by handlers from pet and laboratory hamsters.

The disease is of interest from an immunological point of view, as mice are not uncommonly infected in utero; when this happens they have a generalized infection with high titres of virus in all tissues and organs: however, the mice remain symptomless, although they later succumb to glomerulonephritis owing to immune complex deposition in the kidney.

Clinical features

The most important syndrome in humans is aseptic meningitis; sometimes meningoencephalitis is seen; the virus also causes an influenza-like febrile illness.

Virology of arenaviruses

RNA viruses: the genome is two single-stranded RNA segments; interestingly, replication involves transcription of both minus- and positive-sense RNA (ambisense transcription): the enveloped particles are unusual in that they contain host cell ribosomes as internal granules. Grow in cell culture and are pathogenic for mice and guinea-pigs.

HANTAVIRUSES

Hantaviruses are rodent viruses which can spread to humans. Rodent infection is chronic and symptomless, but in humans the viruses can cause severe febrile illness.

Clinical features

Four main syndromes associated with different virus species are seen:

Hantaan virus: found in Korea, eastern Russia, China; the animal hosts are field mice; causes haemorrhagic fever with renal syndrome (HFRS): a severe disease with fever, renal impairment giving rise to proteinuria and oliguria, and haemorrhages: abdominal pain is common. Recovery is slow, with prolonged convalescence, and the mortality is variable – around 5–15%.

Seoul virus: causes a somewhat milder form of HFRS: the virus is found in rats worldwide.

Puumala virus: endemic in bank voles (and probably in other rodents also) in Scandinavia and western Europe: causes *nephropathia epidemica*, a similar but milder febrile disease than HFRS and characterized by signs of renal failure – proteinuria and oliguria – but with a lower case fatality rate (less than 1%).

Sin nombre (no name) virus: the cause of hantavirus pulmonary syndrome, a very severe disease with a high case fatality rate – around 50%: a febrile illness with severe respiratory failure and cardiogenic shock: gross pleural effusions are seen in some patients; the natural host is the deer mouse; found mainly in the western USA.

Epidemiology

Transmission: mainly airborne from dust etc. contaminated by rodent excreta.

Geographical distribution: hantaviruses are found worldwide, depending on the distribution of their rodent host.

Virology

Bunyaviruses; single-stranded RNA in three segments with replication involving ambisense transcription: grow, but with great difficulty, in cell culture: molecular technology succeeded in discovering the cause of the Sin nombre outbreak in the USA.

Diagnosis

Serology: by immunofluorescence or ELISA.

Treatment

Ribavirin has been used intravenously to treat severe infection, but is of uncertain value.

HENDRA AND NIPAH VIRUS DISEASES

Two newly discovered diseases caused by paramyxoviruses; although similar in properties, the two viruses are serologically distinct.

Clinical features

Acute encephalitis: the three reported patients with Hendra infection presented with respiratory signs of atypical pneumonia, one having meningoencephalitis; two of the patients died. The Nipah cases were predominantly encephalitic, with fever, headache, drowsiness, various focal and other neurological signs with vertigo and disorientation leading to coma: some patients had respiratory signs: several of the patients died and others were left with neurological sequelae.

Pathology: Nipah virus disease is associated with a widespread vasculitis.

Occupation: patients in reported cases have worked with animals – horses in the Queensland outbreak of Hendra disease and pigs in the Malaysian and Singapore Nipah cases (pig farmers and abattoir workers, respectively).

Animal hosts: fruit bats are the reservoir of both Nipah and Hendra viruses with Hendra virus, horses also develop disease, being intermediate hosts and transmitting the virus to human contacts; similarly, pigs became ill with Nipah virus and human infection is by direct contact with the animals; any other reservoir has not so far been identified.

Diagnosis

Serology: detection of IgM by ELISA. *Isolation* of syncytia-producing virus in cell cultures from CSF.

Treatment

Possibly ribavirin.

31 Retroviruses

The discovery of human retroviruses has been one of the most important developments in clinical virology. Retroviruses have long been known as the cause of cancer in various animal species: research into them led to the discovery of the cause of AIDS – the acquired immunodeficiency syndrome.

HUMAN RETROVIRUSES

The four human retroviruses are listed in Table 31.1. HIV-1 and -2 and HTLV-1 infect CD4 helper T lymphocytes, but whereas HTLV-1 transforms and causes the T cells to proliferate, HIV-1 and -2 are cytopathic and kill the cells. The CD4 molecules on the T cells are the receptors for HIV-1 and -2. HTLV-2 primarily infects CD8 lymphocytes.

Table 31.1 Human retroviruses

Virus	Disease
Human immunodeficiency virus	
HIV-1	AIDS (acquired immune deficiency syndrome)
HIV-2	AIDS
Human T-cell lymphotropic viruses	
HTLV-1	Adult T-cell leukaemia/lymphoma; tropical spastic paraparesis
HTLV-2	Unknown

HIV (HUMAN IMMUNODEFICIENCY VIRUS)

HIV causes failure of the immune system, with consequent opportunistic infections and tumours that are the hallmark of the disease.

AIDS appears to be a genuinely new disease. The first infection recorded was in Kinshasa, Zaire, in 1959 (antibody to HIV was later detected in serum taken at that time). Since then, AIDS has become epidemic in Africa and, with a somewhat different epidemiology, in the USA and western Europe, and is now found in virtually every country in the world.

HIV – there are two types of virus:

- **HIV-1**: the main cause of the worldwide AIDS pandemic
- **HIV-2**: found in west Africa and, as yet, not showing significant spread from there.

Clinical features

The natural history of HIV has four stages:

1. ***Primary infection***: may be symptomless, but from 25 to 65% of patients have some illness at the time of seroconversion. This is usually a mild infectious mononucleosis-like illness some 2 weeks to 3 months after exposure, with fever, maculopapular rash, sore throat, night sweats, malaise, lymphadenopathy, diarrhoea, and relative and absolute lymphocytosis in the peripheral blood. There may be mouth and genital ulcers, and neurological signs such as encephalopathy, meningitis or myelopathy. These symptoms are usually mild and subside spontaneously: antibody appears at about this time.

2. ***Asymptomatic infection***: the length of this is is very variable and can last from 1 to 10 years: virus is present in blood but at low levels and with a slow rate of replication: CD4 counts are generally within normal limits or usually above 350×10^6 cells/L.

3. ***Persistent generalized lymphadenopathy***: this involves at least two sites outside the inguinal area and lasts for some months: it is quite often the presenting sign of HIV infection.

4. ***Symptomatic stage***: virus replication starts to increase, with a a concomitant decrease in CD4 counts and a decline in immune function. There is constitutional upset, with malaise, weight loss, fever, night sweats and prolonged diarrhoea. The disease progresses to a variey of opportunistic infections as microorganisms fail to be controlled by the patient's immune system (these include

disseminated infection with atypical mycobacteria such as the *M. avium* complex, illustrated in Fig. 31.1). Tumours – notably Kaposi's sarcoma (Fig. 31.2) – are also a feature of AIDS. These represent the defining conditions of AIDS and are listed in Table 31.2.

Note that many other conditions are commonly associated with AIDS, such as seborrhoeic dermatitis, oral hairy leukoplakia, zoster, mouth ulcers, and tinea infections of the feet.

5. **Progression to full-blown AIDS**: correlates with decrease in CD4 lymphocyte count to below 200×10^6 cells/L and an increase in the viral load in the blood (measured as viral RNA copies per mL by quantitative PCR or bDNA assay).

Table 31.2 AIDS: defining conditions

Condition	Disease
Parasites	
Cryptosporidium	Diarrhoea
Isospora belli	Diarrhoea
Toxoplasmosis of brain	Encephalitis
Viruses	
Herpes simplex	Oral ulceration (prolonged); pneumonitis; oesophagitis
Cytomegalovirus	Pneumonia; retinitis
JC virus	Progressive multifocal leukoencephalopathy
Bacteria	
Mycobacterium avium complex	Extrapulmonary, disseminated disease
Mycobacterium tuberculosis	Tuberculosis: pulmonary, extrapulmonary
Salmonella spp.	Septicaemia, recurrent
Fungi	
Pneumocystis carinii	Pneumonia
Candida albicans	Oesophageal, pulmonary
Coccidiomycosis	Extrapulmonary
Cryptococcus neoformans	Meningitis
Histoplasmosis	Disseminated
Tumours	Cervical cancer – invasive
	Kaposi's sarcoma
	Non-Hodgkin's lymphoma;
	Cerebral B-cell lymphoma
Other	
HIV	Encephalopathy/dementia
	Wasting disease
	Pneumonia, recurrent

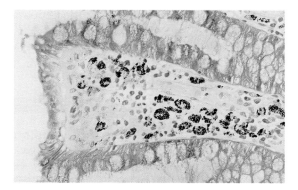

Fig. 31.1   Disseminated *Mycobacterium avium-intracellulare* in the colon of a patient with AIDS. Ziehl–Neelsen stain (approx. × 1000). (Courtesy of Dr C. J. R. Stewart.)

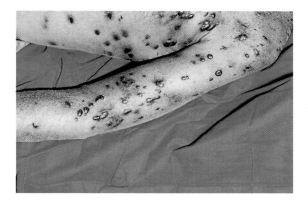

Fig. 31.2   AIDS. The characteristic purplish skin tumours of Kaposi's sarcoma. (Photograph courtesy of The Photography and Illustration Centre, Middlesex Hospital.)

Paediatric AIDS

Infected mothers: transmit HIV to their babies in approximately 15–30% of cases: treatment of the mother with antiretroviral therapy can prevent this in most cases (see Chapter 38).

Virus spreads to the child:

- *Transplacentally* to cause infection in utero
- *During delivery* or in the perinatal period
- *Through breastfeeding.*

Clinically: failure to thrive, fever and diarrhoea, frequent infections, lymphadenopathy, parotitis, hepatosplenomegaly, and a characteristic lymphoid interstitial pneumonia which is progressive and fatal; encephalopathy, convulsions, dementia and motor disorders are also seen.

CD4 counts: tend to be higher than in adults and a less reliable indicator as to disease progression.

AIDS

In both adults and children the disease is uniformly fatal, although treatment with highly active antiretroviral therapy (HAART) and appropriate antimicrobial therapy can greatly prolong and improve the quality of life.

Pathology

AIDS is often described as a disease of CD4 helper T lymphocytes, but although lymphoid tissues are major targets for the virus (which attaches specifically to the CD4 receptors on lymphocytes and on cells such as macrophages), the virus causes disseminated infection and affects many organs, e.g. brain, gut, bone marrow and skin. The pathological processes involved in the course of the infection are still unclear.

Epidemiology

Transmission:

• Sexual
• Parenterally by infected blood or blood products, or by needle-sharing among drug abusers
• In utero from mother to child, perinatally, or via breast milk.

Sources of virus: virus is present in blood, semen, vaginal secretions and breast milk.

High risk: given the routes of infection, certain categories of people are at risk of infection:

• *Promiscuous*, especially male homosexuals
• *Injecting drug abusers*
• *Haemophiliacs*
• *Infants born to infected mothers.*

Healthcare workers: the risk is low (the transmission rate by percutaneous injury with HIV-positive blood is 0.32%).

Geographical distribution: worldwide more than 30 million people are infected with AIDS. The problem is particularly bad in sub-Saharan Africa, where the adult prevalence rate is 8.8% and infection is spread mainly heterosexually. AIDS, and the tuberculosis associated with it, are causing high mortality, with severe effects on the life expectancy, social and economic life of the countries concerned.

Southeast Asia: is now suffering from the epidemic and infection there is increasing at an alarming rate (mostly associated with prostitution). Intravenous drug use is also an important factor in some areas.

USA and western Europe: most infections have been acquired by homosexual anal intercourse between men, but heterosexual spread is increasing and, in 1999, for the first time in the UK, heterosexual transmission was more common than spread between men. Intravenous drug abuse continues to be an important route of infection which is much more prevalent in inner cities – London and the Thames region contain 70% of all HIV cases in the UK. Haemophiliac patients have in the past been infected by contamination of factor VIII from infected donors, but this has been controlled by blood screening and heat treatment.

Virology (see also Chapter 20)

Retrovirus (Fig. 31.3) with single-stranded, dimeric RNA: the *env* gene codes for the main envelope glycoprotein, which is involved in immunity but shows considerable variation owing to spontaneous mutation. In addition to *pol* and *gag* genes, the genome contains regulatory genes: *tat*, *rev*, *nef* etc., and long terminal repeat regions responsible for integration of the provirus.

Grows in T-lymphocyte cultures stimulated with interleukin-2, but with variable CPE.

Diagnosis

Serology: ELISA: if positive, confirm by additional ELISAs and Western blot to analyse antibodies against individual virus proteins which can also distinguish between HIV-1 and HIV-2 infections. The core (*gag*) p24 antigen is detectable in primary infection as well as in late disease.

Detection of virus nucleic acid: DNA or RNA in blood and other body fluids and measurement of virus load – important along with CD4 counts to monitor disease progression.

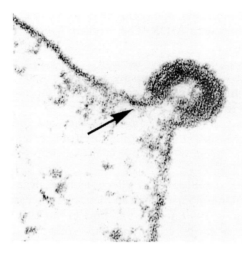

Fig. 31.3 Feline leukaemia virus: a typical retrovirus particle, budding through the plasma membrane on its release from the cell. The continuity between the cell surface membrane and the virion is indicated by the arrow, and the spikes on the surface of the outer virion membrane are clearly seen. × 190 000. (Electronmicrograph courtesy of Dr Helen Laird.)

Infection in infants

Infection in infants is difficult to diagnose serologically because of the persistence of maternal antibody in babies born to infected mothers: HIV antibody persisting beyond 15 months is strong evidence of infection. Test for p24 antigen and for viral DNA or RNA.

Treatment

Aimed at two targets:

- **HIV** (see also Chapter 33): HAART consisting of combinations of nucleoside and non-nucleoside reverse transcriptase inhibitors, together with a protease inhibitor: give also to pregnant and postpartum women to reduce transmission in utero and perinatally. Healthcare workers suffering a percutaneous injury should also be offered a course of antiretroviral therapy.
- **Opportunistic infections and tumours**: treat with antimicrobial drugs and chemotherapy as appropriate.

HTLV-1

HTLV-1 is an endemic infection is certain areas of the world. Usually latent in T lymphocytes but causes adult T-cell leukaemia/lymphoma (most other leukaemias/lymphomas are tumours of B lymphocytes) and other diseases in a small proportion of individuals infected.

Clinical features

Symptomless infection: most infected people do not develop disease and, of the 2–6% who do, disease appears after a very prolonged interval – up to 20 or more years after infection: the risk factors that lead to the onset of disease are unknown.

There are three main syndromes associated with HTLV-1:

• *Adult T-cell leukaemia/lymphoma* (ATLL): an aggressive malignancy of T cells, with lymphadenopathy and hepatosplenomegaly; sometimes cerebral involvement. The disease may present with lymphomatous infiltration of the skin (so that it can be mistaken clinically for mycosis fungoides): atypical transformed T cells are present, sometimes in large numbers, in the peripheral blood. The level of calcium in the blood is increased, possibly related to osteoporotic lesions in bones.

• *HTLV-associated myelopathy/tropical spastic paraparesis* (HAM/TSP): a progressive, demyelinating spastic paralysis caused by lesions of heavy mononuclear infiltrates in the pyramidal tracts of the spinal cord: there are atypical lobulated lymphocytes in the blood; more common in females than males.

• *HTLV-associated uveitis* (HAU): presents with blurred vision, iritis, vitreous opacities and retinal vasculitis.

Virus persists as a latent infection in the T cells of infected individuals, including those who remain asymptomatic. Antibody also persists throughout.

Epidemiology

Geographical distribution: marked; infection is particularly common in southwestern Japan, but also found in the Caribbean, Africa, South America, the Middle East and Polynesia. It is present at a low level in Britain, mostly in immigrants from the West Indies.

Transmission: vertical (mainly via infected breast milk), sexual and by blood – transfused blood is highly infectious, but the virus is strongly cell associated and plasma is not infectious.

Seroprevalence: antibody to HTLV-1 in endemic areas varies in prevalence, generally being around 1–5%, although clusters are found in which the prevalence is much higher, e.g. in southern Japan, where some 30% of the population are antibody positive. The prevalence of antibody in children is low, but rises with increasing age.

Virology

Typical retrovirus: grows in cultures of human T lymphocytes stimulated with interleukin-2: cells are transformed or immortalized without cytopathic effect.

Diagnosis

Serology: ELISA, particle agglutination test, Western blot – available at specialized laboratories.

HTLV-2

Originally isolated from a patient with hairy cell leukaemia, the virus is now thought to be unrelated to this disease. Similar structurally and with some nucleic acid homology to HTLV-1, its epidemiology and pathogenicity are ill understood. Clusters of antibody-positive people have been described among drug abusers in London, UK, and in several cities in the USA, and also in certain other areas of the world, e.g. Africa, where infection seems endemic and unrelated to drug abuse.

HTLV-1 and -2 can be distinguished serologically and by differences in their gene sequences.

RETROVIRUSES AND CANCER

Retroviruses are widespread in the animal kingdom and can produce leukaemia or sarcomas in the host animal: these tumours are due to the activity of cancer-producing genes or oncogenes, which are part of the genome of many retroviruses and also found in the chromosomes of the host animal. Note, however, that HTLV-1 does not contain an oncogene but transforms through *trans*-activation of various cellular genes by its *Tax* gene.

Oncogenes

Some retroviruses cause cancer because their genome has acquired cellular oncogenes by recombination when RNA tumour viruses integrated in the form of provirus DNA into cellular chromosomes. Oncogenes do not always give rise to carcinogenesis. They need to be activated, and different mechanisms can be responsible for this:

- *Virus promoter*, such as that contained in the long terminal repeat regions of the retrovirus genome.
- *Cellular promoter*: possibly by translocation of the oncogene to a site on a chromosome with high activity.
- *Cofactor*, such as a chemical carcinogen.

Interaction with other genes

Oncogenes probably function as regulatory mechanisms in cells: their activation to produce tumours is probably the result of a loss of control of normal gene function, leading to disturbance of the usual regulatory activity.

Inheritance

By genetic or vertical transmission: the virus is inherited as a provirus (i.e. viral DNA transcript) integrated into the chromosomes of the germ cells of the parent animals. The viruses produced from these provirus genes are known as *endogenous* and are typical retroviruses: some are tumour-producing on inoculation into experimental animals, but many are not. Endogenous retrovirus genes are usually repressed, but can be induced or derepressed by various agents, with production of virus in the animal. Endogenous retroviruses have been demonstrated in normal cells of chickens, mice, cats and primates, and have also been identified in human chromosomes.

32 Papilloma and polyoma virus infections

Papillomaviruses and polyomaviruses belong to the family of *Papovaviruses*. Papillomaviruses are the cause of warts and are now recognized as the cause of cervical cancer.

Warts

Warts are amongst the commonest of virus infections and few people reach adult life without suffering from them. Knowledge of their virology has come from modern biotechnology, as papillomaviruses cannot be cultivated in vitro. Warts are benign tumours of the skin, with virus-induced proliferation of keratinized and non-keratinized squamous epithelial cells – i.e. affecting both skin and mucous membranes.

Clinical features

Below are the main clinical types of wart.

Common warts: found mostly on the hands and extremely common in young children.

Plantar warts: deep-seated painful lesions usually affecting the soles of the feet; tend to be seen in older children and adolescents.

Flat (or plane) warts: less common, mostly found on the face of children and especially on the chin and eyelids.

Butchers' warts: common on the hands of butchers, fishmongers and slaughtermen, owing to contamination of small cuts and abrasions.

Condylomata acuminata: sexually transmitted warts in the anogenital region: often small, clinically symptomless, and common in women, especially if young and sexually active; also found in men, affecting the penis and anus; sometimes large – occasionally very large (Fig. 32.1).

Laryngeal warts: rare in UK but relatively common in other countries – notably the southern USA; the juvenile form is acquired during birth from maternal condylomata acuminata.

Epidermodysplasia verruciformis: a rare autosomal recessive inherited disease in which affected patients develop multiple warts with a high risk (around one-third) of malignant change to squamous cell carcinoma, especially in areas of skin exposed to sunlight. Interestingly, the papillomaviruses responsible belong to several different and unusual types of virus.

Immunocompromised patients: especially those with renal allografts or suffering from AIDS commonly reactivate warts, both cutaneous and anogenital; occasionally these can become large and unmanageable and can undergo malignant change.

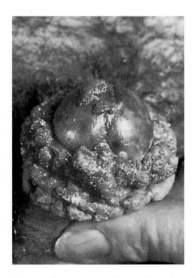

Fig. 32.1   Genital warts: large penile warts caused by papillomavirus. (Photograph courtesy of The Photography and Illustration Centre, Middlesex Hospital.)

Virus types

DNA technology: although papillomaviruses cannot be cultured, analysis and amplification of DNA extracted from infected cells, with tests for homology with other strains, has identified 80 types of virus. Table 32.1 lists the principal clinical types of wart and the papillomaviruses found in them.

Epidemiology

Transmission: by contact, e.g. hand to hand; via water in the surrounds of swimming pools in the case of plantar warts on the feet; sexual transmission in the case of genital warts, and via the infected mother's birth canal in the case of juvenile laryngeal papilloma.

The epidemiology of papillomaviruses is extremely complex: infection is often transient, the viruses can remain latent within tissues for long periods, and individuals can be infected with several different types: it is unclear, for example, how patients with the very rare disease epidermodysplasia verruciformis become infected with types 5 and 8 – types rarely seen in the general population.

Papillomaviruses and cancer

Papillomaviruses are now recognized as a cause – possibly in association with a cofactor – of cervical cancer (see below).

Table 32.1 Human warts and the main papillomaviruses with which they are associated

Wart*	Papillomavirus type
Hand	2, 1
Plantar	1, 4
Flat; juvenile	3, 10
Butchers' warts	7
Condylomata acuminata	6, 11
Laryngeal	6, 11
Carcinoma of cervix	16, 18
Carcinomas in epidermodysplasia verruciformis	5, 8 (and other types not found in other warts)

* *Note*: many other types of virus have been found, although less commonly, in most of these lesions.

Among animals (many, perhaps all, species of which have their own host-specific papillomaviruses) some papillomaviruses certainly cause cancer. In American cottontail rabbits the Shope papilloma, which is virus induced, becomes cancerous in 25% of cases; in domestic rabbits similar experimentally induced Shope papillomas undergo malignant change at a much higher rate. Among cattle, alimentary papillomas – due to bovine papillomavirus type 4 – become malignant when the animals are fed on bracken, which acts as a cofactor.

HUMAN CANCER

Cervical cancer: shows strong epidemiological risk factors, such as early age at first intercourse, multiple sexual partners and high parity, so that the incidence of the disease correlates with high sexual activity (it is virtually unknown in nuns); it therefore has many of the characteristics of a sexually transmitted infectious disease.

Papillomavirus DNA is almost always found in the tumour cells of cervical cancer, most often of types 16 and 18, less often of types 31 and 45 (as well as other less frequent types). In most (but not all) cervical cancers the sequences of the genome coding for virus early proteins E6 and E7 are integrated into the cell chromosome (in some tumours the virus DNA is episomal and not integrated). The types of virus most strongly associated with human cancer correlate with in vitro tests of oncogenicity.

Precancerous lesions: known as *cervical intraepithelial neoplasia (CIN)*, are seen in degrees of histological change to malignancy. Lesions with the highest risk of developing into invasive cancer contain DNA of types 16 or 18; low-risk CIN lesions contain types 6 or 11, the types responsible for benign condylomata acuminata.

Genital cancer in men: penile cancer is not common in the UK, but in countries where it is relatively common (such as Brazil) DNA of types 16 and 18 has been incriminated.

Skin cancer: apart from the warts associated with epidermodysplasia verruciformis, skin warts virtually never become malignant in immunocompetent people. Interestingly, warts are common in immunocompromised patients with renal transplants and, in them, malignant change to squamous cell carcinoma is associated with types 5 and 8 papillomaviruses.

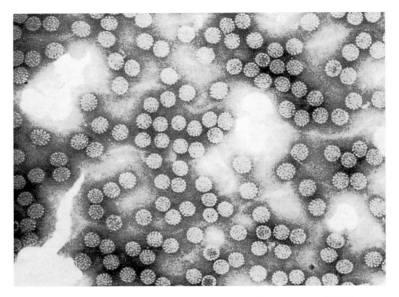

Fig. 32.2 Human papillomavirus. The virus particles have cubic symmetry. × 90 000. (Electronmicrograph courtesy of Dr E. A. C. Follett.)

Virology

Papovaviruses: double-stranded, circular DNA; icosahedral particles (Fig. 32.2): do not grow in cell cultures.

Diagnosis

Laboratory tests are not available for individual patients – the diagnosis is based on clinical examination.

POLYOMAVIRUSES

There are two human pathogenic polyomaviruses:

1. *JC virus*: a neurotropic virus – the cause of progressive multifocal leukoencephalopathy (see Chapter 28).
2. *BK virus*: of low pathogenicity; reactivates symptomlessly in the urinary tract of aproximately one-third of pregnant women; reactivation in the immunocompromised may be associated with haemorrhagic cystitis or ureteric obstruction.

Epidemiology

Both viruses infect humans in childhood and through adolescence, but clearly remain latent within tissues throughout life; both are *opportunistic* in that, in conditions of immunodeficiency, they may reactivate to cause severe neurological disease in the case of JC virus and less serious but unpleasant infections in the case of BK virus.

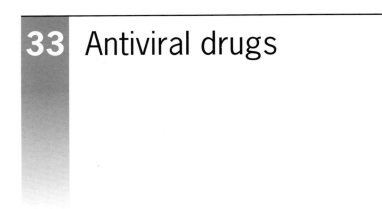

33 Antiviral drugs

A considerable number of drugs that are active against viruses are now available, but it must be admitted that they fall a long way behind antibacterials in their efficacy and in the scope of their application. The majority of antivirals are nucleoside analogues, but some important exceptions are not.

Table 33.1 shows the viruses (with the exception of HIV) for which effective antiviral therapy is available and the drugs with which they can be treated; the numerous antivirals for HIV are dealt with separately.

DRUGS ACTIVE AGAINST HERPESVIRUSES

Aciclovir

A breakthrough in antiviral therapy when introduced in 1982, because it is non-toxic to cells but strongly inhibits herpes simplex and (rather less strongly) varicella-zoster virus replication. Valaciclovir, famciclovir and penciclovir have similar chemical structure and antiviral activity.

Viruses inhibited:

1. Herpes simplex virus types 1 and 2
2. Varicella-zoster – but less sensitive than herpes simplex virus.

Action

Aciclovir – a nucleoside analogue – is activated upon phosphorylation by herpes-specific thymidine kinase and then inhibits virus

Table 33.1   Currently available antiviral drugs*

Virus	Drug	Indications
Herpes simplex types 1 and 2	Aciclovir, famciclovir valaciclovir	Genital, mucocutaneous herpes; encephalitis; prophylaxis in genital herpes; and the immunocompromised
Varicella-zoster	Aciclovir, famciclovir, valaciclovir	Zoster, severe varicella in neonates, the vulnerable and the immunocompromised
Cytomegalovirus	Ganciclovir	Prophylaxis and treatment of infection in the immunocompromised, especially with bone marrow transplants
	Cidofovir	Retinitis
	Foscarnet	Retinitis
Respiratory syncytial virus	Ribavirin	Infant bronchiolitis, pneumonia, infection in the immunocompromised
	Palivizumab[†]	Prophylaxis of vulnerable children
Hepatitis B	α-Interferon Lamivudine	Treatment of chronic hepatitis B
Hepatitis C	α-Interferon with ribavirin	Treatment of chronic hepatitis C
Lassa fever, hantavirus infection	Ribavirin	Treatment of acute disease

* There are numerous anti-HIV drugs currently available: a selection of the most widely used are described separately in the text.
† Palivizumab is not a drug but a monoclonal antibody.

DNA synthesis by competitive inhibition of the viral DNA polymerase with termination of the nascent DNA. Varicella-zoster virus DNA polymerase is also sensitive, but less so. Cellular DNA polymerase is resistant to the inhibition and, as the drug is inactive unless in phosphorylated form, it is inactive in uninfected cells and therefore virtually non-toxic.

Latent virus is not eradicated, so that reactivations are not prevented – although they can be suppressed by long-term prophylaxis.

Indications

Treatment

1. Herpes simplex infections: for example, genital herpes, cold sores, dendritic ulcer of the cornea, encephalitis (but survivors have sequelae often affecting the quality of life), and herpes simplex in the immunocompromised.

2. Varicella-zoster: severe varicella in leukaemic or other immunocompromised children and in neonates; zoster: especially in the immunocompromised. *Note*: aciclovir must be used in higher dosage for varicella-zoster than for herpes simplex.

Prophylaxis: to prevent recurrences and mucocutaneous reactivation of herpes simplex in the immunocompromised (e.g. organ transplant recipients, leukaemia patients etc.).

Administration: oral, intravenous (for severe infections); topical (as a cream).

Side-effects: basically a safe drug with minimal side-effects: occasionally renal impairment – usually transient, but use with care in patients with reduced renal function; minor – rashes, gastrointestinal disturbances.

Valaciclovir

A prodrug of aciclovir with an additional side chain to enhance gastrointestinal absorption. Host enzymes remove the side chain yielding the active drug, aciclovir. With better bioavailability the dosage is lower and less frequent than with aciclovir.

Indications: zoster and herpes simplex infections as above, but especially recommended for zoster, genital herpes and suppression of recurrences of mucocutaneous and genital herpes.

Administration: oral.

Famciclovir

Marketed for the treatment of zoster and genital herpes: the prodrug of penciclovir, an agent similar in action to aciclovir, which is also activated by viral thymidine kinase in infected cells and which has good inhibitory activity against varicella-zoster virus, but which is not an obligate chain terminator.

Indications: zoster and genital herpes, including suppression of recurrences.

Administration: oral.

Note: Penciclovir cream is available for topical application to mucocutaneous herpes simplex.

Ganciclovir

A nucleoside analogue structurally very similar to aciclovir and active against cytomegalovirus (CMV): becomes phosphorylated within cells by CMV phosphotransferase (for which it is a better substrate than aciclovir) and inhibits viral DNA synthesis, but is not an absolute chain terminator.

Indications: treatment of severe, life-threatening cytomegalovirus infections in the immunocompromised, e.g. pneumonia, retinitis; also prophylaxis, especially in bone marrow transplant patients. Contraindicated in pregnancy. Must not be given with zidovudine because of the increased risk of myelosuppression.

Administration: by slow intravenous infusion; orally for maintenance prophylaxis in solid organ (but not bone marrow) transplant recipients.

Side-effects: bone marrow suppression with neutropenia is common, so that blood counts must be monitored during treatment; also fever, rash, impaired renal function and abnormal liver function tests; occasionally, encephalopathy.

Foscarnet

A pyrophosphate analogue which complexes with viral DNA polymerase, so blocking chain extension and inhibiting virus replication; active against CMV, but toxic especially with regard to renal function.

Indications: CMV retinitis in AIDS patients: aciclovir-resistant herpes simplex and varicella-zoster infections; contraindicated in pregnancy.

Administration: by slow intravenous infusion.

Side-effects: renal toxicity, including acute renal failure; nausea, vomiting, malaise, hypocalcaemia, convulsions.

Cidofovir

Inhibits DNA polymerase: use in CMV retinitis where ganciclovir and foscarnet cannot be given.

Administration: by slow intravenous infusion with probenecid to prevent nephrotoxicity.

Side effects: nephrotoxicity, iritis and uveitis, neutropenia.

DRUGS ACTIVE AGAINST HIV

HAART

In recent years there has been a dramatic advance in the treatment of HIV owing to the introduction of effective antiviral drugs used in combination so as to minimize the risk of emergence of drug-resistant mutants. These regimens are known by the acronym HAART, or 'highly active antiretroviral therapy'. The aim is long-term inhibition of viral replication (no virus detected in plasma), and although the infection is not cured, in that latent virus is not eliminated, damage to the immune system is reversed and the mortality rate significantly reduced, enabling long-term survival with a reasonable quality of life.

Patients on HAART should be monitored regularly for clinical progression of HIV disease – i.e. decreasing CD4 counts and increasing virus load (number of RNA copies per mL) in plasma: checks for the emergence of resistant virus should also be carried out.

At least *three drugs* are used in combination: two nucleoside reverse transcriptase inhibitors together with either a protease inhibitor or a non-nucleoside transcriptase inhibitor (see below).

Compliance: a major problem – the side-effects of these drugs are often severe: added to this is the problem that the daily schedule of dosage is extremely taxing, with many pills and often inconvenient accompanying requirements. As a result, compliance is a major problem with HAART. All the anti-HIV drugs are administered orally.

New anti-HIV drugs are continually being developed and the exact details of HAART are frequently updated. The actual drugs prescribed will depend on the stage of the disease, the individual patient's tolerance, how effectively the viral load is reduced, and the appearance of resistance in the infecting virus (resistance to one of the nucleoside analogues increases the chance of resistance to others in the same group, and the same is true for non-nucleoside reverse transcriptase and protease inhibitors).

There are three kinds of anti-HIV drug:

1. *Nucleoside inhibitors of the virus reverse transcriptase (RT)*
2. *Non-nucleoside inhibitors of the virus RT*
3. *Inhibitors of the virus protease* (the enzyme responsible for cleavage of the viral *gag* primary translation product).

Note that there are numerous drugs available within these categories: below are examples of some currently most widely used.

Nucleoside reverse transcriptase inhibitors (NRTI)

For example: • Zidovudine • Lamivudine.

Action: these nucleoside analogues act like aciclovir (except that phosphorylation is carried out by host cell enzymes) and inhibit reverse transcriptase during DNA synthesis with chain termination and so block the production of the DNA provirus.

Non-nucleoside reverse transcriptase inhibitors (NNRTI)

For example: • Nevirapine.

Action: bind to RT near the polymerase active site, which becomes distorted with consequent inhibition of enzyme activity. They have high antiviral effect but with relatively low toxicity. Note that their action is very specific, so that they inhibit the reverse transcriptase of HIV-1 but not that of HIV-2.

Protease inhibitors

For example: • Saquinavir.

Action: peptidomimetic analogues that fit into the site of viral protease – an enzyme that cleaves the precursor protein to yield the core proteins – to block viral assembly by competitive inhibition.

SIDE-EFFECTS

The principal side effects of HAART are listed in Table 33.2.

Table 33.2 Anti-HIV drugs and their toxicity. (Reproduced and modified with permission from Weller I V D and Williams A G 2001 *British Medical Journal, 322*, 1410–1412)

Drug	Toxicity
Nucleoside RT* inhibitors	
Associated with class of drug	Lactic acidosis, hepatic steatosis, lipodystrophy (peripheral fat wasting)
Specific to drug	
Zidovudine	Bone marrow suppression, nausea, vomiting, myopathy
Lamivudine	Few side-effects
Non-nucleoside RT inhibitors	
Nevirapine	Rash, hepatitis, Stevens–Johnson syndrome
Protease inhibitors	
Associated with class of drug	Lipodystrophy (fat wasting or accumulation), hyperlipidaemia, diabetes mellitus
Specific to drug	
Saquinavir	Few side effects

* *RT* = reverse transcriptase.

DRUGS ACTIVE AGAINST OTHER VIRUSES

Ribavirin (tribavirin)

A guanosine analogue active against a wide range of RNA and DNA viruses in vitro, although difficulties in administration and toxicity limit its usefulness.

Action: after phosphorylation, interferes with early transcription and eventually ribonucleoprotein synthesis.

Indications: severe respiratory syncytial virus infection in infants, such as bronchiolitis or bronchopneumonia; also some of the severe haemorrhagic fevers such as Lassa and hantavirus infections. With α-interferon for treatment of chronic hepatitis C (see below).

Administration: for respiratory syncytial virus: by aerosol within a hood (which limits its usefulness); for hepatitis C, oral. Administer intravenously for treatment of Lassa and hantavirus infections.

Side-effects: respiratory depression with aerosol administration; anaemia and reticulocytosis with oral therapy.

Zanamivir

Active against both influenza A and B.

Action: analogue of the sialic (neuraminic) acid which binds to the active site of the viral neuraminidase: it blocks the cleavage by the neuraminidase of sialic acid from the infected cell surface leading to inhibition of the release of new viral particles.

Indications: treatment of influenza in adults at risk during an outbreak of influenza: must be administered within 48 h of onset.

Administration: by inhalation of powder (not a pleasant way to take medication).

Side-effects: gastrointestinal; rarely, bronchospasm.

Amantadine

Active against influenza A but not influenza B. Effective for prophylaxis – and also for treatment if given early in infection; it has never been widely used, but might be useful in an influenza A pandemic if vaccine were not available.

Action: blocks M2 protein ion transport channel: main effect is to inhibit uncoating of the virus in endosomes.

Indications: prevention and treatment of influenza A.

Administration: oral.

Side-effects: dopaminergic, especially in the elderly, in whom lower doses should be used: insomnia, nervousness, dizziness.

Interferon

Interferon-α (see Chapter 20), prepared by recombinant technology or from stimulation of leukocyte cultures, has some limited use against viruses.

Action: blocks virus RNA transcription and protein synthesis.

Indications: *chronic hepatitis B* with active disease and viral replication: not all patients respond and relapse is common: only a minority clear the virus. Monitor response by markers and hepatitis B DNA viral load. Probably best used in combination with oral lamivudine (see above), but the optimal long-term schedules for this are not yet established.

Acute hepatitis C: interferon can be effective in resolving infection and preventing carriage.

Chronic hepatitis C: use in combination with oral ribavirin: not all patients respond, and in those that do, relapse is common. Infections with genotypes 2 and 3 respond better than with genotypes 1 and 4; virus load should be monitored regularly.

Administration: subcutaneously.

Side-effects: nausea, flu-like symptoms, tiredness, depression; sometimes, bone marrow depression.

Peginterferon-α

A recently available preparation conjugated with polyethylene glycol that prolongs the persistence of interferon in the blood. Administer subcutaneously.

Palivizumab

This monoclonal antibody prepared against respiratory syncytial virus can be used to protect vulnerable infants and young children with chronic lung disease: administer intramuscularly.

SPECIAL INFECTION PROBLEMS

34 Sterilization and disinfection

Doctors must know how to render articles safe from the risk of transmitting infection. This does not always require *sterility*, which means the complete destruction of all organisms, including spores. The degree of microbial inactivation that is necessary to prevent infection depends on individual circumstances, particularly the susceptibility of the tissues with which an instrument makes contact and the immune status of a patient.

Sterilization is a process that kills ALL microbial life.

Disinfection is a process that renders items safe with respect to infection transmission without necessarily making them sterile. In general, it is a process that destroys all microbial life except bacterial spores.

The term *decontamination* covers both sterilization and disinfection.

The choice between sterilization and disinfection should be guided by assessing the risk that a particular item poses to a patient:

High risk: items that make contact with body tissues that are normally sterile pose a high risk and should be sterilized. Once the skin has been breached any microbe, including low-pathogenicity bacterial spores, can cause an infection. Examples: syringes and needles, scalpels and other surgical instruments.

Medium risk: items that make contact with intact mucous membrane pose a medium risk and should be disinfected, although they can be sterilized. Intact mucous membranes will resist bacterial spores but can be infected with some bacteria and viruses (mostly via contamination by use on other patients). Examples: respiratory equipment, gastroscopes.

Low risk: items that make contact with intact skin pose a low risk to patients and should be clean, though disinfection may be appropriate in situations of high vulnerability. Examples: stethoscopes and washing bowls.

STERILIZATION

Sterilization – the absolute destruction of microbial life – requires the killing of bacterial spores and need rigorous, specialized conditions. To be of practical use, processes used for sterilization must have a very high quality assurance of the process working effectively on every occasion. Viruses, fungi, protozoa and bacteria in the vegetative – or non-sporing – state are readily killed by comparatively mild heat treatment, e.g. 80°C for a few seconds. Methods of sterilization are shown in Table 34.1.

Spores are survival mechanisms possessed by members of the bacterial genera *Bacillus* and *Clostridium*. They are resistant to heat and disinfectants and need very rigorous conditions to destroy them. (Fungal spores are for dispersal, rather than survival, and are less resistant to heat and disinfectants.)

Table 34.1 Methods of sterilization

Method	Use	Advantages	Disadvantages
Steam under pressure, e.g. 134°C for 3 min	Surgical dressings; instruments; almost any article or fluid which is not heat sensitive	Cheap, easily monitored	Damages non-heat resistant items
Dry heat at 160°C for 2 h	Glassware; powders; ointments	Cheap, easily monitored	Damages non-heat resistant items
Ethylene oxide gas	Plastics, electronic instruments	Sterilizes at room temperature	The gas is toxic, flammable and explosive in air Difficult to monitor
Gamma irradiation	Plastic goods; orthopaedic prostheses	Easy to monitor, sterilizes at room temperature	Very hazardous, expensive to set up and maintain
Filtration through cellulose membranes	Heat-sensitive fluids	Can be used at room temperature	Will not remove viruses

Autoclaves

Steam has energy stored within it as latent heat (boiling water takes in energy to turn water at 100°C to steam at 100°C). Similarly, when steam condenses it transfers this energy to the surface it condenses on. Bacterial spores are killed very slowly at 100°C, but more rapidly at higher temperatures; steam at over 100°C can only be produced under pressure. Such a pressure vessel used for sterilization is called an *autoclave*. Figure 34.1 shows the most simple of the large autoclaves, a *downward displacement autoclave*, where the steam displaces air which flows downwards and out through a valve in the chamber floor.

Steam needs to condense on a surface to transfer its latent heat. Wrapped items, such as theatre instruments, will trap air within them and prevent steam reaching and condensing on the instrument. There are autoclaves that get round this problem by drawing a vacuum in their sterilization chamber to remove all air before replacing it with steam. These are called *porous load autoclaves*.

There are also small, self-contained autoclaves that can be powered from standard electrical supplies. These are known as *table-top autoclaves*. Both downward displacement and porous load versions exist.

Cleaning, inspection, packing and sterilization of medical instruments for hospitals, and increasingly for clinics and general practice, takes place in specialized *Central Sterile Supply*

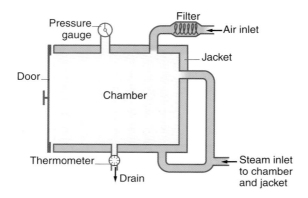

Fig. 34.1   Diagram of an autoclave (simplified).

Departments (CSSDs). These specialized units can be either within hospitals or on remote sites.

Other sterilization methods

The following are used:

- *Dry heat*: for items that cannot withstand exposure to steam, or by microbiology laboratories for glassware
- *Ethylene oxide gas; ionizing radiation*: largely by commercial suppliers, for plastic goods
- *Filtration*: by pharmaceutical firms, for the sterilization of drugs for injection.

Sterile single-use articles

Syringes, catheters, tubing, infusion bags etc. are supplied as presterilized single-use (i.e. disposable) articles. They can be used once and destroyed. They must not be reprocessed and reused.

The agents of spongiform encephalopathies ('prions')

The agents associated with spongiform encephalopathies, 'prions', are highly resistant to inactivation. Six sequential autoclave 'sterilization' cycles will reduce, but not eliminate, infectivity. Control by physical removal by scrupulous cleaning before autoclaving instruments used on known or suspected infected patients or preferably, use disposable instruments.

DISINFECTION

There are two main ways of achieving disinfection: heat and chemical disinfectants.

Heat disinfection is one of the most reliable, long-lasting infection control procedures. Pasteurization, introduced by Louis Pasteur, is a form of heat disinfection. Milk can be pasteurized by heating it to 74°C for 15 seconds and is far from sterile, but it is safe because any human pathogens of bovine origin that it might have contained have been killed. In hospitals, heat disinfection is used in specialized washer–disinfectors that treat tubing and masks used in anaesthesia, or in bedpan washer–disinfectors.

Chemical disinfectants (usually just referred to as disinfectants) will kill most microorganisms, but not necessarily spores. Some will also kill bacterial spores, but they do this slowly and without the high quality assurance needed to assure sterility. Chemical disinfectants are often unpredictable in real-life use (even if they can be shown to work perfectly in carefully controlled laboratory tests) and are inhibited by the presence of organic matter (blood, faeces etc.).

Table 34.2 lists the most common disinfection procedures used in hospitals today.

Hands and skin

The hands of hospital staff are thought to be one of the main vehicles for infection transmission between patients. Contamination picked up on the hands of medical staff by touch (*transient microflora*) is an efficient means of transferring infection from one patient to another. However, such contamination is superficially located on skin and easily removed by washing with soap amd water, or killed by the use of an alcohol handrub. The only situation in which bacteria normally present on staff hands (*resident microflora*) need to be removed or killed, is that of a surgeon's hands. This limits the contamination deposited in a surgical wound in case of glove puncture. Surgical scrubs, usually either chlorhexidine or povidone-iodine based, are used to remove the

Table 34.2 Hospital disinfection procedures

Disinfection purpose	Disinfection procedure
Skin	
Hands – ward staff	Soap and water
	Alcohol rub
Hands – surgeons	Surgical scrubs with chlorhexidine
	or povidone-iodine
Patient skin at operation	Alcoholic chlorhexidine
	Alcoholic povidone-iodine
Environment	
Spills of blood, body fluids	Hypochlorite
Instruments	
Endoscopes	Glutaraldehyde
Thermometers	Single-use sheath
	70% alcohol or non-contact thermometers
Bedpans	Heat disinfection or single use

transient microflora and kill the resident microflora and inhibit their regrowth. Patients' operation sites are disinfected with alcoholic chlorhexidine or povidone-iodine. The alcohol produces a high initial reduction in bacteria and evaporates to leave a good layer of the bactericide behind, to exert continued suppression of overgrowth of the resident microflora in the greenhouse conditions under the dressing.

Treatment of water

The natural habitat of some saprophytic bacteria (e.g. legionellae) is water, and many soil bacteria gain access to water during heavy rain. In addition, microorganisms of faecal origin from the human and animal intestine may find their way into water supplies and cause outbreaks of waterborne infection, causing diseases such as enteric fever, dysentery, cholera, hepatitis A and gastroenteritis.

Before entering the piped supply, reservoir or drinking water is treated by:

• *Filtration* through sand supported on gravel and clinker
• *Chlorination.*

The filtration removes all organic matter and allows very low concentrations of chlorine to disinfect the water.

35 Healthcare-associated infection

Previously called 'hospital infection', this is probably as great a problem today as it was in the pre-antibiotic era: around 10% of hospital patients suffer from infection acquired in hospital, resulting in substantial morbidity, sometimes mortality, and prolongation of hospital stay and consequent increased healthcare costs. Nowadays, with shorter stays in hospitals and more day care, much of the infection acquired in hospitals is seen at home after discharge.

Infection within hospitals is a particular problem because of the interaction between *seed* and *soil* – in this instance the aggression of the organisms compounded by the vulnerability of the patients.

The seed

Antibiotic resistance: the resident flora of hospitals is now heavily contaminated by pathogens resistant to many antibiotics, especially strains of coliforms, *S. aureus* and enterococci. Hospitals worldwide are experiencing outbreaks of infection due to MRSA (i.e. strains of *S. aureus* multiresistant to many antibiotics, including flucloxacillin) and to enterococci resistant to vancomycin (VRE). The heavy and often overuse of antibiotics in hospitals has caused the creation of an environment that selects these organisms. Multiresistant coliforms are a particular problem in intensive care units; MRSA are encountered everywhere; VRE particularly infect immunocompromised patients.

In susceptible patients: organisms normally considered to be virtually non-pathogenic can cause serious infection: often this presents in a clinically atypical form.

The soil

Patients in hospital are particularly vulnerable to infection because:

1. *Pre-existing illness* makes them less able to withstand infection: leukaemic patients with diminished cell-mediated immunity can develop severe and life-threatening virus infections such as varicella-zoster; even diseases less serious than leukaemia can render the patient more susceptible to a variety of bacterial, viral and fungal diseases.
2. *Treatment* such as immunosuppression, radio- or chemotherapy lowers resistance to infection.
3. *Surgery* necessarily involves a skin wound, thereby breaching one of the major barriers to invasion by organisms: infection risk is increased when contaminated organs such as the lower bowel are opened.
4. *Implants* of prostheses such as artificial hips or heart valves, intubation, indwelling catheters or long lines strongly predispose to bacterial infection: even if not left in situ, urinary catheterization is an infection hazard.
5. *Age*: neonates and the elderly are especially liable to severe effects of infection, both bacterial and viral, possibly because of immature or dysfunctional immune systems.

INFECTION ASSOCIATED WITH HEALTHCARE

Sometimes called *nosocomial* infections. Those most commonly encountered are shown in Table 35.1.

Sporadic (endemic) infections are daily occurrences in hospitals: only of concern if they threaten the recovery of an individual patient.

Outbreaks of cross-infection are relatively common – defined as two or more related cases of the same infection *or* when the observed number of infections exceeds the number expected.

Classic contagious diseases (e.g. varicella, rotavirus gastroenteritis, enterovirus infection in neonates) can cause outbreaks in children's wards and can be life-threatening, especially varicella in leukaemic children. Influenza and gastroenteritis can cause outbreaks in geriatric institutions, sometimes with considerable mortality. Epidemics of respiratory syncytial virus infection recur every year, and a sick child who requires inpatient treatment is often the source of a hospital outbreak.

Table 35.1 The most frequently encountered healthcare-associated infections and the organisms that cause them

Infection		Commonest causes
Urinary tract		Coliforms
Wound infection		*S. aureus*, *S. pyogenes*
Respiratory	upper	RSV, parainfluenza, rhinoviruses
	lower	Pneumococci, coliforms, influenza
Gastrointestinal	bacterial	*C. difficile*, rarely, salmonella, *C. perfringens*
	viral	Norwalk-viruses, rotavirus
Septicaemia		*S. aureus*, coliforms, coagulase-negative staphylococci
Childhood fever		Varicella
Bloodborne virus infection		Hepatitis B and C, CMV, parvovirus B19, HIV

SOURCES

Infection may be either:

• *Endogenous*: from the patient's own normal flora
• *Exogenous*: from other people, inanimate objects (fomites) or the environment.

Endogenous infection

1. *Urinary infection*: coliforms from the bowel flora colonize the urethra: catheterization introduces these organisms into the bladder and the urinary tract.
2. *Chest infection*: aspiration into the lungs of the patient's upper respiratory flora often follows tracheal or nasogastric intubation.
3. *Wound infection*: often due to patient's skin flora – especially high risk after colonic surgery owing to contamination with extensive large bowel flora: *S. aureus* infections (flucloxacillin-sensitive) are often acquired from the patient's own endogenous nasal flora.

Exogenous infection

Hospitals harbour numerous and varied sources from which organisms can be transmitted to patients:

1. *People*: the most important source – patients, especially if they have a discharging wound or other source of disseminating organisms; also staff, who may themselves have an infection or who can transfer organisms during nursing care or invasive surgical procedures e.g. MRSA.

2. *The hospital environment* contains its own resident but continuously changing flora of bacteria, found on floors, in blankets, lockers, baths and washbasins, commodes, bedpans, urinals and toilets, food and water, dust, air-conditioning systems.

3. *Some hospital equipment* is especially likely to be a source of infection, particularly of Gram-negative bacilli of normally low pathogenicity:
   - *Ventilators and humidifiers*: difficult to disinfect between patients; now should be either disposable or autoclavable.
   - *Endoscopes*: cannot be heat-sterilized and notoriously difficult to disinfect; risk of transmitting *M. tuberculosis*.
   - *Parenteral solutions*: though usually sterile on preparation can become contaminated after opening, and if used on more than one patient.

4. *Water*: supplied through taps or shower heads and that used to cool air-conditioning systems can become contaminated with legionella.

5. *Air*: construction work near transplant units can cause outbreaks of aspergillosis when the fungi are dispersed from building materials.

6. *Operating theatres*: bacteria that can cause wound infection – or viruses such as hepatitis B – can access the operation area through surgical invasive procedures. Orthopaedic operations where prevention of infection is crucial are often carried out under a system of 'laminar flow' in which filtered air is directed over the operation area.

ROUTES

Contact

Direct: from hands of healthcare workers during patient care such as wound dressing, thereby unwittingly causing cross-infection between patients.

Indirect: via inanimate objects, e.g. theatre equipment, or products such as parenteral fluids.

Airborne

Via aerosols from respiratory and other secretions and excreta; also from inhalation of contaminated dust and air from ventilation equipment.

Ingestion

Faecal–oral or via contaminated food (*C. perfringens*, Norwalk-like viruses): *C. difficile* can contaminate the hospital environment and become part of a patient's intestinal flora, often as a result of antibiotic therapy.

Infection in hospital staff

It must not be forgotten that staff as well as patients can be (and often are) infected during the course of their work. Bloodborne viruses such as hepatitis B and C (and very rarely HIV) can be acquired through sharps injuries (a common accident) and other infections through the various procedures involved in patient care. All hospital staff nowadays must be immunized against hepatitis B (in addition to the other routine immunizations).

CONTROL

Infection associated with healthcare can never be entirely prevented, but with scrupulous attention to infection control procedures can be minimized.

Procedures for infection control

Standard Infection Control Procedures: is a policy universally applied to all patients irrespective of disease status. All healthcare workers must be trained in and must implement policies for the prevention of infection, such as:

- *Hand hygiene*: the single **most important** measure for preventing cross-infection. All staff must be taught to wash or disinfect hands effectively.
- *Careful nursing technique in the ward*: to minimize dissemination of organisms from wounds, endotracheal tubes etc., and to prevent spread of infection from one patient to the next.

- *Strict asepsis in theatre*, with good surgical technique to minimize tissue destruction, avoidance of haematoma; equipment, instruments and dressings must be sterilized (or, as a minimum when heat-sensitive, disinfected): as many as possible of these should be for single patient use.
- *Blood for transfusion*: must be screened for bloodborne viruses.
- *Isolation*: single-bedded rooms (cubicles) available to accommodate infected patients who may be a source of infection to others, with negative-pressure ventilation to prevent airborne infection escaping into the ward; anyone coming into contact with the patient must wear plastic aprons, masks and gloves; these precautions constitute '*source isolation nursing*'. Conversely, immunocompromised patients often require protection from outside, and their isolation rooms should have positive-pressure ventilation using filtered air and strict precautions to avoid introducing infection during healthcare procedures: this is known as '*protective isolation nursing*'.
- *Staff*: exclude staff suffering from infections such as septic lesions, viral respiratory infections, as well as more serious infections such as varicella, from contact with patients. Staff who are hepatitis B positive may continue to work in certain circumstances, but must not take part in invasive procedures.
- *Cleaning*: of hospital wards and theatres – and equipment – is essential to reduce infection risk: policies must be in place to ensure the provision of sterile instruments and proper use of disinfectants.
- *Waste disposal*: there must be a system for the safe disposal of clinical waste, with appropriate accountability.

Antibiotic policies

Every hospital requires antibiotic policies which lay down instructions and guidance for the prescribing of antibiotics. This includes a rational policy for preoperative prophylaxis to reduce postoperative infection, as well as instructions for prescribing for individual infected patients. Such policies have the dual benefit of helping to reduce the emergence of multiply antibiotic-resistant organisms as well as controlling expenditure on the pharmaceutical budget.

Organization of infection control

Hospitals require management structures to enable infection to be monitored, with systems in place to act rapidly and appropriately to detect and control outbreaks. These structures are:

1. *Infection Control Committee*: with representatives from nurses, microbiologists, pharmacist, occupational health, management, clinicians, catering, engineering staff, public health and sterile services department.
2. *Infection Control Team*: the Infection Control Nurse, Infection Control Officer (usually the hospital medical microbiologist): the team's duties include:
   • Day-to-day monitoring of infection
   • Preparing and implementation of policies
   • Audit
   • Liaison with clinicians and public health departments
   • Surveillance
   • Outbreak management
   • Training and education.

Surveillance

Defined as 'the systematic, active, ongoing observation of the occurrence and distribution of disease in a population and response to the information collected': this requires close collaboration between the microbiology laboratory and the Infection Control Nurse and, in turn, feedback to colleagues in the wards and theatres can lead to reduction in infection rates.

Table 35.2 'Alert organisms'

Bacteria	Viruses
MRSA and glycopeptide-resistant *S. aureus*	RSV, parainfluenza, influenza
S. pyogenes	Rotavirus, Norwalk-like viruses
C. difficile	Varicella-zoster virus
Vancomycin-resistant enterococci	Hepatitis B
Multiresistant coliforms	Hepatitis C
Verocytotoxin-producing *E. coli*	HIV
Legionella	
M. tuberculosis	
Penicillin-resistant pneumococci	

Note: the fungus *Aspergillus* can be a major problem in specialist wards with immunocompromised patients, such as bone marrow transplant units.

Table 35.3 'Alert conditions'

Pyrexia of unknown origin

Tuberculosis

Food poisoning or dysentery

Legionellosis

Severe soft tissue infection

Varicella or zoster

Hepatitis B and C

Surveillance methods include:

1. *Continuous monitoring* of 'alert organisms' and 'alert conditions' – see Tables 35.2 and 35.3.
2. *Laboratory-based ward surveillance*, with follow-up of positive microbiological reports in relation to the patient's condition and case records.
3. *Targeted or selective surveillance* to monitor infection trends in certain defined types of patient.

Outbreaks

When an outbreak is detected, an Outbreak Control Group must be set up to include, among appropriate representation from clinicians and other staff, the members of the Infection Control Team. If the outbreak is *major*, then the local Consultant in Communicable Disease Control must be informed. Every hospital must have an Outbreak Control Plan.

36 Pyrexia of unknown origin

Fever results when the release of endogenous pyrogens (e.g. interleukin-1, tumour necrosis factor) raises the setting of the thermoregulatory centre in the hypothalamus. This is usually due to an inflammatory cause, most often infection.

Febrile episodes of short duration are almost always due to infection and are usually easy to diagnose.

Pyrexia of unknown origin (universally known as PUO) is of longer duration and can be extremely difficult to diagnose.

PUO is defined as being:

• Significant (a temperature over 38°C)
• Persistent (lasting at least 1 week – usually longer, often 3 weeks)
• Without a readily identifiable cause.

The main types of disease that can cause PUO are shown in Table 36.1. Note that this list and the others that follow indicate some of the most common causes of PUO: there are many others.

INFECTION

The most important cause of PUO: with a stringent definition, infection accounts for around 40% of cases; with less rigid criteria (i.e. lower-grade fever of shorter duration) it causes at least 70% of cases.

Bacterial infections

Bacteria probably cause PUO more often than other organisms, and the bacteria particularly associated with this are listed in Table 36.2.

Table 36.1 Causes of pyrexia of unknown origin

Cause		Percentage of cases
Infections		40
Neoplasms	Especially lymphoma and leukaemia, but also other forms of cancer, e.g. renal carcinoma, hepatoma, disseminated malignancy	20
Connective tissue diseases	Systemic lupus erythematosus, vasculitis, e.g. polyarteritis nodosa, giant cell arteritis etc.	20
Others	Granulomatous diseases – Crohn's disease, sarcoidosis Drug-induced fevers Malingering ('factitious fever')	20

Table 36.2 Bacterial diseases commonly presenting as pyrexia of unknown origin

Cause	Disease – special features
Systemic infections	
Infective endocarditis	Infection of heart valves
Tuberculosis	Pulmonary, non-pulmonary (e.g. bone, renal) or cryptic miliary
Q fever	Occupational exposure to cattle, sheep
Psittacosis	Acquired from budgerigars, parrots
Enteric fever	Usually acquired abroad
Brucellosis	Usually acquired abroad
Leptospirosis	Exposure to rat-infested water
Localized sepsis	
Hepatobiliary sepsis	Cholecystitis, cholangitis, liver abscess
Intra-abdominal abscess ⎫	Usually follow intestinal or gynaecological
Subphrenic abscess ⎬	sepsis; sometimes postoperative
Pelvic abscess ⎭	
Renal infections	Chronic pyelonephritis; perinephric abscess
Mycoplasma pneumoniae	Atypical pneumonia, community acquired
Sinusitis	
Dental infection	Apical dental abscess
Bone sepsis	Osteomyelitis

Table 36.2 shows that bacteria that cause PUO are many and varied. Some are relatively common – such as tuberculosis, renal infection, dental and other abscesses and even bacterial infective endocarditis. Others are rare in the UK – such as enteric fever

and brucellosis. It is important to be aware of the rarer causes, especially those not found naturally in the UK.

Viruses and other infectious causes of PUO

The viruses, fungi and parasites often found in PUO are listed in Table 36.3.

Many of these are imported diseases: foreign travel is much more frequent now than in former years, and the UK has a large immigrant population who may have acquired infection abroad. Apart from the common viral causes of PUO – such as infectious mononucleosis – the prevalence of HIV is increasing, and the possibility of this infection should always be borne in mind.

Non-infectious causes

Fever is quite often a feature of non-infectious diseases. Some forms of malignant disease are well known to be accompanied by fever, although the classic Pel–Ebstein fever (in which episodes of

Table 36.3 Viral, fungal and protozoal diseases which can present as pyrexia of unknown origin

Cause	Disease
Viruses	
EB virus	Infectious mononucleosis
Cytomegalovirus	Infectious mononucleosis-like syndrome
HIV	AIDS-associated infections
Hepatitis viruses	Especially hepatitis A and B
Lassa, Ebola, Marburg viruses	Severe, haemorrhagic fevers
Dengue	Dengue
Fungi	
Candida spp.	Disseminated candidiasis
Histoplasma capsulatum	Histoplasmosis
Coccidioides immitis	Coccidioidomycosis
Micropolysporum faeni	Farmer's lung – hypersensitivity to contaminated hay
Protozoa	
Plasmodium spp.	Malaria
Toxoplasma gondii	Toxoplasmosis
Leishmania spp.	Visceral leishmaniasis (kala-azar)
Entamoeba histolyticum	Amoebic dysentery and abscess
Trypanosoma spp.	Trypanosomiasis (sleeping sickness)

fever alternate with long periods of 2–4 weeks of normal or low temperature), which is particularly associated with Hodgkin's lymphoma and renal carcinoma, is rare. It is not always appreciated that drug reactions due to hypersensitivity – especially to antimicrobials – also cause fever, as does allergy to the fungus in mouldy hay (farmer's lung). The possibility of connective tissue or granulomatous disorders must also be kept in mind.

INVESTIGATION

Often time-consuming; the main examinations to be undertaken are listed below, with emphasis placed on those that help to establish an infective cause.

History

Patient's previous illnesses, including recent surgery; family illnesses (e.g. tuberculosis); illness in work colleagues or other contacts; foreign travel; contact with pets or farm animals; occupation; currently prescribed drugs; any abuse of drugs.

Physical examination

Especially to detect lymphadenopathy, enlargement of liver or spleen, or areas of tenderness.

Laboratory tests

Microbiology

- *Blood culture*: serial cultures should be taken: isolation of viridans streptococci points to infective endocarditis; isolation of coliforms, enterococci, *Streptococcus milleri* or 'bacteroides' suggests intra-abdominal sepsis.
- *Urine microscopy and culture*: serial specimens may be necessary to detect intermittent bacteriuria in chronic pyelonephritis; microscopic haematuria is often present in infective endocarditis and hypernephroma.
- *Stool culture and microscopy*: especially if there is a history of diarrhoea: microscopy to include examination for protozoa: several specimens should be examined.
- *Serology*: 'screens' for viruses – e.g. EB virus, HIV (remember the patient's permission is necessary for this); bacteria – e.g. enteric

fever; *Mycoplasma pneumoniae* and other causes of atypical pneumonia, leptospirosis, together with others from the lists of infections above. *Note*: A single raised titre must be interpreted with caution, as many people have had previous exposure to some of these organisms; PUO should not be attributed to a rare cause unless there is other supporting evidence.

Haematology

Full blood count, differential white cell count (eosinophilia suggests parasitic infection); blood film to include examination for malaria parasites; erythrocyte sedimentation rate – a very high result (e.g. >100 mm/h) suggests tuberculosis, a connective tissue disease or malignancy; C-reactive protein, an acute-phase protein of which the level is raised in inflammation.

Biochemistry

Liver function tests.

Radiological examination

Straight radiographs of chest, abdomen, sinuses and teeth.

Further investigations

These should be planned at this stage if the diagnosis has not been made. The order in which they are carried out depends on the most likely cause of the PUO. Examples are listed below:

- *Serological tests* for connective tissue diseases, e.g. antinuclear factor, rheumatoid factor, other autoantibody tests; immunoglobulin studies for myeloma.
- *Specialized radiology*: to identify the site of disease, e.g. echocardiogram cholecystogram, excretion urogram, barium studies (in inflammatory bowel disease), isotope scans with technetium, gallium, ultrasound and CT scans, MRI.
- *Endoscopy*: bronchoscopy, laparoscopy, colonoscopy.
- *Biopsy*: of lymph nodes, bone marrow, muscle, liver, kidney, and of any lesion localized by other investigations.
- *Laparotomy*: a last resort if there is evidence of intra-abdominal pathology.

PROGNOSIS

At the end of the investigations, a proportion of patients – reported as varying from 5% to 25% – remain undiagnosed. Some will recover spontaneously, but not all.

37 Infection in the immunocompromised

Modern medicine has resulted in many more patients with increased susceptibility to infection whose immune system is defective because of disease, therapy or age. These patients present special problems to both clinicians and microbiologists.

The microorganisms responsible include recognized pathogens, but also some considered non-pathogenic in the normal host.

IMMUNOCOMPROMISED PATIENTS

Table 37.1 lists the main types of immune deficiency, together with their cause and the principal kinds of infection to which they render patients susceptible. It is important to be aware that deficiency in one part of the immune response is usually accompanied by some degree of depression in others.

Patients with neutropenia and defective antibody response are particularly vulnerable to bacterial infections, whereas depression of cell-mediated immunity is associated with suseptibility to viruses.

The immune response may be compromised by:

- Disease
- Therapy
- Age
- Congenital deficiency.

Table 37.1 Simplified guide to immune deficiencies and the organisms to which they are susceptible

Immune deficiency	Cause	Main infecting organisms
Antibody	Congenital hypogammaglobulinaemia, multiple myeloma, non-Hodgkin's lymphoma	Pneumococci, non-capsulated *H. influenzae*
Cell-mediated	AIDS, leukaemia, chemotherapy for leukaemia and bone marrow and solid organ transplants, Hodgkin's disease	Herpesviruses, respiratory viruses[†], *M. tuberculosis*, *M. avium* complex, PCP*, toxoplasma
Neutropenia	Leukaemia, chemotherapy for leukaemia, organ transplants	*Pseudomonas, Acinetobacter*, enterobacteria[#], *S. aureus*, coagulase-negative staphylococci, 'viridans' streptococci, enterococci, candida, aspergillus
Spleen	Splenectomy (for trauma, thalassaemia, lymphoma), sickle cell anaemia	Pneumococci, *H. influenzae* type b, malaria
Complement	Congenital	*N. meningitidis, S. pneumoniae*

[†] = respiratory syncytial (RSV), parainfluenza and adenoviruses.
* PCP = *Pneumocystis carinii* pneumonia.
[#] Also *Klebsiella, Enterobacter, Serratia* spp.

DISEASE

Many diseases depress the immune response:

1. *AIDS* (see also Chapter 31) is a disease in which the virus HIV specifically attacks the T cells – in fact the CD4 T cells – but with secondary and severe effects on other parts of the immune system. AIDS is associated with a particularly large variety of infections – indeed, these form the main clinical features of the disease.

2. *Neoplasms of the lymphoid system*: in leukaemia there is suppression of cell-mediated immunity because of the nature of the disease itself, and treatment increases the immunosuppressive effect. In *Hodgkin's disease* the major deficiency is in cell-mediated immunity and, like leukaemia, is associated with increased susceptibility to viral infections; in *non-Hodgkin's lymphoma* humoral immunity is particularly affected. A decrease in normal immunoglobulin levels, with an increase in the characteristic monoclonal antibody, is also seen in *multiple myeloma*.

3. *Solid tumours*: these have much less effect, although the generally debilitating effect of cancer also depresses immunity.
4. *Other diseases*: diminish immunity in a variety of ways: the exact mechanisms involved are complex and often incompletely understood. These diseases include *renal failure, diabetes, autoimmune* diseases, e.g. systemic lupus erythematosus, severe burns and systemic infections, e.g. tuberculosis.

THERAPY

Several forms of therapy which depress immune function are now widely used in modern medicine. They include:

- Drugs: such as immunosuppressive regimens for organ transplants, steroids, chemotherapy with cytotoxic drugs
- Radiotherapy
- Splenectomy.

Therapeutic regimens in the categories listed, often in combination, are used to treat malignant disease and to prevent graft rejection after organ transplantation – including bone marrow transplants. Thus both the disease itself and the treatment administered predispose to infection.

Patients with acute leukaemia receiving chemotherapy to achieve remission, and also because of the nature of the underlying disease, often develop neutropenia (neutrophil count less than 0.5×10^9/L) and are at special risk of bacterial infection.

Patients after organ transplantation are maintained on an immunosuppressive regimen designed to reduce the cell-mediated immune response that causes graft rejection: sometimes the anti-infective agents themselves carry a risk of neutropenia – this a well-recognized side-effect of ganciclovir, which is widely used to suppress cytomegalovirus: infection in these patients is a common cause of death.

AGE

Extremes of age can result in a diminished immune response: neonates are prone to infections because of their immature immune system (see also Chapter 38). In the elderly patient there is a decrease in cell-mediated and humoral (antibody) immune function, often accompanied by malnutrition, resulting in infections of the respiratory and urinary tracts, and the skin and soft tissues. A common cause of death.

CONGENITAL DEFICIENCIES OF THE IMMUNE SYSTEM

Rarely, children are born with congenital deficiency of the immune system. This may involve:

1. **Immunoglobulin synthesis**, e.g. B-cell deficiency with depressed production of immunoglobulins. All immunoglobulins may be affected, as in Bruton's agammaglobulinaemia, or only some, as in hereditary telangiectasia with deficient IgA and IgE.
2. **Cell-mediated immunity**: T-cell deficiency, e.g. thymic hypoplasia (DiGeorge's syndrome).
3. **Combined variable immunodeficiency**: lack of differentiation of the common lymphoid stem cell, resulting in both B- and T-cell deficiency, e.g. Swiss-type agammaglobulinaemia, in which there are no lymphocytes or plasma cells in lymphoid organs, and the thymus is very small.
4. **Neutrophil function**: several syndromes affect aspects of phagocytosis, e.g. chronic granulomatous disease; Chediak–Higashi syndrome.
5. **Complement**: congenital deficiency can affect amost any of the components of complement; C2 deficiency is probably the most common, but C7, 8 and 9 defects are particularly associated with enhanced susceptibility to *Neisseria*.

INFECTION IN THE IMMUNOCOMPROMISED

Many of the organisms involved are of known, relatively high, pathogenicity, but in the immunocompromised these can show an unfamiliar presentation and are often unusually severe; examples of this are tuberculosis in AIDS and varicella in leukaemic children. Others are of low pathogenicity and rarely cause disease in immunocompetent patients, but can produce severe life-threatening disease in the immunodeficient: examples of these are cytomegalovirus and adenovirus in bone marrow transplant recipients.

Table 37.2 lists the most frequently encountered organisms – sometimes called 'opportunistic' – together with the principal types of infection they cause. The list of organisms is long and the clinical presentations are shown in more detail in earlier chapters in which the individual organisms are described.

Table 37.2 Some common causes of infection in immunocompromised patients and the diseases produced

Type of infectious agent	Main microorganisms involved	Clinical features of infection
Bacteria	*Escherichia coli*	Urinary infections, sepsis, septicaemia
	Other enterobacteria	Septicaemia, meningitis
	P. aeruginosa	Pneumonia, septicaemia
	M. tuberculosis	Pulmonary, miliary tuberculosis
	M. avium complex	Pulmonary, bowel infection, disseminated disease
	S. aureus	Soft tissue sepsis, pneumonia, septicaemia
	S. epidermidis	Local sepsis, septicaemia
	S. pneumoniae	Pneumonia, septicaemia, meningitis
	'Viridans' streptococci	Mucositis, respiratory distress syndrome
	L. pneumophila	Pneumonia
	L. monocytogenes	Septicaemia, meningitis, arthritis
	C. jeikeium	Local sepsis, septicaemia
	N. asteroides	Pneumonia, metastatic abscesses, especially brain
Viruses	Herpes simplex virus	Severe cold sores
	Varicella-zoster virus	Zoster, sometimes generalized
	Cytomegalovirus	Pneumonitis, retinitis
	EB virus	Lymphoproliferative disease
	Adenoviruses	Respiratory, haemorrhagic cystitis, disseminated disease
	RSV, parainfluenza	Chronic, progressive respiratory disease
	Parvovirus B19	Chronic anaemia
	JC (human polyoma) virus	Progressive multifocal leukoencephalopathy
	Papillomavirus	Warts (sometimes florid)
Fungi	*Candida* spp.	Local thrush, systemic candidiasis
	Cryptococcus neoformans	Meningoencephalitis
	A. fumigatus	Pulmonary, occasionally disseminated infections
	Pneumocystis carinii	Interstitial pneumonia
Protozoa	*Toxoplasma gondii*	Cerebral, retinal toxoplasmosis
	P. falciparum	Malaria
	Cryptosporidium	Chronic diarrhoea, malabsorption

SOURCES OF INFECTION IN THE IMMUNOCOMPROMISED

As with most healthcare-associated infection, this can be acquired:

- *Endogenously*: caused by microorganisms that are part of the normal flora, e.g. septicaemia from colonic bacteria, herpes simplex causing abnormal cold sores from sites of latency, thrush from candida in the mouth; *or*
- *Exogenously*: acquired from the environment, e.g. MRSAs, *C. difficile*, *L. pneumophila*; respiratory syncytial virus (a particular problem in children's wards), parvovirus B19 from other infected people, or blood or platelet transfusion; *Aspergillus fumigatus* from contaminated dust.

Note: An exogenous potential pathogen, often an antibiotic-resistant hospital strain, can colonize the patient and become part of the normal flora before causing infection.

- *Reactivation*: (endogenous) infection in the immunocompromised – often the result of reactivation of asymptomatic latent infection, e.g. tuberculosis, cytomegalovirus pneumonia, toxoplasmosis, pneumocystis pneumonia.
- *Transplanted tissue*: (exogenous) can be the source of a variety of infections, e.g. primary cytomegalovirus infection acquired by a seronegative recipient from a seropositive donor.

PREVENTION OF INFECTION

Surveillance:

- Regular clinical and laboratory examinations to detect infection early and to monitor progress: if indicated, treatment must be started without delay.
- Screening for colonization by potential pathogens: take repeated cultures from a variety of body sites and blood for serology.

PROPHYLAXIS

Various regimens are used to prevent infection in the immuno-compromised. These are complex and also change over quite short periods of time as new and better drugs become available. They cannot be described in detail here, but some of the main principles involved are shown below.

Antimicrobials: avoid indiscriminate use of 'prophylactic' broad-spectrum antibiotics: this promotes an abnormal flora of resistant bacteria. During periods of neutropenia prescribe ciprofloxacin (antibacterial), aciclovir (antiviral) and fluconazole (antifungal). Co-trimoxazole may be given in addition to protect against pneumocystis pneumonia, sometimes with colistin to prevent infection with Gram-negative bacilli. Ganciclovir is widely used prophylactically to prevent cytomegalovirus disease in bone marrow transplant patients.

Immunization: pneumococcal vaccine and Hib (*H. influenza* type b) for splenectomized patients; also killed vaccines such as influenza vaccine and, with care, live attenuated virus vaccines.

Isolation: to protect the patient from infection if severely neutropenic: the measures can be either simple (*protective isolation nursing* to protect the patient from infection in a single room) or elaborate (nursing in a laminar-airflow bed or room with catering using sterilized food).

38 Infection and pregnancy

Infection in pregnancy carries a risk to the mother, but even more to her fetus or newborn infant. The fetus and the neonate are especially vulnerable to infection, probably because of the immaturity of the immune system and other defence mechanisms. Viruses pose the greatest risk but bacterial infections, especially in the neonatal period, can be life-threatening and require prompt diagnosis and treatment.

Transmission

1. *In utero*: many viruses – and, more rarely, bacteria and at least one species of parasite – cross the placenta, possibly through infecting it, and invade the tissues and organs of the fetus: in most cases the disease in the infant will be apparent at birth – and, if not, can be detected by laboratory tests.
2. *Intrapartum*: during the passage of the infant through the birth canal organisms can be acquired from infected or colonized maternal genital tissues.
3. *Postpartum*: infection can be acquired in the neonatal period from the mother via breastfeeding or, by contact, from her or from nursing or medical staff in the maternity ward.

Neonatal infection (i.e. within the first 4 weeks of life): both intrapartum and postpartum transmission cause neonatal infection.

VIRUS INFECTION IN PREGNANCY AND POSTPARTUM

Viruses associated with infection in the fetus or newborn are listed in Table 38.1.

Table 38.1 Principal viruses causing fetal and neonatal infection

Virus	In utero	Neonatal
Rubella	Congenital rubella	No
Varicella/zoster	Congenital varicella	Severe varicella
Herpes simplex	Rare	Severe generalized infection
Cytomegalovirus	Cytomegalovirus inclusion disease	No
Parvovirus B19	Non-immune hydrops fetalis	No
HIV	Fetal infection	Neonatal infection
HTLV-1	No	Carrier state
Hepatitis B	Rare	Carrier state
Enteroviruses	No	Generalized infection

Congenital infection

Virus infection in utero can give rise to congenital defects in the fetus owing to the destructive effect of viral replication in developing tissues and organs; affected infants often also show signs of generalized infection, such as hepatosplenomegaly, CNS involvement, choroidoretinitis and thrombocytopenic purpura: a newborn baby with rash or skin lesions should always arouse suspicions of congenital virus infection. The viruses which infect in utero are described below.

1. *Rubella*: before the advent of immunization rubella was the most important cause of virus-induced congenial abnormalities, despite being one of the mildest of childhood fevers. The congenital rubella syndrome consists of generalized infection with a triad of congenital anomalies – cataracts, heart defects and deafness; mental retardation is a common sequel: babies asymptomatic at birth may develop a significant degree of deafness in later childhood; rubella in the first trimester poses the greatest risk, and deafness is usually the sole clinical manifestation of fetal infection in the second trimester. The earlier the infection in the first 3 months, the higher risk of fetal abnormalities (see also Chapter 26).

2. *Varicella*: congenital varicella can be a complication of maternal varicella: affected infants have signs of generalized infection, including limb hypoplasia, cicatrices (skin scars) and

cerebral and psychomotor retardation – but this is rare (incidence 1%). The risk is greatest in the second trimester, but it is also seen after maternal varicella in the first 3 months. Late on in pregnancy, varicella before delivery is especially dangerous as the child is at risk of severe, life-theatening varicella. Varicella is occasionally unusually severe in pregnant women.

3. *Cytomegalovirus*: unlike the viruses above, maternal infection with cytomegalovirus is not uncommon in pregnancy, often due to reactivation but much more dangerous to the fetus if infection is primary – but note that reactivations also commonly result in virus spread to the fetus: 1% of women experience primary infection during their pregnancy, and about one-third of them transmit the infection to their baby. The majority of affected babies are asymptomatic at birth, but around 7% have severe generalized infection (also known as *cytomegalic inclusion disease*) and, in them, the prognosis is poor, with mental deficiency sometimes associated with microcephaly, and deafness. In asymptomatically infected babies approximately 15% will develop deafness or show impaired intellectual function in later years. Infection can be transmitted in utero throughout pregnancy and does not show the gradient of disease seen with rubella. Congenital cytomegalovirus infection also differs from rubella in that the virus has a destructive effect on fetal tissue, rather than the teratogenicity of rubella virus.

4. *Parvovirus B19*: has strong tropism for dividing erythrocyte progenitor cells in the bone marrow, causing aplastic crisis, e.g. in sickle cell disease. Infection in utero does not give rise to congenital defects but can become manifest in the second or third trimester to cause a catastrophic fall in fetal haemoglobin and a severely anaemic fetus, with gross oedema and congestive cardiac failure (non-immune hydrops fetalis): interestingly, this condition sometimes corrects spontaneously during the course of the pregnancy.

5. *HIV*: can be transmitted in utero, although perinatal infection is more common (see below).

Rare: *hepatitis B* and *herpes simplex virus types 1 and 2* can – although rarely – cross the placenta and infect in utero, causing severe generalized infection with visceral and CNS involvement in the case of herpes simplex, or the carrier state in the case of hepatitis B; there is some doubt about the timing of infection, and perinatal infection with either virus is certainly much more common.

Abortion: *rubella* and *B19 infection* – especially in early pregnancy – cause an increased incidence of spontaneous abortion. *Mumps*, not a cause of congenital fetal disease, is also associated with increased risk of abortion.

Neonatal infection

The neonate can acquire infection either *intrapartum* during passage through the infected birth canal, or *perinatally* from its mother's breast milk, or through close contact with her or with nursing attendants or visitors in the puerperium. In either case, symptomatic infection in the neonate does not become manifest until some time after birth – sometimes a few days later, but often longer.

Rubella and *cytomegalovirus* do not seem to be a problem postpartum.

Varicella: in an infant born to a mother suffering from varicella around the time of delivery, varicella can present with severe, even life-threatening, infection: this is because of the absence of protective maternal antibody. Infection may be acquired either in utero or postpartum from the mother with varicella, or postpartum from another person with varicella or zoster. This is an urgent indication for the prophylactic administration of ZIG (zoster immune globulin).

Herpes simplex, especially type 2 (but also type 1) can also cause severe generalized infection, with severe neurological damage in the neonate and often large, vesicular skin lesions: usually acquired if the mother suffers from primary infection in the third trimester, and transmitted from her genital tissues during delivery.

HIV: unfortunately, a variable proportion of infected mothers – around 17% in Europe, 30% in Africa – if untreated, transmit the virus to their offspring: virus is present in breast milk, and breast-feeding is an important source of infection; the virus can also be transmitted intrapartum and perinatally by close contact with the mother; affected infants are asymptomatic at birth, but are chronically infected and have a high risk of disease later on in childhood. Retroviral therapy in pregnancy can prevent transmission: HAART can reduce the viral load to undetectable levels, with consequent low risk of transmitting HIV to the child. The key to prevention of transmission is antenatal screening of all women for HIV and timely initiation of therapy.

HTLV-1: this retrovirus is endemic in populations in Japan and in the Caribbean and is transmitted mainly by breastfeeding through virus in mothers' milk: infection is usually silent, often throughout life, but may – although rarely – result in the development of adult T-cell lymphoma/leukaemia or tropical spastic paraparesis in later life.

Hepatitis B: carriage in the mother, especially if she is HBeAg positive, carries a high risk of transmitting infection to the child. The child does not develop acute hepatitis B but becomes a carrier, and this form of vertical transmisssion is largely responsible for the high rates of carriage seen in many parts of the world. Transmission is mainly intrapartum, but perinatal infection may also play a part.

Enteroviruses: spread to the infant may be intrapartum, but infection is usually acquired perinatally from the mother – although epidemics due to case-to-case spread have been reported in neonatal nurseries; infection in the neonate may be mild, even symptomless, but can be life-threatening, with meningoencephalitis, myocarditis, pneumonia and severe hepatitis: the types of virus most commonly involved are echovirus 11 and Coxsackie viruses B2 and 4.

Hepatitis C: from 5 to 10% of carrier mothers transmit the virus to their child: the long-term effects of this are as yet unclear.

Papillomaviruses: are commonly transmitted during delivery: types 16 and 18 are usually symptomless in the child, but types 6 and 11 may (rarely) cause juvenile laryngeal papillomas.

Rotavirus: diarrhoea can become epidemic in neonatal nurseries, causing severe dehydration and collapse, although infection in the neonate is often symptomless.

Diagnosis

Congenital infection is usually first suspected by recognition of infection in the mother; however, rubella and B19 infection are clinically similar and *all* cases of suspected maternal infection must be investigated by laboratory test. Acute maternal infection is confirmed by detection of virus-specific IgM antibodies. However, cytomegalovirus infection in pregnancy is nearly always symptomless and so is not usually detected antenatally. Antenatal patients are routinely tested for hepatitis B and (with permission) for HIV, so that appropriate preventive measures or therapy can be instituted. Virus culture or amplification techniques to detect virus nucleic acid are used on cells from fetal tissues or from amniocentesis. Tests on fetal blood for IgM may be helpful.

Neonatal infection and infection detected in the child after birth is diagnosed by the laboratory tests appropriate to the suspected virus infection: IgM tests are helpful (as maternal IgM does not cross the placenta) but are occasionally difficult in neonatal sera. PCR can be used to detect viral DNA or RNA in the infant's tissues or urine culture.

Management

Congenital infection: antiviral therapy and passive immunization cannot generally be used to treat the fetus in utero. But passive administration of virus-specific immunoglobulin to the newborn child at birth can prevent or modify infection from a mother with primary varicella near the time of delivery, or prevent transmission of hepatitis B from an e-antigen positive carrier mother. Babies born to all hepatitis B-positive mothers (even if e-antigen negative) must also be vaccinated at birth. Consider caesarian section in mothers suffering primary genital herpes after 34 weeks. Mothers infected with HIV should be treated with appropriate antiretroviral therapy during and after pregnancy. Mothers positive for HIV or HTLV-1 should be advised not to breastfeed their infants. In cases where infection in the mother in early pregnancy is associated with a high risk of fetal abnormality, termination is an option but requires careful and consensual consideration of individual circumstances.

Neonatal infection: should be treated with the appropriate antiviral drug – such as aciclovir, which is well tolerated by infants.

VIRUSES PRESENTING INCREASED RISK TO THE MOTHER

Pregnant women show increased susceptibility to certain viruses during their pregnancy. Below are listed some of the virus diseases that can be unusually severe, or even lead to death if contracted in pregnancy:

- Varicella
- Hepatitis E
- Lassa fever
- Japanese encephalitis
- Poliomyelitis
- Measles.

BACTERIAL INFECTION IN PREGNANCY AND POSTPARTUM

Bacteria associated with infection in the fetus and newborn are listed in Table 38.2.

Congenital bacterial infections

In contrast to viruses, few bacteria are capable of crossing the placenta to infect the fetus in utero.

SYPHILIS

Transmission of syphilis (*Treponema pallidum*) from mother to fetus is most likely if the woman becomes pregnant during the first year of her infection. Transmission can occur early (16th week) until late in the pregnancy.

Clinical features

Abortion or stillbirth if the congenital syphilis is acquired very early in the mother's disease.

1. **Latent infection**: more than half of the infants have no symptoms – but they are serologically positive.
2. **Early**: up to the end of the second year of age. Most infants appear healthy at birth; symptoms develop in the first few weeks of life, starting with failure to thrive, followed by generalized infection, with skin rashes, snuffles, nasal deformity (saddle nose), hepatitis, bone lesions, meningitis, anaemia.

Table 38.2 Principal bacterial infections of the fetus and neonate

Bacteria	Congenital	Neonatal
T. pallidum	Congenital syphilis	No
Listeria monocytogenes	Fetal death, severe disease	Meningitis, septicaemia
N. gonorrhoeae	No	Ophthalmia neonatorum
Group B streptococcus (Streptococcus agalactiae)	No	Septicaemia, meningitis, pneumonia
C. trachomatis	No	Conjunctivitis, pneumonia

3. *Late*: manifestations appear after the second year of life: interstitial keratitis, bone sclerosis, joint effusions and arthritis, juvenile general paralysis of the insane and tabes, notching of incisor teeth (Hutchinson's teeth), deafness.

Diagnosis

Serological tests at birth and after 6 weeks. Spirochaetes may be detected in early skin and mucous membrane lesions.

Prevention and treatment

Fetal infection is unlikely to occur if the mother's infection is detected and treated before the fourth month of pregnancy. Follow-up of the infant is essential in case the infection has become latent.

LISTERIOSIS

This was a relatively rare disease in the UK until the late 1980s, when a large number of cases were recorded. The causative organism, *Listeria monocytogenes*, is widely distributed in nature: in soil, silage, water and a wide range of animals. Infection is food-borne: often sporadic, but food-associated outbreaks with coleslaw, milk, paté and soft cheeses have been reported. *Listeria* spp. can grow at 6°C and survive in chilled foods.

Clinical features

Usually a mild or inapparent infection presenting as a non-specific febrile illness with flu-like symptoms. Particular at-risk groups are the immunocompromised, the elderly and pregnant women. Listeriosis contracted in early pregnancy results in maternal bacteraemia, which can cross the placenta to result in abortion or stillbirth. If contracted later in pregnancy the baby may be born alive but have a systemic illness associated with abscesses in internal organs, a rash, and perhaps meningoencephalitis. Perinatal infection can occur associated with maternal genital infection and is manifested by septicaemia and meningitis.

Diagnosis

Listeria monocytogenes cultured from meconium in congenital infections and from CSF and blood in perinatal infections.

Prevention and treatment

Ampicillin with gentamicin are effective drugs to treat bacteraemia. Recognition of risk in pregnancy and advice given to avoid soft cheeses, patés and cook–chilled foods has significantly reduced the incidence of listeriosis in pregnancy.

NEONATAL BACTERIAL INFECTIONS

GROUP B STREPTOCOCCUS

The group B streptococcus (GBS), or *Streptococcus agalactiae*, is now the most common life-threatening neonatal infection in the industrialized world. The bacterium is a normal commensal of the female genital tract and can be recovered from 10–20% of pregnant women, regardless of the stage of pregnancy.

Clinical features

Neonatal invasive disease can be divided into early- and late-onset disease. *Early-onset disease* occurs within the first week of life, usually within 24 h of birth. Disease is manifest by septicaemia or meningitis and/or pneumonia. This accounts for 80% of cases and is due to vertical transmission.

Late-onset disease occurs after the first week of life and can be due to vertical transmission, but is mainly due to nosocomial spread from other infants or hospital personnel.

Incidence in UK is 0.5–1.15 per 1000 live births. Mortality is around 20% and is higher in preterm infants.

Prevention of neonatal disease

Intrapartum antibiotics prophylaxis (IAP), together with postpartum antibiotics for the infant, can significantly reduce early-onset GBS disease. Penicillin is the agent of choice and should be administered intravenously prior to delivery. Women allergic to penicillin should be given clindamycin. IAP will not prevent late-onset disease.

The question of which women should be selected for treatment is not easy. Risk factors include GBS in a previous baby; GBS found incidentally in urine or vagina during pregnancy; prolonged preterm rupture of membranes; fever in labour; preterm labour; and prolonged rupture of membranes in labour. There are two possible strategies for selecting women for IAP, a risk-based strategy or microbiological screening-based strategy. Guidelines on prevention, based on either strategy or a combination of the two, have been published in the USA but are not yet available in the UK.

SEXUALLY TRANSMITTED DISEASES

Neisseria gonorrhoeae, a common sexually transmitted disease, can cause ophthalmia neonatorum, a rare conjunctival infection of the neonate acquired from the maternal genital tract during birth. Severe purulent conjunctivitis can develop within 36–48 h of birth. Can be prevented by instillation of 1% silver nitrate solution into the eyes at birth. Gonococcal vulvovaginitis is an uncommon infection of female infants contracted during birth.

Chlamydia trachomatis: an obligate intracellular bacterium and the cause of the most common sexually transmitted disease. Intrapartum infection of the infant occurs from maternal infection of the cervix; the main infection seen is neonatal ophthalmia – a purulent conjunctivitis which responds to treatment with erythromycin; sometimes afebrile pneumonia with cough, patchy infiltrates on X-ray, often following a prodromal illness of rhinitis and conjunctivitis.

OTHER BACTERIAL INFECTIONS

Tuberculosis

Tuberculosis in pregnancy is now rare in the UK and is most likely to occur in recent immigrants. The treatment is the same as for non-pregnant individuals. First-line therapeutic drugs have no risk to the fetus. Congenital tuberculosis is very rare indeed: a baby born to an infected mother may be more at risk after birth.

Bacterial vaginosis

Bacterial vaginosis is a clinical syndrome of unknown aetiology and is associated with adverse pregnancy outcome and infectious morbidity after gynaecological surgery. Microbiological studies have shown that there is alteration of the normal vaginal flora, reflected in an overgrowth of anaerobes and a rise in pH ≥ 4.5 in the vagina. Systemic therapy with metronidazole or clindamycin can restore the normal flora. Bacterial vaginosis is associated with complications of pregnancy, including miscarriage, perterm birth and postpartum endometriosis. Further studies are needed.

Chlamydophila abortus: primarily a disease of sheep, but can infect pregnant farm workers at lambing, causing abortion and severe generalized infection in the mother.

Some other common infections that may affect a woman at the time of delivery include *E. coli* or other urinary tract infections, and enteric infections, e.g. *Salmonella* spp. These organisms can colonize the maternal genital tract and be transmitted to the neonate. As with GBS disease, a long interval between rupture of membranes and start of labour can increase the opportunities for these organisms to cause infection in the neonate.

PARASITIC INFECTION IN PREGNANCY AND POSTPARTUM

Parasites associated with infection in the fetus and newborn are listed in Table 38.3.

Toxoplasmosis

The protozoan parasite *Toxoplasma gondii* is an established cause of fetal loss and severe neonatal disease. Pregnant women acquire toxoplasmosis by ingesting the sporocysts of the parasite excreted in the faeces of cats, which are the primary host. Infection in the mother is usually symptomless and is relatively rare in the UK (~0.1–0.2%), although as many as 85% of pregnant women are susceptible. Infection is commoner in France.

Transmission: infection is most often transmitted in the third trimester, but the risk of fetal damage is higher in early pregnancy, when termination may be considered. Infection is transmitted in approximately one-third of affected pregnancies.

Table 38.3   Principal parasitic infections of the fetus and neonate

Parasite	Congenital	Neonatal
Toxoplasma gondii	Intracranial calcification, hydrocephalus, choroidoretinitis	Ocular defects, mental retardation
Plasmodium falciparum	Hepatosplenomegaly	

Congenital toxoplasmosis

Infants infected in early pregnancy may be severely affected. The classic triad of the disease is intracerebral calcification, hydrocephalus and choroidoretinitis, with or without other signs of generalized infection in utero: later in pregnancy fetal infection tends to be milder or asymptomatic.

Diagnosis

Detection of specific IgM (or a rising antibody titre) in the mother; test for IgM in fetal blood after 20 weeks; culture of amniotic fluid for parasites using special media; culture of blood and CSF in the neonate; test blood for IgM.

Prevention and treatment

Primary prevention, aimed at reducing the number of women who acquire toxoplasmosis in pregnancy, is achieved by health education and reducing the infective load in the environment. Secondary prevention is termination of pregnancy or antiparasitic therapy, e.g. spiramycin to reduce parasitaemia in the mother; the combination of pyrimethamine plus sulphadiazine is effective for both prenatal and postnatal therapy, but pyramethamine is teratogenic and should not be given in the first 16 weeks of pregnancy.

Malaria

Plasmodium falciparum malaria in pregnancy is a potentially life-threatening condition.

Clinical features

Depends on the immune status of the woman – determined by previous exposure to malaria. In malaria-endemic areas, pregnant women are the main groups of adults at risk. On a global basis, 40% of pregnant women are exposed to malaria. Non-immune pregnant women with malaria are more likely to die from severe disease than are non-pregnant women. Studies from sub-Saharan Africa have estimated that the disease is associated with significant numbers of both maternal and neonatal deaths.

Effects on mother: fever (in non-immune women is associated with miscarriage and preterm labour), severe anaemia, hypoglycaemia, coma and pulmonary oedema.

Effects on fetus: fetal heart-rate abnormalities, premature delivery and fetal distress.

Congenital malaria

It is not clear how commonly parasites cross the placenta in the antenatal period. Babies born to non-immune women with untreated or incompletely treated malaria can manifest with overwhelming infection. Hepatosplenomegaly is common. Mortality is high.

Antimalarial therapy in pregnancy

Drug therapy is dependent on the local antimalarial resistance, the severity of the disease and the degree of pre-existing immunity. The danger of malaria to the mother and fetus will be far greater than any potential adverse drug reactions.

Pregnant women should be discouraged from travelling to a malaria-endemic area. A particular risk group are women who have moved to a non-endemic area and return to an endemic area during pregnancy.

PREVENTION OF MICROBIAL DISEASE

39 Immunization

Immunization against infectious disease has been one of the most successful developments in medicine. Widespread vaccination of human populations – the aim is usually to achieve acceptance rates of at least 90% – has caused a dramatic fall in the incidence of many infectious diseases, e.g. diphtheria, poliomyelitis. However, in some instances the introduction of other measures (e.g. improved housing, sanitation or nutrition, or antimicrobial therapy which reduces the duration of infectivity) at the same time as a vaccine may have had more effect on the prevalence of the disease than vaccination, e.g. tuberculosis.

Immunization aims to produce *immunity* to a disease, artificially and without ill effects, and can be either active or passive:

1. **Active**
   - (a) *Natural*: follows clinical or subclinical infection
   - (b) *Natural*: due to transplacental maternal IgG antibody, which protects the child for first 6 months of life.
2. **Passive**
   - (a) *Artificial*: induced by vaccination
   - (b) *Artificial*: by injection of preformed antibody derived from serum of humans or animals.

Active immunity

1. Associated with the *production of antibody*, and often cell-mediated immunity as well.
2. The *onset* of immunity is delayed but, when established, lasts for years, sometimes for life.

3. *Antibody*: protects in different ways, depending on the type of disease: most effective in virus diseases because antibody neutralizes virus infectivity. In bacterial disease due to exotoxin, antibody neutralizes the toxin. In both bacterial and virus infections, antibody enhances phagocytosis.

4. *Cell-mediated immunity (delayed hypersensitivity)*: stimulated independently of antibody: particularly important in resistance to chronic bacterial infections characterized by intracellular parasitism (e.g. tuberculosis, leprosy, brucellosis), and in some virus diseases, e.g. herpes simplex.

Passive immunity

Naturally acquired by fetus from mother, or artificially induced by injection of preformed antibody present in human or animal serum. *Immediate* immunity is conferred but it is short lived, usually for only a matter of weeks. There is no associated induction of cell-mediated immunity.

Antibody production

Figure 39.1 shows antibody levels after immunization, passive or active, with either live attenuated or killed organisms.

ACTIVE IMMUNIZATION

Aims to produce immunity with adequate antibody levels and a population of cells with immunological memory. *Long-lasting* once produced, the immunity persists and, even after many years, infection can still stimulate an accelerated antibody response.

TYPES OF VACCINE

1. Live attenuated organisms
2. Killed (inactivated) organisms or cell components
3. Toxoids.

Live attenuated organisms

Cultivated under conditions in which they lose virulence but retain antigenicity, i.e. the ability to stimulate a protective immune response: multiply in the body and mimic natural

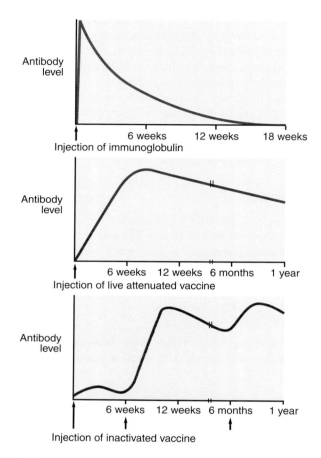

Fig. 39.1 Antibody levels following different methods of immunization.

infection, so producing antibody but usually without symptoms: reactions are mild and are similar to the natural disease. A *single dose* gives long-lasting immunity, which can be reinforced with subsequent booster doses.

Killed (inactivated) organisms or cell components

Usually require three doses (because there is no multiplication in the body) – the first and second doses 4 or 6 weeks apart, the third dose 6 months later; subsequent booster doses often necessary. Reactions do not resemble those of the natural disease, and usually follow soon after inoculation.

Older vaccines contained whole cells, but those recently introduced are often made from cell components such as purified proteins, e.g. obtained by genetic engineering (as in hepatitis B vaccine), or polysaccharides conjugated to proteins (as in *Haemophilus influenzae* vaccine).

Toxoids

Very successful vaccines in diseases due to a single exotoxin, e.g. diphtheria, tetanus. Toxoids are toxins rendered harmless – usually by formaldehyde – but retaining antigenicity. This can be increased by adsorption to a mineral carrier (such as aluminium salts) or by mixture with a suspension of other bacteria containing lipopolysaccharide endotoxin, e.g. the pertussis component of triple vaccine (pertussis, diphtheria, tetanus).

Future vaccines

Using molecular technology, novel vaccines are being developed, e.g. vaccinia virus, whose DNA includes a gene coding for an immunogenic protein derived from a different organism, and vaccines consisting of DNA – which, rather surprisingly, stimulates antibody production.

ASSESSING PROTECTION

Immunization must give a significant degree of protection against infection. Live attenuated organisms and toxoids are better than killed organisms. Vaccines require extensive testing in large-scale trials before introduction.

Field trials, studying the effect of a vaccine in a population which is 'at risk', are of crucial importance: look for a significant reduction in the *attack rate* or in the *severity* of the disease in vaccinees. Trials involve:

1. The estimation of *antibody levels (titres)* after vaccination: but note, the ability to stimulate antibody production does not guarantee effective prophylaxis.
2. Sometimes tests for the *appearance of cell-mediated immunity* (e.g. tuberculin conversion after BCG vaccination).
3. Detailed studies in *human volunteers* indicate the likelihood of the vaccine providing worthwhile protection and allow detection of possible side-effects.

Vaccine failure: the reasons are complex: the vaccine may be of *poor antigenicity* (e.g. meningococcal B strains): sometimes *inappropriate antibody* is formed – after injection of killed vaccine, IgM and IgG but not secretory IgA are formed when the latter is the main protective antibody at mucosal surfaces and necessary for protection against respiratory virus infections (e.g. influenza) and gut infections (e.g. poliomyelitis and cholera).

CONTROL OF VACCINE PREPARATION

The manufacture of each batch of vaccine is subject to stringent legal control to ensure safety and potency.

Safety

The main problems are:

• *Contamination*: by extraneous bacteria or viruses (derived from the cell cultures used in vaccine production)
• *Inadequate inactivation* of killed vaccine
• *Reversion* to virulence of attenuated vaccine: still an occasional problem in vaccinees and in contacts who excrete vaccine virus which has undergone partial reversion to virulence on passage
• *Residual toxicity* of toxoids.

With modern control of vaccine production these are less of a problem than formerly.

Potency

Ensured by the following measures:

• *Live vaccines*: prepared from organisms grown for only a few passages from the parent strain, to ensure that antigens essential for protection are not lost and that virulence remains low.
• *Killed vaccines*: prepared from organisms with a full complement of the antigens involved in the protective immune response. The antigenic composition of the vaccine organisms may have to be altered if new variants of wild organisms appear in the population.
• *Tests of potency*: measure the antibodies produced on inoculation into experimental animals; other tests assess the survival of

immunized animals after challenge with virulent organisms, but the method of the test may bear little relationship to the human disease, e.g. tests of pertussis vaccine measure the protection of mice against intracerebral injection with *Bordetella pertussis*: this correlates with the ability of the vaccine to prevent human disease.

ADMINISTRATION

Age

Target the age group at greatest risk. Some vaccines (e.g. typhoid, cholera) are indicated regardless of age for anyone entering an endemic area; others (e.g. influenza) are given primarily to the elderly or those with chronic cardiac or respiratory disease.

Childhood: most vaccines, however, are given to children because most of the diseases they prevent are encountered in childhood: e.g. more than two-thirds of deaths from pertussis are of infants under 1 year old.

There are two problems with starting immunization early in life:

• *The infant immune system is not fully developed* at birth, so the capacity to make antibody is limited; nevertheless, it is probably adequate if the vaccine is potent.
• *Transplacental maternal antibody* may prevent a response to live virus vaccines, and reduce that to some killed vaccines.

Official policy in Britain is to start immunization at 2 months of age: a compromise, because delay until the child is 6–9 months old would produce better responses but the chance of establishing immunity when it is most needed would be lost.

Combined vaccines

Attractive because they reduce the number of injections required, and therefore increase acceptability by both parent and child.

Combined vaccines may enhance antibody production (e.g. the presence of the pertussis component acts as an adjuvant for the toxoids in triple vaccine): there were fears in the past that the response to one organism might diminish that to others, but this has not been a problem in practice.

Complications of immunization

Side-effects: not uncommon after administration of some vaccines, e.g. many killed bacterial vaccines cause mild reactions, both local (pain and redness at the injection site) and general (fever and constitutional upset): although unpleasant, they are usually trivial.

Serious complications: rare, but seen with some vaccines and include anaphylaxis, bronchospasm and laryngeal oedema: sometimes involving the CNS (febrile convulsions); occasionally encephalitis, which can cause permanent brain damage.

The small but definite risk of serious reactions in a tiny proportion of vaccinees must be balanced against the benefits: the controversy some years ago over pertussis vaccine illustrates the difficulty that this may present. The controversy is increased when the natural disease all but disappears – usually due to vaccination.

Contraindications to vaccination

- **Previous reactions** – either *severe local or generalized* to that (or a similar) vaccine, or a history of *hypersensitivity* to some of its components, e.g. egg allergy in the case of virus vaccines grown in chick cells, antibiotic hypersensitivity with many virus vaccines.
- **Live vaccines** should **never** be given to:
  - *immunocompromised* patients because of the risk of severe generalized infection
  - *pregnant women*: because of the danger of transplacental spread to the fetus.

VACCINES IN CURRENT USE

Table 39.1 lists the main vaccines in current use in the UK.

LIVE BACTERIAL VACCINES

BCG vaccine

Contains: live attenuated *Mycobacterium bovis* (Bacille Calmette–Guérin). Killed vaccines are of no value as immunizing agents against tuberculosis: they do not produce a cell-mediated response.

Indications: policy in the UK is to vaccinate all children between their 10th and 14th birthdays, *after* a tuberculin test has shown that they are non-reactors. Infants should be immunized at

Table 39.1 Vaccines currently available in the UK

	Bacterial vaccines	Viral vaccines
Live	BCG (tuberculosis)	Measles–mumps–rubella (MMR)
	Typhoid	Poliomyelitis (Sabin)
		Rubella
		Yellow fever
Killed or cell components	Cholera	Hepatitis A
	Haemophilus influenzae b (Hib)	Hepatitis B
	Meningococcal	Influenza
	Pertussis	Poliomyelitis (Salk)
	Pneumococcal	Rabies
	Typhoid	
Toxoids	Diphtheria	
	Tetanus	

birth if there is high risk of contact with tuberculosis, e.g. a close relative with the disease. Others at high risk of exposure to tuberculosis should be immunized if not already protected (e.g. healthcare staff, contacts of known cases, immigrants from countries with a high prevalence of the disease).

Administration: one dose *intradermally* at the insertion of the deltoid muscle, near to the middle of the upper arm. Normally a red papule develops at the injection site some 2–6 weeks later, and soon subsides.

Adverse reactions: the papule may progress to an indolent ulcer and discharge pus: associated axillary lymphadenopathy is not uncommon. Keloid formation at injection site.

Protection: MRC field trials in the UK (1950–71) and studies in North America both showed durable (10–15 years) protection. The incidence of clinical disease in vaccinees was reduced by 80%. However, other field trials have yielded less encouraging results.

Typhoid vaccine (live)

A recently introduced live attenuated vaccine.

Contains: the attenuated Ty 21a strain of *S.* Typhi.

Indications: for those travelling to or living in areas where typhoid fever is endemic; healthcare staff at risk.

Administration: orally in enteric-coated capsules, in three doses on alternate days. Repeat course at yearly intervals.

Adverse reactions: mild and transient nausea, vomiting, abdominal cramps and diarrhoea; occasionally urticaria.

Protection: efficacy similar to parenteral vaccine but may be less durable.

LIVE VIRAL VACCINES

Warning: must not be given to pregnant women or the immunocompromised.

Measles–mumps–rubella (MMR) vaccine

Introduced in 1988 as a combined live attenuated vaccine against the three childhood fevers.

Contains: live attenuated strains of all three viruses.

Indications: give to all children in the second year of life, to prevent complications such as respiratory infections, encephalitis (measles), meningitis (mumps) and congenital infection (rubella).

Administration: two doses by deep subcutaneous or intramuscular injection: the first at age 12–15 months; the second at 3–5 years on school entry. The second dose protects those who did not develop immunity after the first injection and ensures a high enough level of herd immunity to prevent future epidemics.

Adverse reactions: few: fever, malaise and transient rash may follow 6–12 days after vaccination; occasionally, febrile convulsions. Around 1% of children have mild parotitis. Rarely, meningo-encephalitis was reported owing to an earlier component of the mumps vaccine, now replaced by a more attenuated strain.

Protection: good – of the order of 90% – and apparently long lasting.

Note: Alarmist allegations first made in 1998 claimed a link between MMR vaccination and autism and inflammatory bowel disease. Trials have disproved this, but public anxiety has resulted in a decline in uptake of MMR and, with this, the likelihood of a resurgence of measles outbreaks.

Poliomyelitis (Sabin) oral vaccine

Contains: live attenuated strains of poliovirus types 1, 2 and 3 (Salk vaccine, developed earlier, contains inactivated strains).

Indications: all infants, starting at 2 months old.

Administration: orally on a sugar lump, in three doses, to ensure multiplication in gut with both local gut IgA and serum antibody production to each virus type. Booster doses at school entry and on leaving school.

Adverse reactions: minimal: rare cases of paralysis in adults due to Sabin type 3 virus: the type 3 strain is less stable than the other two and has undergone a degree of reversion to virulence, causing outbreaks of poliomyelitis in Egypt, Haiti and the Dominican Republic.

Protection: excellent: it also eliminates wild poliovirus from circulation in the community; now used worldwide by WHO to eradicate poliomyelitis.

Rubella vaccine

Contains: live attenuated virus.

Indications: now used mainly for pregnant women (but only after delivery) detected as seronegative on routine antenatal testing – usually because they are unimmunized or have failed to develop an adequate immune response to earlier vaccination. Also used for seronegative women of childbearing age and healthcare workers in contact with pregnant women.

Pregnancy must be avoided for 1 month after vaccination: the vaccine should never be given during pregnancy.

Administration: one dose by injection.

Adverse reactions: uncommon, but there may be mild rubella-like symptoms, including arthralgia, some 9 days after vaccination.

Protection: good, with long-lasting immunity.

Varicella virus vaccine

Not licensed for routine use in the UK and other countries, but used in the USA (and elsewhere) for routine infant vaccination between 12 and 18 months. Available for use in the UK on a named-patient basis.

Contains: live attenuated virus (the Oka strain).

Administered: in one subcutaneous injection; in susceptible adults (and in children or adolescents with lymphatic leukaemia) two doses 4–8 weeks apart.

Adverse reactions: rash resembling mild varicella is seen in around 5–15% of vaccinees, who are infectious.

Latency: vaccine virus becomes latent in ganglia but reactivation appears to be less frequent than with naturally acquired wild-type virus.

Protection: around 70–90% effective.

Yellow fever vaccine

One of the most successful and effective vaccines ever produced – traditionally regarded as one of the safest (but see below) and conferring long-lasting immunity.

Contains: the attenuated 17D strain of yellow fever virus.

Indications: travellers to endemic areas, laboratory workers handling the virus.

Administration: deep subcutaneous injection.

Adverse reactions: mild – headache, myalgia, low-grade fever; very rarely encephalitis: recently, the vaccine's reputation for safety has come into question by reports of a few cases of fatal yellow fever and of severe multisystem organ failure in four elderly patients, in each case due to vaccine virus.

Protection: solid immunity for at least 10 years.

KILLED BACTERIAL VACCINES

Cholera vaccine

Contains: heat-killed *Vibrio cholerae* O1, serotypes Inaba and Ogawa.

Indications: formerly for those travelling to areas where cholera is endemic, but evidence of vaccination is no longer a requirement for entry into any foreign country.

Administration: two spaced doses by injection.

Adverse reactions: local and general reactions are quite common; serious reactions are rare.

Protection: poor, and use of the vaccine is no longer recommended in the UK.

Attempts to produce a better vaccine have so far failed.

Hib vaccine

Contains: capsular polysaccharide from *Haemophilus influenzae* type b, conjugated to protein carrier to enhance immunogenicity. *H. influenzae* is an important cause of invasive disease, especially meningitis and acute epiglottitis in children under the age of 13 months.

Indications: introduced in 1992 in the UK for routine immunization of babies with a dramatic reduction in the incidence of invasive *H. influenzae* infection. Also for post-splenectomy prophylaxis.

Administration: three doses at 2, 3, 4 months old, at the same time as triple vaccine. Hib vaccine is available mixed with triple vaccine for simultaneous administration by a single injection.

Adverse reactions: minor – most common after the first dose.

Meningococcal vaccine

An effective group B vaccine is not yet available.

1. Group C conjugate vaccine

Contains: meningococcal C polysaccharide conjugated to protein.

Indications: now part of the course of childhood immunization: also for post-splenectomy patients. When introduced in 1999 a 'catch-up' programme targeted those at special risk, notably teenagers.

Administration: three doses for children aged 2–4 months by intramuscular injection.

Adverse reactions: minor at injection site.

Protection: excellent and long term, but only against group C disease.

2. Polysaccharide A and C vaccine

Contains: outer capsular polysaccharide of groups A and C *Neisseria meningitidis*.

Indications: those travelling overseas in areas where the disease is endemic, especially if living rough.

Administration: one dose, by intramuscular injection, to both children and adults.

Adverse reactions: local and sometimes fever.

Protection: antibody response detected in more than 90% of those immunized after 1 week: infants respond less well; lasts 3–5 years.

Pertussis vaccine

Contains: killed, freshly isolated, smooth strains of *Bordetella pertussis*. The vaccine should contain all the surface antigens of *B. pertussis* associated with epidemics: these antigens designate the three common serotypes – 1,3; 1,2,3; and 1,2.

Indications: official policy in Britain is the active immunization of all children, starting at 2 months old.

Administration: three doses at 2, 3 and 4 months old: the vaccine is always given with diphtheria and tetanus toxoids, as triple vaccine. Booster doses are not recommended because pertussis is not a problem after 5 years of age.

Adverse reactions: usually local and trivial: a few infants develop excessive crying and irritability. Severe reactions attributed to the vaccine are convulsions and, rarely, permanent brain damage. Subsequent work has cast doubt on whether the severe reactions are, in fact, attributable to the vaccine.

Protection: mass vaccination was started in the UK in 1957. During the following years there were conflicting claims about the efficacy and safety of the vaccine. After a decline in uptake owing to unwarranted concern about the risks of vaccination in the 1970s, there were major outbreaks and control of whooping cough was not achieved until public confidence in immunization returned in the mid-1980s.

Pneumococcal vaccine

Contains: a saline solution of 23 highly purified capsular polysaccharides, extracted from pneumococci of the most prevalent pathogenic types.

Indications: to prevent pneumococcal pneumonia, bacteraemia and meningitis in individuals at special risk, especially those who have had a splenectomy, but also patients with chronic lung, heart, liver and kidney disease.

Administration: one dose, by injection.

Adverse reactions: local in about half of those vaccinated: revaccination within 3 years may produce severe reactions.

Protection: apparently good – but only against infections caused by the serotypes present in the vaccine. Efficacy in preventing pneumococcal pneumonia is about 60–70%, but the vaccine is less effective in young children and the immunosuppressed.

Typhoid vaccines

The classic whole-cell vaccine has now been replaced by other preparations. It contained a heat-killed phenol-preserved suspension of *S*. Typhi.

Capsular polysaccharide typhoid vaccine

This has recently been licensed in the UK.

Contains: the Vi capsular polysaccharide antigen of *S.* Typhi.

Indications: for those travelling to or living in areas where typhoid fever is endemic, and healthcare staff at risk.

Administration: one dose, by injection; booster dose every 3 years.

Adverse reactions: mild and transient local reactions.

Protection: 70–80%, lasting for 3 years or more.

INACTIVATED (KILLED) VIRUS VACCINES

Hepatitis A vaccine

Contains: formaldehyde-inactivated virus, grown in cell culture and adsorbed to aluminium hydroxide.

Indications: for non-immune travellers to areas where hepatitis A is endemic, i.e. most tropical and semitropical regions; haemophiliacs, patients with high-risk sexual behaviour; laboratory workers who handle the virus.

Administration: single dose by intramuscular injection into the deltoid, with booster at 6–12 months.

Adverse reactions: local transient soreness; rarely, malaise, fatigue, arthralgia, myalgia.

Protection: long-lasting, after booster, for up to 10 years.

Note: Now available combined with hepatitis B vaccine or with polysaccharide typhoid vaccine.

Hepatitis B vaccine

Contains: hepatitis B surface antigen (HBsAg) expressed in yeast cells using recombinant DNA technology; adsorbed on aluminium hydroxide.

Indications: those at special risk, e.g. parenteral drug misusers; homosexual and bisexual males; prostitutes; haemophiliacs; healthcare personnel and patients in hospitals for the mentally deficient and renal units; staff in casualty departments and laboratories; infants born to mothers who are HBsAg carriers.

Administration: in three doses intramuscularly into deltoid (*not* buttock), separated by 1 month and 6 months, respectively; can be more rapid with third booster at 2 months if required, e.g. by travellers.

Babies: born to HBsAg-positive mothers; require immunization immediately after birth; if mother is HBeAg-positive, if eAg status is unknown or if eAb-negative, give with hepatitis B immunoglobulin (HBIG).

Adverse reactions: local pain and redness.

Protection: apparently good, lasts at least 15 years: but note that routine immunization of healthcare staff results in a significant proportion of non-responders.

Combined hepatitis A and B vaccine

Contains: both hepatitis A and B vaccines.

Administered: in three doses into the deltoid, the second 1 month and the third 6 months after the first: boosters may be given after 5 years for those at continuing risk and may be with single-component vaccine.

Indications: those at special risk.

NB: Not to be used for postexposure prophylaxis or exposure via mucous membranes to hepatitis B.

Influenza vaccine

Contains: inactivated virus, usually two of the currently circulating strains of influenza A virus plus the current influenza B strain. Vaccines contain either 'split' virus (i.e. partially purified, disrupted particles) or surface antigen (purified haemagglutinin and neuraminidase). Virus for vaccine production is grown in eggs.

Indications: people aged 65 or over; patients with pre-existing cardiorespiratory or renal disease; diabetes or immunosuppression; if pandemic imminent, key personnel in essential services, e.g. hospital staff, the police force.

Administration: one dose by injection; vaccination needs to be repeated each winter.

Adverse reactions: few and mild; there may be severe reactions in those hypersensitive to eggs, in whom the vaccine is contraindicated.

Protection: short-lived, i.e. about 1 year: the protection conferred is of the order of 70%.

Poliomyelitis Salk inactivated vaccine

The first poliovaccine that gives good protection and produces serum antibody but not the gut immunity conferred by Sabin vaccine.

Contains: the three types of poliovirus inactivated by formaldehyde.

Administered: three doses intramuscularly, 4 weeks apart.

Indications: useful for immunocompromised patients.

Availability: on named-patient basis only in UK.

Protection: long-lasting.

Note: Although now largely replaced worldwide by oral Sabin vaccine, Salk is still the preferred vaccine in some countries, e.g. in Scandinavia.

Rabies vaccine

First developed by Pasteur in 1885 using spinal cords of infected rabbits attenuated by drying for different lengths of time.

Contains: inactivated virus grown in human diploid cells.

Administered: by deep subcutaneous or intramuscular deltoid injection in three doses at 0, 7 and 28 days for pre-exposure immunization; for travellers to enzootic areas, two doses 4 weeks apart; for those at continuous risk, give a booster at 6–12 months with further boosters every 2–3 years.

Side-effects: usually mild local reactions; rarely, systemic with urticaria, anaphylaxis.

Indications: workers in animal quarantine centres, zoos, or with animals abroad; others with possible exposure through their occupation, e.g. laboratory staff handling the virus; travellers to areas where exposure is possible, or to remote regions where medical treatment is not immediately available.

Protection: good, with high levels of neutralizing antibody produced.

Postexposure: five doses at 0, 3, 7, 14 and 30 days; with rabies-specific immunoglobulin; if previously immunized, two doses at 0 and days 3–7.

TOXOIDS

DIPHTHERIA TOXOID

Contains: diphtheria formol toxoid (i.e. toxin treated with formaldehyde) – usually adsorbed on a mineral carrier.

Indications: children and selected adults at risk, e.g. hospital or laboratory staff.

Administration: three spaced injections starting at 2 months old, as for pertussis vaccine, with which it is usually combined as part of the triple vaccine. Booster dose at school entry and on leaving school.

Older children (i.e. aged 10 years or more) and adults, use a *low-dose* vaccine: administer by deep subcutaneous or intramuscular injection.

Adverse reactions: mild and transient under 10 years of age; older children and adults may experience more severe side-effects.

Protection: excellent – the disappearance of diphtheria in the UK between 1941 and 1951 was due to immunization, and the disease is now extremely rare in this country.

Tetanus toxoid

Contains: tetanus formol toxoid adsorbed on a mineral carrier.

Indications: the aim is active immunization of the entire population: although tetanus is rare, it may develop after common, trivial wounds. Those at greatest risk are the non-immunized – now usually elderly people, and more often women.

Administration: three spaced injections, starting in infancy as part of the triple vaccine. In the unvaccinated a course should begin when a situation of risk presents, e.g. after injury, at the casualty department. Booster doses are given at school entry, on leaving school, and in the event of injury.

Adverse reactions: rare and minor; severe reactions may be seen in patients with hypersensitivity to a component, and occasionally in adults who have been hyperimmunized with too many booster injections.

Protection: excellent.

Triple vaccine

Contains: killed *Bordetella pertussis*, diphtheria toxoid and tetanus toxoid.

Indications: active immunization of all infants.

Administration: three doses by injection, at 2, 3 and 4 months of age. At school entry and leaving: booster doses of diphtheria and tetanus toxoids only.

Adverse reactions: see sections on individual vaccines.

Protection: see sections on individual vaccines.

SCHEDULE OF CHILDHOOD IMMUNIZATION RECOMMENDED IN THE UK

This is shown in Table 39.2.

TRAVEL ABROAD

Additional vaccinations – and sometimes booster doses of previous vaccines – are often advisable for travel abroad. These are shown in Table 39.3.

Arthropod-borne and other tropical virus vaccines: although not generally available (except for those against yellow fever and Japanese encephalitis), other vaccines have been developed for some of these viruses – eastern, western and Venezuelan equine encephalitis viruses; Rift Valley and Omsk haemorrhagic fevers; and tickborne encephalitis viruses. All contain inactivated virus. An attenuated virus vaccine has been produced against Junin haemorrhagic fever in Argentina. Note that some of these vaccines are at the experimental stage.

Smallpox vaccine: small quantities of this are available for those with special indications, e.g. working with vaccinia or other poxviruses in the laboratory. *Anthrax vaccine*: also available for those with occupational exposure.

Table 39.2   Schedule of vaccination and immunization recommended in the UK

Age	Vaccine	Notes
During the first year of life	Triple vaccine, polio vaccine, Hib Meningococcal	Give in three doses at 2, 3 and 4 months
During the second year of life (at age 12–15 months)	Measles–mumps–rubella	Administer to both boys and girls
3–5 years (school entry)	Diphtheria and tetanus toxoids	Booster dose
	Polio vaccine	Booster dose
	Measles–mumps–rubella	Booster dose
Between 10th and 14th birthdays	BCG vaccine	For tuberculin-negative children
13–18 years (on leaving school)	Polio vaccine	Booster dose
	Tetanus toxoid	Booster dose
	Diphtheria toxoid	Booster dose with low-dose vaccine

Table 39.3 Vaccines to be considered for travel

Vaccine	Indications; area of travel
Polio ⎫ Typhoid ⎬	Anywhere except Europe, North America, Australia, New Zealand
Cholera	Some countries in Asia, Africa, Middle East, South and Central America
Tetanus	If the traveller is unprotected and liable to be at risk
Yellow fever*	Some countries in South America and Africa
Rabies	Anywhere except Australia, New Zealand and various island communities (e.g. Cyprus) – if occupational exposure to animals
Meningococcal groups A, C	Endemic areas in North India, Nepal, Central Africa, Middle East
Tickborne encephalitis	Endemic areas in Eastern Europe
Japanese encephalitis	Endemic areas in Nepal, Thailand, Korea, China
Plague	For workers in rat-infested, poor conditions, e.g. refugee camps
Hepatitis A	For travel to tropical or semitropical regions
Hepatitis B	For workers exposed to blood and its products in areas of Asia and Africa with high carriage rate of HBsAg

* Vaccination certificate essential for travel to certain countries.

PASSIVE IMMUNIZATION

Produces *immediate* immunity by the injection of preformed anti-bodies in human sera. The immunity that follows wanes in a matter of weeks or a few months. Antisera are also used in treatment.

SPECIFIC IMMUNOGLOBULINS

Human immunoglobulins have replaced those made in animals, which often caused hypersensitivity reactions. Prepared from plasma pools containing high levels of appropriate antibody. Donations are taken from individuals recovering from infection (convalescent serum) or who have recently been actively immunized against the disease and are first screened for antibody content.

Protection: temporary; human immunoglobulins have a half-life of 26 days after injection: significant protection may last up to 3 months, sometimes longer.

Preparations

- *Hepatitis B immunoglobulin (HBIG)*: for babies born to mothers who are HBs and eAg positive; postexposure prophylaxis after accidental injury from high-risk or known HBsAg positive patients – rarely indicated because all health workers are now vaccinated against hepatitis B.
- *Rabies*: for postexposure prophylaxis in a non-immunized individual from a high-risk area.
- *Tetanus immunoglobulin*: for prophylaxis and treatment of tetanus.
- *Varicella-zoster immunoglobulin (ZIG)*: *prophylaxis of chickenpox*: important for seronegative pregnant women if in contact with case of varicella or zoster, especially in first 20 weeks or near the time of delivery: give to babies born to mothers who develop chickenpox 7 days before or within 28 days of delivery: also indicated for prevention or treatment of the disease in immunocompromised patients, who are likely to develop severe varicella or generalized zoster.

NORMAL IMMUNOGLOBULIN

Human immunoglobulin prepared from donations of pooled normal plasma: contains antibodies to the wide range of infective agents likely to have been encountered by most people, although often at only low level.

Indications

Prophylaxis of hepatitis A: no longer recommended for travel but still used for protection of household contacts of confirmed cases and to control outbreaks.

Prophylaxis of measles: given within 6 days of exposure to prevent or modify disease in immunocompromised children and adults.

To boost immunoglobulin levels in children with hypogamma-globulinaemia.

MEDICAL
MYCOLOGY

40 Fungal infections

Fungi, unlike bacteria, are *eukaryotic*: the cell nucleus contains multiple chromosomes enclosed by a membrane, and in the cytoplasm there are mitochondria and 80s ribosomes (see Chapter 2). Unlike plants, fungi do not contain chlorophyll and must therefore obtain their nutrients from their surroundings. Many fungi have a sexual stage that involves meiosis; for others only an asexual form is known. Most fungi grow as filaments (*hyphae*), which intertwine to form a network (the *mycelium*), and are known as moulds. Yeasts are unicellular and reproduce by budding.

Of the thousands of species of fungi, only a few are pathogenic for humans: some others cause disease in other animals or plants. However, with the increase in immunocompromised patients due to underlying disease or treatment, the last two decades have seen an unprecedented increase in the incidence and diversity of life-threatening invasive fungal infection (see Chapter 37).

Habitat: fungi, like bacteria, are ubiquitous. In the soil they play an important role in the degradation of organic compounds: they may produce antibiotics (e.g. penicillin) which inhibit the growth of competitive bacteria.

Culture: all fungi are aerobic: most are not fastidious and grow readily on simple media.

Classification: is complex and based on the method of spore production (sexual or asexual); the morphology of the colony; the vegetative hyphae that form the mycelium; and the specialized aerial hyphae that bear the spores. Fungi of medical importance can conveniently be divided into three groups:

- *Yeasts* – unicellular fungi which replicate by budding
- *Filamentous fungi* or moulds, which include the dermatophytes
- *Dimorphic fungi* – which grow as moulds in the environment and as yeasts in vivo.

DISEASES CAUSED BY FUNGI

Fungi cause three types of disease:

- Infections (mycoses)
- Mycotoxicoses
- Allergic reactions.

Infections (mycoses)

1. *Superficial infections* of the mucous membranes with yeasts (thrush) and of the keratinized tissue of skin, nail and hair with dermatophyte fungi (ringworm) are among the most widely suffered in the UK. However, although troublesome, they are usually trivial and do not involve deeper tissues.

2. *Subcutaneous infections*: the result of the traumatic implantation of spores of environmental fungi, leading to progressive local disease with considerable tissue destruction and sinus formation (eumycetoma): rare in the UK, but common in the tropics.

3. *Systemic infections*: with haematogenous spread throughout the body, are serious and often fatal: increasing in incidence in the UK in immunocompromised patients with impaired host defences (see Chapter 37), who may develop widespread disease due to yeasts or filamentous fungi such as *Aspergillus* species. In other parts of the world, certain forms of deep disseminated mycoses caused by dimorphic fungi are endemic and can occur in otherwise healthy individuals.

Mycotoxicoses

The result of ingesting food contaminated with moulds, in which the fungus has produced toxic metabolites, or poisoning following ingestion of poisonous toadstools. Many fungi can produce a variety of toxic metabolites. Probably the most significant is aflatoxin produced by *Aspergillus flavus*, which is a common contaminant of poorly stored food. Aflatoxin is carcinogenic and repeated ingestion can lead to liver cancer. Ingestion of *Claviceps purpurea* growing on infected wheat is the cause of ergotism.

Allergic reactions

Inhalation of fungal spores, notably those of *Aspergillus fumigatus*, may provoke a type I and/or a type III hypersensitivity reaction. Sometimes the antigenic stimulus is prolonged because the fungal hyphae grow in the lumen of the bronchi: invasion of lung tissue does not take place.

YEASTS

Yeasts are round to oval unicellular fungi, which reproduce by budding: some may develop *pseudohyphae* – chains of elongated budding cells – but only a few are able to form true hyphae.

CANDIDA

Infection with *Candida* spp. (candidosis) continues to play a predominant role among the invasive mycoses, and recent advances in medical and surgical procedures have increased the pool of susceptible patients. There has been a pathogen shift away from *Candida albicans* towards other *Candida* spp. Although *C. albicans* is still responsible for about half of the cases of candidaemia, other species, such as *Candida glabrata*, *Candida tropicalis*, *Candida parapsilosis*, *Candida krusei* and *Candida lusitaniae*, are isolated from blood cultures with increasing frequency, and specific yeast species appear to be particularly linked with different patient groups. Infection is usually acquired by cross infection.

CANDIDA ALBICANS

Habitat: the normal flora of the upper respiratory, gastrointestinal and female genital tracts.

Laboratory characteristics

Morphology and staining: two forms, both Gram-positive, are recognized in clinical material and on culture:

- Spherical to oval budding cells ($3–5 \times 5–10$ μm): the yeast or blastospore form.
- Elongated filamentous cells, joined end to end (*pseudohyphae*) and producing buds (*blastospores*); also true hyphae. These constitute the mycelial form. *C. albicans*, *C. tropicalis* and the recently recognized *Candida dubliniensis* all have the capacity to produce hyphae and pseudohyphae in vivo (see Fig. 6.1).

Culture: aerobic and easy to cultivate, but isolation from clinical material may be impeded by faster-growing bacteria:

1. *Sabouraud medium*: a simple glucose–peptone agar, pH 5.6, often made more selective by the addition of antibiotics (e.g. chloramphenicol): useful for primary isolation. Incubation at 37°C for 48 h may be necessary.
2. *Nutrient agar* and *blood agar*: colonies may be observed more easily around antibiotic discs which have inhibited bacterial growth.
3. *Chromogenic agar:* there are various agars that incorporate a chromogenic substrate to allow differentiation of some yeast species by the colour of the colonies they produce. Such agars are particularly useful for detecting mixed infections.

Colonial morphology: colonies are cream to white, flat or domed, and have a dry, glistening or waxy surface. The yeast cultures are predominantly blastospores, but mycelial forms may develop in older cultures, with pseudohyphae projecting from the edge of the colonies.

Identification: *C. albicans* can be readily differentiated from other species except *C. dubliniensis* by:

1. *Formation of germ tubes* by incubation in serum for 3 h at 37°C. A wet film reveals the presence of filamentous outgrowths – *germ tubes*, which can be distinguished from the pseudohyphae produced by other yeast species by the absence of pinching at the base of the tube.
2. *Formation of chlamydospores* on a dalmau plate which consists of a streak inoculum, on a nutritionally poor medium such as corn-meal agar, covered with a coverslip to produce microaerophilic conditions and incubated for 24 h at 28°C. The presence of round, thick-walled resting structures – *chlamydospores* – usually found at the ends of pseudohyphae, deep in the agar, is diagnostic for *C. albicans* and *C. dubliniensis*.

Abundant chlamydospore production is a particular feature of *C. dubliniensis* and can help to differentiate this species from *C. albicans*.

Biochemical activity: the results of fermentation (anaerobic metabolism) and assimilation (aerobic metabolism) of a range of carbohydrates are used in the identification of *Candida* species. Various commercial kits, some of which have chromogenic substrates to help to distinguish growth, can be used in conjunction with examination of morphology on a dalmau plate to identify the common pathogenic species.

Antigenic structure: strains fall into two serotypes: A – antigenically similar to *C. tropicalis*; and B. Low levels of candida antibodies can be demonstrated in most human sera. Delayed-type hypersensitivity is common, and a positive candida skin test is almost universal in normal adults.

Pathogenicity

Source: usually endogenous, but cross-infection may occur, e.g. from mother to baby, from baby to baby in a nursery; oral transfer of resistant strains has been demonstrated between HIV-infected individuals.

Host: infections are most common in babies who are premature and in adults debilitated by general ill health, notably diabetes. Other at-risk groups are composed of patients immunocompromised by either the nature of their disease (e.g. AIDS; malignancy, in particular leukaemias or lymphomas) or the treatment they have received (e.g. long courses of broad-spectrum antibiotics, immunosuppressive or cytotoxic drugs) and patients undergoing surgical procedures.

Clinical features

Infection is known as *candidosis*. The form of candidosis is determined by the nature of the underlying predisposition of the host. Thus minor predisposing factors lead to mild or superficial infection of the mucous membranes and skin, whereas more serious disturbances lead to deep, invasive infections.

Superficial: *mucous membranes*: thrush: white adherent patches on buccal mucosa or vagina.

Skin: red weeping areas, usually where skin is moist and traumatized, e.g. intertrigo in the obese.

Chronic mucocutaneous candidosis: an intractable, disfiguring condition, especially affecting the face and scalp, which usually becomes apparent within the first 2 years of life. The condition is due to a congenital defect in the immunological response, in which T-cell function is reduced but antibody response to candida remains normal. There are also associated abnormal hormone responses.

Deep: candidaemia may be transient and associated with a contaminated line, or may result in more serious consequences, with localization in various tissues, including eye, endocardium, meninges, kidney, liver and bone. Urinary infections may be easily treated or may be an indication of more serious kidney involvement.

Diagnosis

- By demonstration of yeasts in a wet film or Gram-stained smear, followed by isolation of candida when the specimen is cultured.
- By detection of mannan antigen in serum or other body fluid.
- By detection of antibody in serum. A variety of methods are available, e.g. countercurrent electrophoresis and ELISA. These tests are of limited value because antibody is present in more than half of the healthy adult population but is not produced by neutropenic patients with invasive disease. In an immunocompetent patient, high (>1:8) or rising titres can be indicative of active infection, and such tests are of particular value in patients with candida endocarditis.
- Investigational techniques include the detection of elevated levels of various metabolites, including arabinitol, by gas–liquid chromatography. The detection of β-1–3-D-glucan by the limulus lysate test and the detection of genomic sequences in body fluids by PCR.

Treatment

Candida are eukaryotic microorganisms, and the number of potential targets for antifungal agents is smaller than that for prokaryotic cells: thus there are considerably fewer drugs with the selective toxicity required for use in vivo than for bacterial infections.

Superficial infections can be treated topically with a polyene (nystatin, amphotericin B) or an imidazole (miconazole, clotrimazole, econazole, tioconazole).

Systemic infections may be treated with intravenous amphotericin B, either given alone or with 5-fluorocytosine: the combination may be synergistic in some cases. Lipid or conventional formulations of amphotericin may be used, but the former are associated with reduced toxicity. Oral administration of fluconazole (not for *C. glabreta* or *C. krusei*) or itraconazole is effective in mucosal and systemic candida infections: they may also be used prophylactically in susceptible (e.g. neutropenic) patients. There are several new azole antifungals (posaconazole, ravuconazole and voriconazole) and a cancidin (caspofungin) in late stages of clinical development, all of which have good activity against yeasts.

CRYPTOCOCCUS

The major pathogenic species in the genus is *Cryptococcus neoformans*. Two varieties have been distinguished, *C. neoformans* var. *neoformans* and *C. neoformans* var. *gatii*.

CRYPTOCOCCUS NEOFORMANS

Habitat: *C. neoformans* var. *neoformans* is a ubiquitous saprophyte: often found in soil contaminated with pigeon guano. The natural distribution of *C. neoformans* var. *gatii* follows that of the River Red Gum tree *Eucalyptus camaldulensis* and is therefore limited to tropical and subtropical climates.

Laboratory characteristics

Morphology and staining: a capsulated, budding yeast with spherical cells 5–15 μm in diameter; does not form a pseudomycelium. Gram-positive, although the capsule may prevent staining.

Culture: aerobic: grows on a wide variety of common media at 37°C, but also at room temperature. Isolation from clinical material is best achieved by culture at 30°C: several days' incubation may be required before colonies develop.

Colonial morphology: on Sabouraud medium forms glistening mucoid cream colonies, which become duller and darker on extended incubation.

Identification: make a wet preparation of a portion of the colony in Indian ink to demonstrate the capsule. *Note*: the capsule, which is usually pronounced in clinical material, may be rudimentary in culture.

Biochemical activity: produces a urease; assimilates a number of compounds, including inositol, but is unable to metabolize by fermentation; produces phenol oxidase, detected by the formation of brown colonies on birdseed agar.

Pathogenicity

Pathogenic for humans and a variety of animals.

Source: from the environment, usually by inhalation, especially of dust containing pigeon excreta.

Clinical features

A lung granuloma, usually symptomless, is the primary lesion. This resolves spontaneously and, in the vast majority of patients, without dissemination. Haematogenous spread results in subacute or chronic meningoencephalitis – the classic disease presentation – and sometimes involvement of skin, lungs, lymph nodes and other organs. Clinical disease is usually found in immunocompromised patients, especially those with AIDS – cryptococcal meningitis is a common AIDS-defining illness.

Diagnosis

- By demonstration in CSF, exudate, urine or other appropriate specimen of an encapsulated yeast, confirmed by isolation on culture. A drop of Indian ink mixed with a drop of infected body fluid may reveal budding yeasts surrounded by a clear area or halo, which occurs when the ink particles are displaced by the capsule. *Note*: CSF changes resemble those in tuberculous meningitis, and the yeast may be confused with red blood cells or lymphocytes.
- By detection of antigen in CSF, blood or urine, using a latex agglutination test.
- By detection of antibody in serum: a variety of tests are available, including agglutination and immunofluorescence.

Treatment

Intravenous amphotericin B combined with 5-fluorocytosine. This combination is synergistic and results in faster sterilization of the CSF than amphotericin alone. Fluconazole is an alternative treatment for less severe infections. After primary therapy, particularly in AIDS patients, maintenance therapy with fluconazole should be continued to prevent relapse.

MALASSEZIA

Malassezia furfur (*Pityrosporum furfur*, *P. orbiculare*, *P. ovale*, *P. sympodialis*) and *Malassezia pachydermatis* are both implicated in human infection.

Habitat: skin; *M. pachydermatis* is particularly associated with the ears of dogs.

Laboratory characteristics

Morphology: oval yeast, reproducing by unipolar budding on a broad base to reveal a characteristic shoe-print-like appearance.

Culture: dull, buff colonies on agar supplemented with lipids, e.g. olive oil. *M. pachydermatis* grows poorly on unsupplemented Sabouraud medium.

Pathogenicity

Superficial: *M. furfur* is the cause of pityriasis (tinea) versicolor, in which large scaling patches develop on the skin of the trunk: brownish on light-skinned people, lighter on dark-skinned people; usually asymptomatic. This yeast is also associated with seborrhoeic dermatitis and dandruff.

Systemic: catheter-related fungaemia due to *M. furfur* and *M. pachydermatis* has emerged as a well recognized complication of the administration of total parenteral nutrition. Such infections are most commonly encountered in low-birthweight infants, and there are numerous reports of outbreaks on neonatal intensive care units often involving *M. pachydermatis*.

Diagnosis

Although the yeast can be isolated on culture, diagnosis of pityriasis versicolor is usually made by the demonstration of short, curved, non-branching hyphae and yeasts in skin scales.

Systemic infection is diagnosed by the presence of a poorly growing yeast isolated from blood culture with the typical morphological appearance of a *Malassezia* species.

OTHER YEASTS

In recent years there has been an increase in the number of invasive infections in immunocompromised patients caused by yeasts that were previously regarded as contaminants or harmless commensals. Many are yeasts found in foodstuffs or as commensals of the mouth or gastrointestinal tract. Trichosporonosis, caused by *Trichosporon beigelii* (formerly *cutaneum*) and *Blastoschizomyces capitatus* (formerly *Trichosporon capitatum*), is a deep or disseminated infection of immunocompromised patients associated with a high mortality. *Saccharomyces cerevisiae*, better known as brewers' and bakers' yeast, has been implicated in increasing numbers of fungaemias in compromised patients. Other species encountered on a regular basis are *Geotrichum candidum*, *Hansenula anomola*, *Pichia* spp. and *Rhodotorula* spp.

FILAMENTOUS FUNGI

DERMATOPHYTES

The dermatophytes comprise a group of fungi which cause infection – *tinea* or *ringworm* – of the keratinized tissue of the skin, nails and hair. They belong to three different genera, *Trichophyton*, *Microsporum* and *Epidermophyton*, and can be further subdivided into those species that are anthropophilic, zoophilic or geophilic. The common species and the types of ringworm they cause are listed in Table 40.1. There are also some dermatomycotic moulds capable of causing skin or nail infections. Tinea nigra, caused by *Phaeonnellomyces werneckii*, and *Scytalidium dimidiatum* (*Hendersonula toruloidea*) can cause infection of the skin. There are a large number of moulds that can cause infection in traumatized nails, the most common being *Scopulariopsis brevicaulis*, *Aspergillus versicolor* group and *Fusarium* spp.

Habitat: the keratin of humans and animals.

Source: by person-to-person spread, sometimes via fomites, or from contact with animals, as a zoonosis. A few species are present in the soil (Table 40.1).

Clinical features

These are summarized in Table 40.2.

Table 40.1 Dermatophytes and ringworm

| | | | Type of ringworm caused | | | |
| | | | | *Tinea* | | |
Fungus	Source	capita	corporis	cruris	pedis	unguium
Trichophyton rubrum	Human		+	++	+++	+++
Trichophyton mentagrophytes var. interdigitale	Human			+	++	+
Trichophyton mentagrophytes var. mentagrophytes	Animal: cattle, horses, rodents	+	++			
Trichophyton tonsurus	Human	++	+			
Trichophyton schoenleinii	Human	+ (Usual cause of favus)				
Microsporum audouinii	Human	+	+			
Microsporum canis	Animal: cats, dogs	+++	++			
Microsporum gypseum	Soil	+	+			
Epidermophyton floccosum	Human			++	+	+

+++: most commonly caused by; ++: commonly caused by; +: sometimes caused by.

Diagnosis

Specimen: scrapings of skin or nail, sellotape strippings of skin or short lengths of plucked hair.

Preparation: make a wet preparation of the specimen in 20% potassium hydroxide: leave for 10–20 min to digest the keratin. Use of an optical brightener such as Calcofluor and a fluorescence microscope may enhance the detection of fungal hyphae, particularly in nail tissue.

Observe: filamentous branching hyphae: arthrospores may also be seen. In tinea capitis, fungal elements and arthrospores may be seen either outside the hair – *ectothrix* infections, e.g. with *Microsporum canis* or, less commonly, inside the hair – *endothrix* infections, e.g. with *Trichophyton tonsurans* and *Trichophyton schoenleinii*.

Table 40.2 Clinical manifestations of ringworm

Site	Affects	Clinical features
Tinea capitis	Scalp and hair	Small scaling papules which spread to leave areas of baldness: infected hairs break, to leave stumps. Skin may suppurate. *Favus* is a variety characterized by yellow lesions which later develop cup-shaped crusts that heal, leaving atrophic bald skin
Tinea corporis	Skin, excluding scalp, bearded areas and feet	Circular spreading lesions: as the centre scales and heals, the periphery advances, with vesicles and pustules in inflamed skin
Tinea cruris	Skin of groin and perineum	Spreading scaly dermatitis, with vesicopustular edge: little central healing
Tinea pedis	Soles of feet and between toes	Inflamed skin with vesicles, leading to peeling and fissure formation (athlete's foot)
Tinea unguium	Nails of hands or feet	Affected nails appear opaque, thickened, and distorted: they may separate from nailbed and be totally destroyed

Culture: necessary to identify the causal fungus: *inoculate* the specimen on to a plate of Sabouraud agar containing chloramphenicol: this antibiotic suppresses the growth of contaminating bacteria. It is also important to include an agent such as actidione to suppress mould growth, unless mould infection is suspected. With nail specimens where mould infections are more common specimens should be inoculated on to agar with and without actidione. *Incubate* aerobically at 25–30°C. *Examine* daily up to 21 days, for fungal colonies.

Colonial appearance: observe pigmentation and texture of the surface of the colony, and pigmentation of the reverse side, seen through the bottom of the plate. Colonial morphology can vary considerably.

Microscopic features of colony: gently remove and tease out a small portion of the colony using needles, suspend in a drop of lactophenol cotton blue or lactofuchsin, and place a cover slip over the preparation, *or*, using a small piece of double-sided sticky tape gently press on to the surface of the colony, remove and mount fungus-side uppermost in a drop of mounting fluid, place a second drop on the surface and cover with a coverslip. This technique results in better preservation of the structural arrangement of spores. *Observe*: hyphae and *conidia* – asexual spores. Two types of conidia are formed by dermatophytes: small unicellular *microconidia* and larger, septate *macroconidia*. Microscopic morphology aids identification.

Treatment

Mild infections: topical imidazole (e.g. clotrimazole, miconazole, ticonazole), or topical terbinafine.

Severe infections: oral terbinafine and itraconazole are effective, as is oral griseofulvin: prolonged treatment is required if hair, and especially nails, are involved.

ASPERGILLUS

Invasive aspergillosis has become a well recognized complication of prolonged immunosuppression and is the leading cause of infective death in patients undergoing allogeneic bone marrow transplantation. *Aspergillus fumigatus* is the main pathogen (85% cases): other species associated with infection include *A. flavus* (5–10%), *A. niger* (2–3%) and *A. terreus* (2–3%), and others only rarely.

Habitat: soil and dust: spores are ubiquitous.

Laboratory characteristics

Culture: after 3–4 days' incubation on Sabouraud agar at 25–37°C the colonies have a velvety to powdery surface and are characteristically coloured: *A. fumigatus* is dark blue-green; *A. niger* black on white, *A. flavus* yellow-green and *A. terreus* cinnamon.

Microscopic colonial appearance: a wet preparation stained with lactophenol cotton blue demonstrates septate hyphae and *conidiophores* – specialized structures that bear phialides which produce conidia (i.e. spores). The conidiophores have swollen, rounded ends and the spores are formed in dry chains which are suited to air dispersal. The general morphology is characteristic of the genus, and there are also interspecies differences that are useful in identification (Fig. 40.1).

Clinical features

Aspergillus species can cause a variety of clinical syndromes:
- *Allergic bronchopulmonary aspergillosis*: inhaled spores provoke a hypersensitivity reaction, which may be of:
  - type I (asthma)
  - type III (extrinsic alveolitis)
  - types I and III combined.

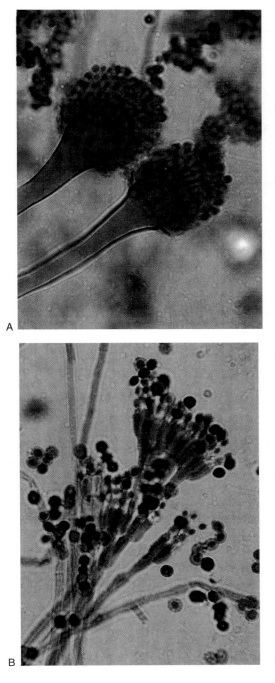

A

B

Fig. 40.1 *(continued overleaf)*

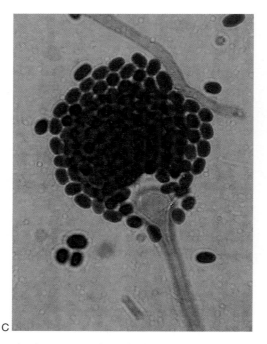

Fig. 40.1 Spore-bearing structures of some fungi. A. *Aspergillus fumigatus* – spores are formed in chains from phialides on a conidiophore. B. *Penicillium chrysogenum* – spores are formed in chains from phialides produced by a branching conidiophore structure. C. *Absidia corymbifera*, a zygomycete – spores are formed within a sporangium, which ruptures to release them.

- *Aspergilloma,* in which a fungal ball grows within, and is usually restricted to, an existing lung cavity, e.g. due to tuberculosis, sarcoidosis, bronchiectasis.
- *Invasive aspergillosis,* in which the fungus establishes a pneumonia and later disseminates to involve other organs, e.g. brain, kidneys, heart: mortality is high. Patients who develop this type of disease are usually immunocompromised (see Chapter 37).
- *Superficial infections* of the external ear (*otomycosis*) and, less commonly, the eye (*mycotic keratitis*) and nasal sinuses.

Diagnosis

Computerized tomography (CT) scans have proved invaluable in the early diagnosis of invasive aspergillosis, as lesions are apparent on CT earlier than they are on chest radiographs. The halo sign, in which a hazy area due to haemorrhage can be seen around the lesion, is visible in the first 1–10 days; the crescent sign, in which a crescent-shaped air space forms within the lesion, is not useful diagnostically as it classically appears later in the course of infection and is a sign of neutrophil recovery.

Direct microscopy to demonstrate septate hyphae: suggestive, but not diagnostic of, aspergillus infection.

Specimens

Sputum: make a wet preparation in 20% potassium hydroxide. Bronchoalveolar lavage (BAL) is a particularly useful specimen and preferable to sputum.

Tissue, e.g. biopsy or post-mortem material: stain sections by PAS (periodic acid–Schiff) method – hyphae are poorly stained by haematoxylin and eosin or Grocott's stain, which is a specific fungal stain. Septate hyphae branching at right-angles are highly suggestive of invasive aspergillosis but cannot be distinguished from the other less common causes of hyalohyphomycosis.

Isolation by culture: on Sabouraud agar at 25–37°C. Colonies grow after 48 h, but longer incubation may be required before characteristic morphological features develop.

Note: Because aspergillus spores are ubiquitous, colonies of the fungus are often found growing on cultures as the result of aerial contamination. Thus it may be difficult to interpret the significance of isolating a few colonies from a clinical specimen. Significance is enhanced if the fungus was seen on direct microscopic examination.

Serology: precipitating antibodies to aspergillus antigens can be demonstrated by a number of laboratory methods, including countercurrent immunoelectrophoresis, immunodiffusion and ELISA. Antibodies are usually absent from the sera of healthy individuals, but can be detected in the majority (70%) of patients with allergic aspergillosis; are found at high levels in patients with endocarditis but are rarely found in neutropenic patients with invasive disease. In immunocompromised patients it may be more helpful to look for circulating antigens. There is a commercial ELISA test for galactomannan, a cell-wall component of *Aspergillus* spp., and a test known as G-test, which is a limulus lysate test for 1-3-β-D-glucans from the fungal cell wall. There is also extensive development of PCR tests for the detection of circulating genomic sequences.

Treatment

Invasive aspergillosis is treated with intravenous amphotericin B: newer lipid preparations have toxicity benefits over the conventional formulation. Oral itraconazole may also be effective: commonly used in prophylaxis of high-risk patients and for maintenance therapy following initial treatment. Mortality of invasive aspergillosis remains high and may be as high as 90% in patients with persistent neutropenia. There are newer drugs for the treatment of invasive aspergillosis: cancidin, which targets the 1-3-β-D-glucans in the fungal cell wall, liposomal nystatin and the triazoles: posaconazole, ravuconazole and voriconazole are all currently undergoing clinical trials.

ZYGOMYCETES

The genera associated with human infection are *Mucor*, *Absidia* and *Rhizopus*.

Habitat: ubiquitous in the soil: spores in air and dust.

Laboratory characteristics

All three genera are similar in that they produce a fast-growing non-septate mycelium which produces spores in specialist structures known as sporangia.

Culture: after 3–4 days' incubation on Sabouraud agar at 30–37°C the colonies are grey-white or brown, with a thick cottony, fluffy surface that rapidly fills the available air-space of the plate.

Microscopic colonial appearance: non-septate broad hyphae which produce aerial *sporangiophores* from which a *sporangium* is formed – a sac containing spores (sporangiospores) (see Fig. 40.1).

Clinical features

Zygomycosis (mucormycosis, phycomycosis) occurs as a systemic infection following inhalation of spores and dissemination from a primary focus in the lung or nasal sinus: almost all patients are immunocompromised or suffering from ketoacidosis associated with diabetes (see Chapter 37). The rhinocerebral form, in which the nose, nasal sinuses and orbit are involved, is a well recognized and usually fatal complication of diabetes: infection may penetrate to involve the frontal lobe of the brain. Cutaneous zygomycosis follows infection of a wound site, especially burns.

Diagnosis

Direct microscopy: to demonstrate broad, non-septate hyphae.

Specimens

Exudate: make a wet preparation in 20% potassium hydroxide.

Tissue: hyphae stain readily with haematoxylin and eosin (unlike aspergillus) and are easily distinguished in a Grocott's stain as broad aseptate hyphae which differ from the narrower, septate hyphae of aspergillus and other agents of hyalohyphomycosis.

Isolation by culture on Sabouraud agar: may be difficult to achieve from necrotic material, even when abundant hyphae are seen. It is important that tissue samples are not homogenized, as this will result in disruption of the hyphae into small, non-viable fragments.

Note: These common environmental moulds are not infrequent contaminants of culture plates.

Treatment

Surgical debridement as far as is possible forms an important component of the therapy, and should be combined with high-dose intravenous lipid amphotericin B. Good medical control of the underlying diabetes or resolution of neutropenia are also important. The developmental azoles may have a role in control of some of the causative agents of this disease.

EMERGING MOULD PATHOGENS

HYALOHYPHOMYCOSIS AND PHAEOHYPHOMYCOSIS

The recent increase in the number of immunocompromised individuals has led to an increase in the number and spectrum of moulds recognized as capable of causing deep infection. Two terms have been coined: *hyalohyphomycosis* describes infection with moulds that adopt a hyaline or colourless, septate filamentous form in tissue, and *phaeohyphomycosis* describes infection with pigmented, septate filamentous moulds. Most of the moulds currently encountered as emerging pathogens come under the collective term of hyalohyphomycosis. The most common emerging pathogens are *Fusarium* and *Scedosporium* species, which are often responsible for devastating and refractory infections. Deep infections with *Acremonium* and *Paecilomyces* are seen less frequently, and others only rarely.

Treatment

Infections with *Fusarium* species and *Scedosporium* species are difficult to treat and a favourable outcome is often only associated with neutrophil recovery together with antifungal chemotherapy. *Scedosporium apiospermum* responds better in vitro to azole antifungals, including voriconazole, than amphotericin B, but *Scedosporium prolificans* demonstrates in vitro resistance to all the currently available agents.

PNEUMOCYSTIS CARINII

At the start of the AIDS era the opportunistic fungus *Pneumocystis carinii* emerged as the predominant cause of pneumonia in HIV-infected individuals. It is currently encountered as an AIDS-defining illness in those intolerant to, or non-compliant with, prophylaxis or antiretroviral therapy, and also remains a significant cause of morbidity and mortality in other groups of immunosuppressed individuals.

Lifecycle: unknown, as is the *route* of human infection, although this is most likely to be via the respiratory tract.

Pathogenesis: pneumocystis pneumonia is the result of reactivation of latent infection.

Subclinical infection in early life is probably widespread.

Immunocompromised: symptoms are rarely (if ever) seen in immunologically competent people: pneumocystis pneumonia is a major indicator disease of AIDS.

CLINICALLY

Symptoms are of a severe pneumonia, with progressive dyspnoea and cyanosis leading to respiratory failure. On X-ray, bilateral diffuse infiltrates.

Diagnosis

Demonstration of the morphologically characteristic cysts or 'trophozoites' in bronchial aspirates, specimens of bronchial

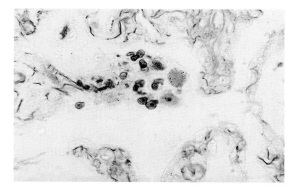

Fig. 40.2 *Pneumocystis carinii* in bronchial washing; methenamine silver stain (approx. × 1000). Courtesy of Dr C. J. R. Stewart.

lavage or lung biopsy: stained by methenamine silver (Fig. 40.2) or by immunofluorescence with monoclonal antibody. There has been recent development of molecular diagnostic methods.

Treatment

Most antifungal agents do not have activity against *P. carinii*, which lacks ergosterol in its cell membrane; an exception is the recently developed cancidin, caspofungin. Infections are usually treated with co-trimoxazole or pentamidine isetionate, also atovaquone, dapsone and trimethoprim, clindamycin or primaquine, but mortality is high despite treatment; in AIDS patients, trimetrexate with folinic acid. Sometimes inhaled pentamidine in mild disease.

Prophylaxis: co-trimoxazole, pentamidine, dapsone or atovaquone.

PENICILLIUM MARNEFFEI INFECTION

A variety of *Penicillium* species abound in the environment and grow on bread, jam, fruit, cheese etc. In the laboratory *Penicillium* is a common airborne contaminant of culture media. *Penicillium marneffei* is the only dimorphic member of the genus, growing as a mould at 30°C and in the environment, and as a yeast in vivo and at 37°C in the laboratory. This agent is increasingly implicated in systemic infection in AIDS patients who are resident in or have travelled to areas of endemicity in northern Thailand, Vietnam, India and southern China. As it is also able to cause infection in individuals with no recognized predisposing factors it is handled as a containment-level 3 pathogen in the UK.

Colonies are blue-green or yellow with a white border, and have a powdery surface. A particular feature is a red-diffusing pigment. If the cultures are incubated at 37°C there is conversion to the yeast form, in which the yeast can be seen to divide by binary fission.

Microscopy demonstrates septate hyphae with branched conidiophores bearing chains of spores, the appearance likened to a 'brush or broom' (Fig. 40.1). Histology reveals yeasts splitting by binary fission.

Treatment

Treatment with amphotericin B or itraconazole is usually effective. The newer developmental agents may also have potential.

OTHER DIMORPHIC FUNGI

Dimorphic fungi grow as either yeasts or filaments. The *yeast form* (parasitic phase) is found in infected tissues and on artificial media at 37°C. The *filamentous form* (saprophytic phase) is present in the soil and on artificial media at 22–25°C.

Habitat: soil: some have a characteristic geographical distribution (Table 40.3).

Pathogenicity

Cause disease in humans (Table 40.3) and in wild and domestic animals.

Infection is usually acquired by inhalation, with the primary lesions in the lungs. In most cases these heal, often without causing illness, and delayed hypersensitivity develops, with a positive skin-test reaction to the appropriate antigen. Progressive disease may affect the lungs, sometimes causing cavitation, and/or

Table 40.3 Dimorphic fungi and disease

Fungus	Disease	Geographical distribution
Blastomyces dermatitidis	North American blastomycosis	North America, especially Mississippi and Ohio valleys
Paracoccidioides brasiliensis	South American blastomycosis	South America; less commonly, Central America
Coccidioides immitis	Coccidioidomycosis	USA from California to Texas; South and Central America
Histoplasma capsulatum var *capsulatum*	Histoplasmosis	Eastern and Central USA; occasionally other parts of the world
Histoplasma capsulatum var *duboisii*	African histoplasmosis	Equatorial Africa
Penicillium marneffei	Penicilliosis	Southeast Asia, Southern China
Sporothrix schenckii	Sporotrichosis	Worldwide

disseminate widely to involve the skin, mucous membranes and internal organs. The lesions are chronic granulomas. *Note* the similarity of this disease process to tuberculosis.

Sporotrichosis is different: it follows traumatic implantation of the fungus into the skin and results in a chronic local pyogenic infection, with lymphatic spread and ulceration of the lymph nodes: disseminated disease is rare.

Diagnosis

Direct demonstration of the yeast-like form in suitably stained preparations of exudate (e.g. sputum, pus) or biopsy specimens or, in the case of coccidioidomycosis, the demonstration of spherule production. Spherules are large, thick-walled structures containing multiple endospores.

Isolation on appropriate culture media, incubated at the correct temperature: some of the fungi grow slowly in culture. One of the features of these dimorphic fungal pathogens is that many of them will grow on medium containing actidione, which usually suppresses mould growth.

Serology: useful in the diagnosis of histoplasmosis, coccidioidomycosis and South American blastomycosis, but of uncertain value in the other diseases because of difficulties in interpreting the significance of antibody levels.

Treatment

Amphotericin B is the drug of choice for invasive disease. Itraconazole or fluconazole are alternative treatments, especially for long-term therapy.

FUNGI CAUSING MYCETOMA

Mycetoma usually affects the foot (Madura foot) and can be caused by a variety of fungi and actinomycetes (usually *Nocardia* species: see Chapter 3). Important filamentous fungi which cause mycetoma include *Madurella mycetomatis*, *Madurella grisea* and *Phialophora verrucosa*.

Habitat: soil.

Pathogenicity

Fungi implanted into subcutaneous tissue following trauma (e.g. by a splinter) produce destructive granulomatous lesions, with suppuration and abscess formation in soft tissue and bone, which drain through multiple sinus tracts. There is local spread but no dissemination. A common condition in tropical and subtropical areas where people go barefoot.

Treatment

Chemotherapy is less effective when mycetoma is due to filamentous fungi, but some of the newer agents may have potential. Radical surgical debridement is an important component.

CHROMOBLASTOMYCOSIS

Chromoblastomycosis is a chronic, localized infection of the skin and subcutaneous tissue, mainly of the limbs, and is characterized by raised crusted lesions. It is caused by brown-pigmented (dematiaceous) fungi such as *Phialophora verrucosa*, *Fonsecaea* spp. and *Cladophialophora carionii*.

Habitat: soil, wood and plant material.

Pathogenicity

Infection follows traumatic inoculation of the fungus, and commonly affects the limbs. Lymphatic spread may follow, with satellite lesions around the initial lesion that develop into hyperkeratotic plaques.

Treatment

This condition is difficult to treat. Local application of heat may be beneficial, and a long course of oral itraconazole.

MEDICAL PARASIT- OLOGY

Parasitic infections

Parasites are larger and more complex organisms than bacteria. Classified as:

- Protozoa: single-celled parasites
- Metazoa: multicelled parasites.

Infection with parasites is a major cause of morbidity and mortality in tropical and semitropical countries. In Britain infections are increasing, partly because of increasing foreign travel; also, large immigrant communities have resulted in the import of tropical parasites. This chapter can only describe a few of the more important encountered in Britain, although this includes several kinds that must have been acquired abroad.

Transmission

- *Faecal–oral*: the most common route
- *Arthropod vectors*
- *Intermediate hosts*, e.g. snails, fish, are required for the lifecycle of certain parasites.

PARASITIC INFECTIONS INDIGENOUS TO THE UK

Table 41.1 lists the main parasites that can be acquired in Britain.

Table 41.1 Parasites indigenous to Britain

Parasite	Host	Source of infection	Principal symptoms*
Nematodes (roundworms)			
Toxocara canis	Dog	Dog faeces	Often asymptomatic sometimes visceral larva migrans
Toxocara cati	Cat	Cat faeces	Cerebral or ocular damage
Enterobius vermicularis	Human	Faecal–oral	Asymptomatic, anal pruritus
Cestodes (tapeworms)			
Echinococcus granulosus	Dog, sheep	Animal faeces	Hydatid cysts, especially liver and lung
Trematodes (flukes)			
Fasciola hepatica	Sheep	Contaminated watercress	Hepatitis, cholecystitis, cholangitis
Protozoa			
Trichomonas vaginalis	Human	Sexual transmission	Vaginal discharge
Toxoplasma gondii	Cat	Cat faeces; raw or undercooked meat	Lymphadenopathy; congenital infection
Giardia lamblia	Human	Contaminated water	Diarrhoea
Acanthamoeba species	Human	Corneal abrasions, contaminated contact lens solutions	Keratitis, uveitis, corneal ulceration

* Symptomless infection is common with all parasites.

TOXOCARA CANIS AND *TOXOCARA CATI* (TOXOCARIASIS)

T. canis and *T. cati* are the common roundworms of dogs and cats, respectively. Humans are the *paratenic* (or incidental) hosts, in whom the parasite does not develop fully (i.e. beyond the second larval stage).

Adult worms: length: 5–15 cm. *Habitat*: small intestine of dogs or cats (the definitive hosts).

Pathogenesis: after ingestion, the eggs hatch in the small intestine into larvae, which then migrate, often widely, into other tissues.

Clinical features

Infection: most often symptomless.

Disease: *visceral larva migrans*, owing to larval migration in the body and most often seen in children: accompanied by eosinophilia, hepatomegaly, chronic pulmonary infection or pneumonitis – with cough and fever.

Ocular lesions: retinitis, usually unilateral and due to migrating larvae, is the commonest manifestation – usually seen in children.

Diagnosis: *ELISA test*, with secretory/excretory products (derived from second-stage larvae maintained in vitro) as antigen.

Treatment: albendazole (of doubtful efficacy); photocoagulation of ocular lesions.

Control: de-worming of pets.

ENTEROBIUS VERMICULARIS (THREADWORM)

Known as *pinworms*. Common in children: often asymptomatic, but pruritus ani is a frequent complication, and can perpetuate autoinfection because infection is via the faecal–oral route.

Adult worms: length: about 1 cm. *Habitat*: caecum and colon.

Females: migrate to the anus and lay eggs on perianal skin.

Diagnosis

Demonstration of eggs (ova) on perianal sellotape smear, or of adult worms in faeces.

Treatment: mebendazole, piperazine.

ECHINOCOCCUS GRANULOSUS (HYDATID DISEASE)

A disease of sheep-rearing communities, but rare in Britain. Dogs – the definitive hosts – acquire infection by feeding on sheep offal containing hydatid cysts.

Adult worms (tapeworms): length: about 1 cm. *Habitat*: small intestine.

Pathogenesis: in the dog, adult worms mature in the small intestine, producing eggs which are excreted in the faeces.

Infection of humans is by ingestion of eggs, but humans are accidental and intermediate hosts.

Eggs hatch in the human duodenum or small intestine into embryos, which migrate via the portal blood supply to the liver and, less often, the lungs.

In liver and lungs (and rarely other tissues, such as muscle, brain, bones), larvae develop into *hydatid cysts*. The cysts may be large, are filled with clear fluid and contain characteristic protoscolices (immature forms of the head of the parasite): the protoscolices mature into developed scolices, which are infective for dogs.

Clinical features

Asymptomatic infection is common, especially with hydatid disease of the lungs; humans are surprisingly tolerant, even of large cysts in the liver.

Symptoms include *hepatomegaly*, with abdominal pain and discomfort; *cough*, sometimes with haemoptysis in lung hydatid disease; *pressure*, resulting from expanding cysts, may cause signs and symptoms in any of the affected organs and tissues.

Rupture of cysts can cause a severe allergic reaction, such as type I anaphylaxis.

Diagnosis

- *Scan*: ultrasound or CT
- *Serology*
- *Demonstration* of characteristic protoscolices in cysts removed at operation: histology of cyst wall.

Treatment: for active cysts, albendazole followed by surgery. If inoperable, albendazole alone.

FASCIOLA HEPATICA (FASCIOLIASIS)

The common liver fluke of sheep and cattle.

Replicative cycle involves an intermediate host, the snail *Lymnaea truncatula*. Fasciola eggs from sheep (or cattle) develop into *miracidia*, which infect the snails: after a complex multiplication process, *cercariae* are shed from the snails on to surrounding vegetation, forming *metacercariae*. These are infectious for sheep and cattle, and also for humans.

Route of infection for humans: most often, by eating contaminated watercress.

Adult worms: length: 3 cm; width: 1.5 cm. *Habitat*: the larger biliary passages and gall bladder.

Pathogenesis: After ingestion, metacercaria burrow through the wall of the duodenum and cross the peritoneal cavity to the bile ducts and liver tissue.

Clinically: human disease is often mild.

Symptoms include: fever; dyspepsia; anorexia; vomiting; pain in epigastrium or right upper abdomen.

Hepatomegaly, with tenderness over the liver and sometimes with disturbance of liver function; occasionally, jaundice.

Allergic reactions, such as urticaria or eosinophilia, are common.

Diagnosis

Demonstration of eggs in faeces or bile.

Treatment: triclabendazole.

TRICHOMONAS VAGINALIS (TRICHOMONIASIS)

A flagellated protozoon and the major cause of vaginitis in women.

Transmission: mostly sexually transmitted from males with inapparent infection; possibly also via contaminated articles.

Clinically: vaginal discharge, characteristic greenish-yellow, foamy discharge, with an offensive smell.

Diagnosis

Demonstration of motile parasites in wet preparations of vaginal secretion.

Culture in Fineberg's medium.

Treatment: metronidazole, tinidazole.

TOXOPLASMA GONDII (TOXOPLASMOSIS)

A protozoon which is a parasite of all warm-blooded animals. Cats are the only definitive hosts.

In the cat: the parasite develops as sexual forms in the small intestine, and eventually oöcysts are excreted in the faeces. Trophozoites – characteristically crescent-shaped – can spread widely in cat organs and tissues, with subsequent development into cysts.

Transmission: ingestion of oöcysts shed in cat faeces, or of trophozoites or cysts in undercooked meat, e.g. pork or mutton from infected animals.

Pathogenesis: humans – like other warm-blooded animals – are intermediate hosts. After ingestion, the protozoon, which is an obligate intracellular parasite, disseminates widely via the bloodstream. Cysts form – especially in the brain and muscles, and also in the eye.

Clinical features

Primary infection: usually symptomless, although probably always results in a generalized infection. Symptoms include fever, myalgia, headache, fatigue and lymphadenopathy. Rarely: hepatitis, encephalitis, myocarditis, chorioretinitis.

Congenital infection: acquired in utero, as a complication of primary infection in the mother during pregnancy, this can also cause abortion or stillbirth. Unlike infection in later life, congenital infection is generally severe. Typically presents with *a triad* of disorders:

• Chorioretinitis
• Hydrocephalus or microcephaly
• Cerebral calcification.

Congenitally infected babies also have signs of generalized infection, e.g. fever, rash, jaundice and hepatosplenomegaly.

Later sequelae of congenital infection may appear months or years after infection: most often chorioretinitis, sometimes mental retardation, ocular palsy, deafness.

Immunocompromised

Reactivation of infection involves the rupture of cysts, long after primary infection, with the release of parasites. Reactivation is a serious complication of immune deficiency: not uncommon in AIDS, and also reported as a complication of heart transplantation.

Clinically: most often reactivation involves the brain – *cerebral toxoplasmosis*.

Heart transplants: myocarditis has been reported after cardiac transplantation. Apparently most often due to reactivation of cysts in a donor heart transplanted into a seronegative recipient.

Diagnosis

Serology: ELISA for IgM; latex agglutination, dye and haemagglutination tests for IgG.

Demonstration of protozoan in tissues or body fluids is sometimes possible.

Treatment rarely necessary: most infections are self-limiting, except for toxoplasmosis in AIDS or the immunocompromised, or in choroidoretinitis: treat with pyrimethamine, sulphadiazine and folinic acid in combination.

GIARDIA LAMBLIA (GIARDIASIS)

A flagellated protozoon and an important cause of diarrhoea worldwide. *Outbreaks* due to waterborne infection have been described in which cysts have been demonstrated in the water.

Route of infection: faecal–oral.

Pathogenesis: ingestion of cysts – the resistant, infective stage – is followed by the production of *trophozoites* in the upper small intestine. Trophozoites cause irritation, which leads to gastrointestinal symptoms.

Clinical features

Symptoms: diarrhoea, mild to severe, with characteristic light-coloured fatty stools; abdominal pain: cramps, with flatulence and epigastric tenderness; anorexia.

Malabsorption: steatorrhoea is not uncommon and may lead to the full-blown malabsorption syndrome.

Diagnosis

Demonstration of cysts or the characteristic trophozoites, in faeces. *Trophozoites*, in duodenal aspirates or biopsies.

Treatment: tinidazole, metronidazole, albendazole.

PARASITIC INTESTINAL INFECTIONS IN AIDS PATIENTS

Some parasites – such as the tiny coccidia – were first recognized as common and important when they were found to be responsible for severe, prolonged and debilitating diarrhoea in AIDS patients. Most also infect the immunocompetent, although less severely. The most important are listed in Table 41.2.

CRYPTOSPORIDIUM PARVUM (CRYPTOSPORIDIOSIS)

A zoonosis but also a human pathogen, its frequency and importance were realized in AIDS patients: now known to be a common and important cause of diarrhoea in normal populations, especially children.

Animal hosts: several species of domestic animal, especially calves, are commonly infected with cryptosporidia: human infection is often acquired as a result of animal slurry contaminating water supplies.

Transmission: the infective stage is the oöcyst, passed in faeces: transmitted person-to-person, animal-to-person or via contaminated water.

Waterborne outbreaks: common and often involve large numbers of people.

Clinically: self-limiting diarrhoea in the immunocompetent: severe in AIDS.

Table 41.2   Intestinal parasites in AIDS patients

Parasite	Symptoms
Coccidia	
Cryptosporidium parvum	Severe, protracted diarrhoea
Isospora belli	Severe, protracted diarrhoea
Cyclospora cayetanensis	Severe, protracted diarrhoea
Microsporidia*	
Enterocytozoon bieneusi	Severe, protracted diarrhoea
Encephalitozoon intestinalis	Severe, protracted diarrhoea

* Some species, notably *Encephalitozoon cuniculi* and *Enc. hellem*, cause eye disease (small corneal ulcers and keratoconjunctivitis) in AIDS patients.

Diagnosis

Demonstration of oöcysts in faeces, stained with phenol auramine, modified Ziehl–Neelsen method, or by immunofluorescence with monoclonal antibody.

Treatment: no really effective treatment is available: none is indicated in the immunocompetent; paromomycin may be helpful in AIDS: nitazoxanide has recently shown some activity.

ISOSPORA BELLI

Humans seem to be the only host of this parasite, which infects the small intestine. It is difficult to diagnose in the laboratory and is now realized to be considerably more common worldwide in the normal population than originally thought.

Transmission: faecal-contaminated food and water.

Clinically: in the immunocompetent infection is often asymptomatic and the diarrhoea, when present, tends to be mild: in AIDS, the diarrhoea is severe and prolonged, sometimes with malabsorption.

Treatment: co-trimoxazole.

CYCLOSPORA CAYETANENSIS (CYCLOSPORIASIS)

First recognized in 1979 but not named until 1992, this coccidian protozoon infects the small intestine.

Transmission: the infective stage is the oöcyst passed in faeces. Human infection is food- or waterborne.

Clinically: diarrhoea, remitting and relapsing, sometimes lasting as long as 6 weeks; malabsorption in some cases; weight loss.

Treatment: co-trimoxazole: disease may be self-limiting and treatment unnecessary.

MICROSPORIDIA (MICROSPORIDIOSIS)

Obligate intracellular protozoa, characterized by resistant spores – the infective stage. Usually found as opportunistic infection in patients with AIDS, although occasionally cause disease in the immunocompetent.

Transmission: human infection is thought to be by ingestion or inhalation, or direct inoculation in the case of ocular infection.

Clinically: severe diarrhoea in AIDS patients; infection can become disseminated, involving most often the biliary tract and liver: ocular infection with small ulcers on the cornea and conjunctival involvement are seen with the *Encephalitozoon* species *cuniculi* and *hellem* (and in immunocompetent patients with *Nosema ocularum* and *Vittaforma corneae*).

Diagnosis: *Histology* of tissue biopsies; *microscopy* of modified trichrome-stained faecal smears.

Treatment: albendazole: topical treatment with fumagillin or itraconazole, or propamidine isethionate for treatment of ocular microsporidiosis.

DIAGNOSIS

The coccidian parasites are best diagnosed by examination of stools for oöcysts – or spores in the case of microsporidia.

PARASITIC INFECTIONS NOT INDIGENOUS TO THE UK

Parasitic diseases are major causes of morbidity and mortality in tropical countries. Malaria is described in some detail below, because of its importance if the diagnosis is missed in travellers returned from abroad. *Falciparum malaria* can be rapidly fatal if not treated promptly. Also included are other parasite infections seen in returned travellers and immigrants.

PLASMODIUM SPECIES (MALARIA)

Malaria is an important cause of death and debility throughout the tropics and subtropics.

The four species of plasmodia that cause malaria are shown in Table 41.3.

Transmission: by the bite of female anopheline mosquitoes.

Lifecycle is complex, with sexual multiplication in the mosquito and asexual multiplication in human hepatocytes (exoerythrocytic schizogony) and erythrocytes (erythrocytic schizogony).

Pathogenesis: symptoms are due to:

- *Haemolysis*, and the release of metabolites and pigment from malarial parasites
- *Plugging* of capillaries by parasitised erythrocytes.

Table 41.3 The four main malaria parasites

Species	Distribution
Plasmodium vivax	Very common: found in all endemic areas and extending into subtropical and temperate zones
Plasmodium falciparum	Very common: found in most endemic areas but not in temperate zones
Plasmodium malariae	Much less common: mainly found in subtropical and temperate regions
Plasmodium ovale	Predominant in West Africa; rare in other endemic areas

Clinical features

Main symptoms are fever and flu-like symptoms, e.g. headache, muscle pains, anorexia. Malaria may mimic other illnesses, which leads to misdiagnosis, sometimes with fatal results.

Periodicity

P. falciparum	36–48 h (malignant tertian)
P. vivax	48 h (benign tertian)
P. malariae	72 h (quartan)
P. ovale	48 h (ovale tertian).

Note: The classic regular pattern of recurrent fever can be modified by the immunological status of the patient, previous exposure to malaria, inadequate antimalarial prophylaxis, and drug resistance in the infecting strain. In practice, the classic pattern is seldom seen.

Incubation period: variable, depending on the species of *Plasmodium* and the strain within the species, and on the patient's history of previous exposure: usually 8–40 days, but can be as long as 1 year or more.

Malarial paroxysm

Coincides with lysis of infected erythrocytes, and liberation of merozoites.

Rigor or shaking chill – the patient complains of feeling cold, but is in fact febrile.

Followed by feeling hot, flushed, agitated.

Severe headache and aching limbs and back are common.
Relapse: at the appropriate interval usually follows.

Complications

1. *Cerebral malaria*: a complication only of *P. falciparum* infection. Symptoms: headache and disorientation, leading to coma and, if untreated, death. Cerebral infection is due to sequestration of parasites in the capillaries of the CNS.
2. *Blackwater fever*: also most often seen in falciparum malaria. Symptoms: haemoglobinuria, due to sudden intravascular haemolysis: renal failure sometimes ensues, due to acute tubular necrosis as a result of renal anoxia.
3. *Proteinuria*: sometimes seen in infection with *P. malariae* when the kidneys of children are affected, producing 'quartan nephrosis', with oedema of face and limbs. This serious complication has a prolonged course.
4. *Infection of placenta* with *P. falciparum*, leading to abortion, stillbirth and low-weight babies; seen in tropical Africa.
5. *Tropical splenomegaly*: grossly enlarged spleen.

Diagnosis

Malaria should be suspected in any febrile patient who has been in a malarious area within the previous year; sometimes even more than a year.

Demonstration of parasites in thick and thin blood films, using Field's or Giemsa stains (Fig. 41.1).

Treatment: *falciparum malaria*: quinine, mefloquine or 'Malarone' (i.e. proguanil with atovaquone).

Benign malaria (due to *P. vivax*, *P. ovale* and *P. malariae*): chloroquine: supplement with primaquine (if glucose-6-phosphate dehydrogenase level normal) after initial therapy in the case of *P. vivax* and *P. ovale* infections to eradicate parasites in liver.

Prevention: the principles of prevention are:

1. **Awareness** of the risk of malaria.
2. Avoidance of mosquito **bites**.
3. **Chemoprophylaxis**: this is complex and depends on resistance in areas being visited, the species of endemic *Plasmodium* and the condition of the patient. Up-to-date guidelines are given in the British National Formulary: includes chloroquine, proguanil (sometimes in combination), mefloquine,

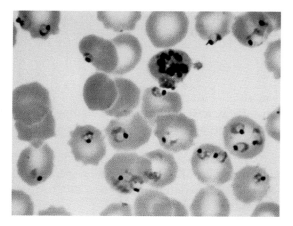

Fig. 41.1 *Plasmodium falciparum* ring forms in blood film. Courtesy of Dr Monika Kettelhut, Hospital for Tropical Diseases, London.

pyrimethamine with dapsone, doxycycline, atovaquine with proguanil.

4. Seeking early **diagnosis**.

5. Rapid assessment of febrile or flu-like illness *within 1 year* (sometimes longer) of leaving an area where malaria is endemic, even if precautions were taken.

Control: attempts by WHO and other agencies to control malaria have been largely unsuccessful owing to:

• Widespread and increasing development of resistance of the plasmodia to antimalarial drugs
• Increased resistance of the vector mosquitoes to insecticides
• Lack of financial and political stability, preventing implementation and monitoring of control programmes.

Vaccination: various preparations, using different antigens of *P. falciparum*, are under trial.

LEISHMANIA SPECIES (LEISHMANIASIS)

Leishmaniasis is a protozoal infection found in many parts of the world, including Asia, Africa, Latin and Central America and the Middle East, but also in Europe – in Spain, France and Italy.

The geographical distribution of the different species of *Leishmania* is shown in Table 41.4.

Table 41.4 Parasites causing leishmaniasis

Species	Distribution
Old World	
Leishmania tropica	Mediterranean, Asia, Middle East
Leishmania major	Middle East, Africa, Asia
Leishmania aethiopica	Ethiopia, Kenya, Southwest Africa
Leishmania donovani	Asia
New World	
Leishmania braziliensis*	Latin America
Leishmania mexicana	Mexico, Central America, Texas
Leishmania chagasi	Latin America

* Now recognized as a subgenus: Viannia.

Reservoirs: humans, dogs, rodents and other small mammals.

Transmission: via the bite of infected sandflies.

Pathogenesis: Leishmania survive within macrophages in the human body as intracellular parasites: cell-mediated immunity determines the host response to infection and the clinical manifestations of the disease.

Clinical features: there are three main forms of leishmaniasis:

- *Visceral* (kala-azar)
- *Cutaneous*
- *Mucosal.*

Visceral leishmaniasis (kala-azar)

Incubation period: long (3–8 months).

Symptoms: fever, weight loss with splenomegaly, hepatomegaly, anaemia, leukopenia and hypergammaglobulinaemia – protozoon-carrying macrophage infiltration is widespread throughout the reticuloendothelial system. Also seen in immunocompromised patients, e.g. with AIDS.

Causes: particularly associated with *L. donovani* (Old World) and *L. chagasi* (New World).

Cutaneous leishmaniasis

Known as 'oriental sore' in the Old World.

Symptoms: initially a papule at the site of the sandfly bite, which enlarges and ulcerates: lesions can be very large (2 cm or more in diameter) and disfiguring: a hard excrescence in the middle of the lesion is characteristic (Montpellier sign).

Diffuse cutaneous leishmaniasis is a more serious form in which satellite lesions spread locally and to distant skin areas.

Main causes: Old World: *L. major, L. tropica*; New World: *L. braziliensis, L. mexicana*.

Mucosal leishmaniasis

Known as '*espundia*'.

A severe complication of cutaneous leishmaniasis, with mutilating destruction of the nose, oral cavity and pharynx where the infective process has extended to the mucous membranes of nose and mouth.

Main cause: New World: *L. braziliensis*.

Diagnosis

Demonstration of intracellular protozoa in stained film from lesions.

Culture: of bone marrow aspirate or splenic puncture, for extracellular forms, on special media.

PCR on skin biopsies.

Skin test: intradermal inoculation of antigen from extracellular parasites (Montenegro test) to detect hypersensitivity: usually positive in established disease. Not useful in diagnosis, but helpful in epidemiological investigations.

Treatment: sodium stibogluconate, amphotericin – preferably as 'AmBisome' in liposomal form; pentamidine isethionate as a second-line drug.

AMOEBIASIS

A common infection abroad especially in tropical countries where sanitation is poor. Seen not infrequently in the UK owing to its importation when acquired by travellers or immigrants: often presents with severe disease, but many infections are mild or asymptomatic.

Cause: *Entamoeba histolytica*.

Host: humans.

Route of infection: faecal–oral, owing to contamination of water and food by sewage.

Clinical features: diarrhoea, progressing rapidly to bloody diarrhoea accompanied by fever and painful abdominal cramps, and so to stools consisting largely of mucus with blood. The symptoms may persist into a chronic relapsing state. Sometimes progresses to dilatation of the colon, with risk of intestinal perforation.

Complications: amoebic abscess owing to spread to the liver, causing painful enlargement and accompanied by high fever, raised white cell count and high ESR. Sometimes there are minimal signs and symptoms and the diagnosis depends on CT scan. Although rare, amoebic abscesses are found in other sites, notably the lung or brain.

Diagnosis

Examine stool: for active amoebic trophozoites containing ingested erythrocytes.

Serology: for extraintestinal disease by immunofluorescence.

Treatment: metronidazole or tinadazole, then diloxanide furoate; in asymptomatic cases, diloxanide furoate.

ASCARIS LUMBRICOIDES (COMMON ROUNDWORM)

A major problem: infects around 1 billion people worldwide.

Adult worms: length: about 15–35 cm. *Habitat*: the small intestine.

Pathogenesis: infection is by ingestion of eggs. *Lifecycle*: larvae hatch in the small intestine, whence they migrate to liver and lungs (while growing and undergoing moults) and return to small intestine as adult worms via trachea and oesophagus.

Clinical features: symptoms accompany the infestation in two phases:

1. *Migratory phase*: about 6 weeks: often accompanied by hepatitis, pneumonitis and allergic symptoms: eosinophilia is usually present.
2. *Intestinal infection*: the presence of worms in the small intestine can cause intestinal obstruction, especially in small children, and with nutritional deficiencies.

Diagnosis

Demonstration of adult worms or – more usually – ova in faeces.

Treatment: mebendazole, piperazine.

TAENIA SAGINATA (TAENIASIS)

Humans are the only *definitive* hosts for this, the *beef* tapeworm: cattle are *intermediate* hosts.
   Adult worms: *length*: often very long – up to 10 m.
   Structure:

* *Head* or *scolex*: with suckers, which attach to jejunal mucosa
* *Body*, made up of segments or *proglottids*: in *T. saginata* these are characteristically elongated. Each proglottid contains both male and female organs, from which eggs are shed into the faeces. *Habitat*: small intestine.

Pathogenesis: ingestion of cysticerci – an intermediate, larval form of the parasite – found in undercooked or 'measly' beef. The cysticerci mature into adult worms in the small intestine. Cattle develop cysticercosis of muscles after ingestion of eggs.
   Clinically: usually symptomless: sometimes weight loss.

Diagnosis

Demonstration of proglottids or eggs in faeces.
   Treatment: niclosamide, praziquantel (both on named patient basis).

OTHER INFECTIONS NOT INDIGENOUS TO THE UK

Other important parasitic infections found in countries other than Britain are listed in Table 41.5.

Table 41.5   Other tropical parasites

Parasite	Host	Intermediate host/vector	Symptoms
Nematodes			
Hookworms			
Ancylostoma duodenale	} Human	–	Anaemia, gastrointestinal haemorrhage
Necator americanus			
Strongyloides stercoralis	Human	–	Serpiginous skin lesions, pneumonitis, enteritis
Trichuris trichiura	Human	–	Diarrhoea
Trichinella spiralis	Pigs	Human	Fever, muscle pain
Wuchereria bancrofti	} Human	Mosquito	Lymphangitis, elephantiasis
Brugia malayi			
Onchocerca volvulus	Human	Blackfly	Skin nodules, ocular blindness
Loa loa	Human	Fly	Calabar swellings, subconjunctival adult worms
Cestodes			
Taenia solium	Human	Pig	Cysticercosis
Trematodes			
Schistosoma mansoni	} Human	Snails	Rectal bleeding, pipestem fibrosis of the liver, portal hypertension, haematuria
Schistosoma japonicum			
Schistosoma haematobium			
Paragonimus westermani	Cats, dogs	Shellfish	Haemoptysis
Clonorchis sinensis	Cats etc.	Fish	Cholangitis, liver abscess
Protozoa			
Trypanosoma rhodesiense	} Cattle, game animals	Tsetse flies	Sleeping sickness
Trypanosoma gambiense			
Trypanosoma cruzi	Various domestic/ wild animals	Bugs	Chagas' disease

Recommended reading

1. Adler M W (ed). ABC of AIDS, 5th edn. London: BMJ Books, 2001
2. Bannister B A, Begg N A, Gillespie S H Infectious disease, 2nd edn. Oxford: Blackwell Science, 2000
3. Chin J (ed). Control of communicable diseases manual, 17th edn. Washington: American Public Health Association, 2000
4. Mandel G L, Bennett J E, Dolin R. Mandell Douglas and Bennett's Principles and practice of infectious diseases, 5th edn. Philadelphia: Churchill Livingstone, 2000
5. Spicer W J Clinical bacteriology, mycology and parasitology: an illustrated colour text. London: Harcourt Sciences, 2000
6. Zuckerman A J, Banatvala J E, Pattison J R Clinical virology, 4th edn. Chichester: John Wiley, 2000

Index

Page numbers in *italic* refer to Figures and Tables.